Copyright 2020 by Susan Stubbs -All rights reserved.

No part of this publication may be reproduced, distributed, or transmitted in any form or by any means, including photocopying, recording, or other electronic or mechanical methods, without the prior written permission of the publisher, except in the case of brief quotations embodied in reviews and certain other non-commercial uses permitted by copyright law.

This Book is provided with the sole purpose of providing relevant information on a specific topic for which every reasonable effort has been made to ensure that it is both accurate and reasonable. Nevertheless, by purchasing this Book you consent to the fact that the author, as well as the publisher, are in no way experts on the topics contained herein, regardless of any claims as such that may be made within. It is recommended that you always consult a professional prior to undertaking any of the advice or techniques discussed within.This is a legally binding declaration that is considered both valid and fair by both the Committee of Publishers Association and the American Bar Association and should be considered as legally binding within the United States.

CONTENTS

INTRODUCTION 9
BREAKFAST 10
    01. Beef & Kale Casserole 10
    02. Korean Beef 10
    03. Beef & Broccoli 10
    04. Beef and Cabbage 10
    05. Instant Pot Beef Cabbage Rolls 11
    06. Beef & Mushroom Soup 11
    07. Spicy Beef & Cashew Curry 11
    08. BBQ Pot Roast with Garlic Sauce 12
    09. Cheesesteak Casserole 12
    10. Cabbage Stew and Beef Shank 12
    11. Shredded Beef with Avocado Salsa ... 12
    12. Cheeseburger Soup 13
    13. Beef Sirloin Lettuce Wraps 13
    14. Ropa Vieja 13
    15. Italian-style Beef 13
    16. Asian Shredded Beef 13
    17. Instant Pot Beef Ragu with Herbs 14
    18. Hot Roast Machaca 14
    19. Korean-style Beef Tacos 14
    20. Instant Pot Beef Stew 14
    21. Caribbean Ginger Oxtails 14
    22. Coconut Yogurt Mix 15
    23. Artichokes Pudding 15
    24. Scotch Eggs and Tomato Passata 15
    25. Parsley Cauliflower Mix 15
    26. Pork Pie 15
    27. Ginger Cauliflower Rice Pudding 16
    28. Bok Choy Bowls 16
    29. Mushroom and Avocado Salad 16
    30. Salmon and Eggs Mix 16
    31. Italian Beef and Green Beans Mix 16
    32. Herbed Mushroom Mix 17
    33. Creamy Zucchini Pan 17
    34. Leeks and Pork Mix 17
    35. Cardamom Walnuts Pudding 17
    36. Basil Eggs Mix 17
    37. Creamy Blueberries and Nuts 17
    38. Kale and Bok Choy Muffins 18
    39. Spinach and Artichokes Muffins 18
    40. Mozzarella and Kale Muffins 18
    41. Chicken Bowls 18
    42. Coconut Pudding 18
    43. Zucchini Spread 19
    44. Blackberries Jam 19
    45. Delicious Poached Eggs 19
    46. Spinach & Tomato Breakfast 19
    47. Banana Cake 19
    48. Breakfast Hash 20
    49. Blueberry Bliss Bowls 20
    50. Quinoa and Granola Bowls 20
    51. Tofu and Potato Casserole 20
    52. French Toast Casserole 21
    53. Tomato Spinach Quiche 21
    54. Mushroom Oatmeal 21
    55. Healthy Oats 21
    56. Lemon Marmalade Recipe 22
    57. Tasty Sausage 22
    58. Pecan Sweet Potatoes 22
    59. Mixed Mushroom Pate 22
    60. Chocolate Steel Cut Oats 23
    61. Breakfast Quiche 23
    62. Eggs Breakfast 23
    63. Chickpeas Spread 23
    64. Maple Millet 23
    65. Barbeque Tofu 24
    66. Apple Porridge 24
    67. Feta Spinach Egg Cups 24
    68. Cheesy Chili Eggs 24
    69. Nutty Blueberries Mix 24
    70. Veggie Pastry 24
    71. Artichoke And Spinach Scones 25
    72. Nutty Coconut Mousse 25
    73. Creamy Zucchini 25
    74. Cheesy Radish And Tomatoes Jumble 25
    75. Garlic Pork Meat With Kale 25
    76. Creamy Zucchini With Walnuts 26
    77. Bacon And Turkey Frittata With Avocado And Tomatoes 26
    78. Creamy Nuts And Strawberries 26
    79. Garlic Turkey With Leeks And Egg 26
    80. Coconut and Berries Mix 26
    81. Chili Mushrooms with Okra Egg Dish ... 26
    82. Creamy Cocoa Vanilla Coconut Meal ... 27
    83. Creamy Almonds And Broccoli With Coconut 27
    84. Creamy Cinnamon And Coconut With Strawberries 27
    85. Creamy Coconut Frittata 27
    86. Spicy Leek And Veggie Egg Dish 27
    87. Cauliflower Rice With Broccoli And Tomatoes 27
MAINS 28
    88. Stuffed Bell Peppers 28
    89. Ginger Stew 28
    90. Chickpeas with Onions 28
    91. Portobello Mushrooms with Green Peas .. 28
    92. Lentil Stew 28
    93. One Pot Quinoa 29
    94. Instant Pot Hot Dogs 29
    95. Curried Potato and Cauliflower (Indian Aloo Gobi 29
    96. Sloppy Joe in Instant Pot 29
    97. Pizza Alla Puttanesca 30
    98. Seitan Fajitas 30
    99. Zesty Stuffed Bell Peppers 30
    100. Moroccan Stuffed Peppers 30
    101. Corn Chorizo pie 31
    102. Cheesy Tomato Gratin 31
    103. Sweet Potatoes and Onions with Jerk Sauce 31
    104. Ziti Mushroom Stew 32
    105. Tofu Cheesecake 32
    106. Garlic Pimento Fondue 32
    107. Sweet and Nutty Fondue 32
    108. Beefy Cajun Po Boy 32
    109. Meatless Philly Cheesesteak Hoagie ... 33
    110. Sloppy Tempeh Sandwich 33
    111. Tex Mex Tofu Taco 'Meat' 33
    112. Black Bean and Potato Burrito Filling 33
    113. Pesto Butternut Grilled Sandwiches ... 33
    114. Soy Ginger Lettuce Wraps 34
    115. Quinoa Pecan Stuffed Squash 34

116. Chicken Noodles Soup 34
117. Taco Soup 34
118. Chicken Transparent Soup 35
119. Egg Loaf 35
120. Lentil Soup 35
121. Chicken Pilaf 35
122. Creamy Pappardelle 36
123. Parmesan Mac&Cheese 36
124. Garlic Pasta 36
125. Ramen Noodles 36
126. Carrot Chicken Soup 37
127. Cabbage Casserole 37
128. Lunch Fritatta 37
129. Chili Black Rice 37
130. Fettuccine Alfredo 37
131. Baked Sweet Potato Soup 38
132. Hawaiian Rice 38
133. Butternut Squash and Coconut Soup 38
134. Spanish Rice 38
135. Tuscan Chicken Pasta 39
136. Egg&Bacon Salad 39
137. Caesar Wrap 39
138. Frito Pie Bowl 39
139. Cheddar Soup 40
140. Lasagna 40
141. Fish Casserole 40
142. Bacon Chowder 40
143. Stuffed Pepper Rings 41
144. Zucchini Meat Cakes 41
145. Fragrant Tomato Soup 41
146. Oregano Soup 41
147. Filipino Sinigang 42
148. Taco Pie 42
149. Nutritious Rice Bowl 42
150. Lentils&Rice Mix 42
151. Chicken Mole 43
152. Mushroom Risotto 43
153. Lunch Saute 43
154. Chickpeas&Noodles Soup 43
155. Lo Mein 43
156. Cajun Rice Bowl 44
157. American Goulash 44
158. Rice Casserole 44
159. Ham Casserole 44
160. Ham Rotini 45
161. Tortilla Soup 45
162. Jacket Potato 45
163. Tomato Kielbasa 45
164. Cauliflower and Mushroom Soup 46
165. Onion Cheesy Soup 46
166. Green Soup 46
167. Vegan Soup 46
168. Lentil Curry 46
169. Lazy Penne 47
170. Chicken Alfredo Pasta 47
171. Chicken Chili Soup 47

SIDES 48
172. Cantonese Winter Squash 48
173. Italian Tomatoes and Zucchini 48
174. Vegan Braciole 48
175. Marmalade Beets 48
176. Creamy Wild Asparagus 48
177. Smashed Potatoes 48
178. Easy Green Peas 49
179. Quick Mushrooms 49
180. Perfect Stuffing 49
181. Instant Pot Refried Beans 49
182. Autumn Stuffed Squash 50
183. Sweet and Sour Cabbage Rolls 50
184. Collard Rolls 50
185. St Patrick's Cabbage Rolls 51
186. Steamed Artichokes 51
187. Sprouts and Chestnuts 51
188. Sweet and Sour Cabbage 51
189. Mediterranean Cauliflower 51
190. Gobi Manchurian 52
191. Zucchini Puttanesca 52
192. Stuffed Artichokes 52
193. Collards and Pot Likker 52
194. Creamed Corn 52
195. Golden Ratatouille 53
196. Country Green Beans and Tomato 53
197. Taters And Sweets 53
198. Garlicky Mash 53
199. Granny Smith Sweet Potatoes 53
200. Scalloped Potatoes 53
201. Tomatoes, Potatoes, and Beans ... 54
202. Maple Glazed Root Veg 54
203. Lemon Herb Beets 54
204. Rutabagas with Apples and Pears 54
205. Mashed Cauliflower and Parsnips 54
206. Garlic Potatoes Au Gratin 55
207. Sesame Ginger Kale 55
208. Mashed Sweet Potatoes with Sweet Pecan Topping 55
209. Herb Roasted Mixed Vegetables ... 55
210. Corn with Creamy Truffle Sauce ... 55
211. Seared Maple Balsamic Brussels Sprouts 56
212. Smoky Cajun Green Beans 56
213. Dill Carrots in White Wine 56
214. Sriracha Ginger Eggplant 56
215. Mint Rum Black Beans 56
216. Basic Baked Potatoes 56

SEAFOOD 57
217. Keto Lobster Tails in Butter Sauce 57
218. Delicious Mussels with Thyme 57
219. Keto Tuna Steak with Mushrooms 57
220. Tasty Cod Chowder with Bacon ... 57
221. Onion Prawn Stew 58
222. Keto Fish Stew 58
223. Keto Salmon Macaroni 58
224. Shrimp Cauliflower Risotto 59
225. Easy Creamy Mussel Soup 59
226. Keto Chili Lime Salmon 59
227. Spicy Keto Shrimp Pasta 59
228. Lobster Tomato Stew 60
229. Teriyaki Shrimps 60
230. Tilapia Curry Recipe 60
231. Spicy and Sweet Trout 60
232. Salmon with Vegetables 61
233. Mussels with Asparagus 61
234. Quick Shrimp Soup 61
235. Delicious Pepper Salmon 62
236. Keto Green Pesto Tuna Steak 62
237. Simple Catfish Stew 62
238. Steamed Salmon Recipe 62
239. Tilapia Fillets 63

240. Keto Seafood Stew...................................63
241. Jamaican Jerk Fish..................................63
242. Adobo Shrimps Recipe............................64
243. Tasty Trout Casserole.............................64
244. Surprising Shrimp Delight.......................64
245. Tuna & Pasta Casserole..........................64
246. Almond Cod..65
247. Mussels and Spicy Sauce........................65
248. Tomato Mussels.....................................65
249. Cheesy Tuna Dish...................................65
250. Poached Salmon Dish.............................65
251. Salmon and Veggies Dish........................66
252. Salmon Dish...66
253. Crispy Salmon Fillet................................66
254. Steamed Fish Recipe..............................66
255. Spicy Salmon Dish..................................66
256. Tuna and Noodle....................................66
257. Delicious Shrimp Paella..........................67
258. Crispy Skin Salmon Fillets......................67
259. Salmon Burger.......................................67
260. Miso Mackerel.......................................67
261. Shrimp with Herbs and Risotto...............68
262. Fish with Orange Sauce.........................68
263. Simple Clams..68
264. Crab Legs and Garlic Butter Sauce.........68
265. Shrimp and Potatoes Dish......................68
266. Shrimp and Fish....................................69
267. Shrimp and Sausage Boil.......................69
268. Tuna and Crushed Crackers Casserole...69
269. Shrimp Coconut Soup............................69
270. Shrimp Teriyaki Recipe..........................70
271. Instant Shrimp Boil................................70
272. Cheesy Tilapia.......................................70
273. Mediterranean Fish...............................70
274. Delicious Salmon and Raspberry Sauce.70
275. Sesame Honey Salmon..........................71
276. Crab Quiche..71
277. Shrimp with Tomatoes, Spinach.............71
278. Seafood Stew..72
279. Fresh Catfish with Herbs.......................72
280. Steamed Scallion Ginger Fish.................72
281. Delicious Cod and Peas.........................72
282. Instant Pot Steamed Mussels................73

POULTRY...74
283. Creamy Basil Chicken Breasts................74
284. Lemon Chicken.....................................74
285. Coq Au Vin..74
286. Coconut Chicken Curry..........................74
287. Chicken Taco Bowls...............................75
288. Sweet Spicy Shredded Chicken..............75
289. Chicken in Tomato Sauce......................75
290. Spinach Feta Stuffed Chicken................75
291. Meatballs Primavera.............................76
292. Buffalo Chicken Soup............................76
293. Balsamic Chicken..................................76
294. Tuscan Chicken.....................................77
295. Barbecue Chicken.................................77
296. Quick Chicken Fajitas............................77
297. Stuffed Full Chicken..............................78
298. Chicken Wings......................................78
299. Whole Chicken......................................78
300. Broccoli Chicken...................................78
301. Simple Chicken Wings...........................78
302. Asian-Style Chicken Thighs....................79
303. Chicken with Sesame oil.......................79
304. Hot Garlic Chicken Breasts....................79
305. Chicken Tenders with Garlic..................79
306. Tropic Shredded Chicken......................79
307. Hot Butter Chicken................................79

MEAT..80
308. Cheesy Pork Chops................................80
309. Portobello Pork Butt Recipe..................80
310. Ground Pork Burgers.............................80
311. Sweet Coconut Pork..............................80
312. Pork Shoulder Recipe............................81
313. Meatloaf Recipe....................................81
314. Mushroom Pork Recipe.........................81
315. Pork Loin with Leeks Recipe..................82
316. Classic Pork Ribs...................................82
317. Steamed Pork Neck Recipe...................82
318. Slow Cooked Pork.................................82
319. Pork Neck with Soy Sauce and Sesame Seeds..83
320. Sweet Pork Ribs....................................83
321. Pork Steak in Mushroom Sauce Recipe..83
322. Garlic Pork Recipe.................................84
323. Thai Style Pork with White Pepper Gravy...84
324. Pork with Cauliflower............................84
325. Pork Chops with Onions........................84
326. Pork Curry...85
327. Asian Pork Strips Recipe.......................85
328. Marinated Pork Recipe.........................85
329. Mushroom and Pepper Pork.................85
330. Pork Shoulder with Sweet Potatoes......86
331. Keto Pork Fillets....................................86
332. Pork in Tomato Sauce...........................86
333. Pork Leg Roast Recipe..........................86
334. Pork Chops and Cabbage......................87
335. Pork Ribs Recipe...................................87
336. Dijon Pork with Turmeric......................87
337. Quick Pork Chops..................................88
338. Buttery Pork Chops...............................88
339. Keto Pork with Eggs..............................88
340. Italian Style Pork Roast.........................88
341. Spring Onion Pork Recipe.....................89
342. Tomato Pork Chops..............................89
343. Pork Belly Recipe..................................89
344. Apple Cider Pork Ribs Recipe................90
345. Spicy Pork with Celery..........................90
346. Pork Chops with Peppers......................90
347. Balsamic Pork with Broccoli..................90
348. Zucchini Pork..91
349. Mint Lamb Chops..................................91
350. Lamb Chops, Fennel and Tomatoes......91
351. Italian Leg of Lamb................................91
352. Hot Curry Lamb and Green Beans........92
353. Lamb and Sun-dried Tomatoes Mix......92
354. Cumin Lamb and Capers......................92
355. Herbed Crusted Lamb Cutlets..............92
356. Pine Nuts Lamb Meatballs...................92
357. Lamb Shoulder Roast...........................93
358. Moroccan Lamb...................................93
359. Spinach Pork Meatloaf.........................93
360. Ginger Lamb and Basil.........................93
361. Coconut Lamb Chops...........................93
362. Spicy Beef, Sprouts and Avocado Mix...94
363. Beef and Creamy Sauce.......................94

364. Pork and Chives Asparagus 94
365. Oregano and Thyme Beef 94
366. Almond Lamb Meatloaf 94
367. Pork and Bok Choy 95
368. Smoked Paprika Lamb 95
369. Cajun Beef and Leeks Sauce 95
370. Beef and Savoy Cabbage Mix 95
371. Pork and Mint Zucchinis 95
372. Beef and Walnuts Rice 96
373. Bangers and Mash with Onion Gravy 96
374. Herby Cuban Pork Roast 96
375. Pork Stew 96
376. Lemony Pork Belly 97
377. Ham with Collard Greens 97
378. Pork in Mushroom Gravy 97
379. Pork Tenderloin with Ginger Soy Sauce . 97
380. Beef Bourguignonne 98
381. Beef Burger 98
382. Pork Carnitas Lettuce Cups 98
383. Easy BBQ Ribs 98
384. Braised Pork Neck Bones 99
385. Pork Roast Sandwich 99
386. Balsamic Pork Tenderloin 99
387. Tender Greek Pork 100
388. Pork in Vegetable Sauce 100
389. Creamy Pork with Bacon 100
390. Pulled Pork in Lettuce Wraps 100
391. Coconut Ginger Pork 101
392. Sweet Spicy Pork Chops 101
393. Green Chile Pork Carnitas 101
394. Pork in Peanut Sauce 101
395. Carrot and Pork Stew 102
396. Beef Steak in Balsamic Sauce 102
397. Rosemary Beef Roast Recipe 102
398. Instant Lamb Shoulder Hash 103
399. Beef Shoulder Roast 103
400. Beef with Greens 103
401. Fried Beef Roast 103
402. Shiitake Beef Sirloin 104
403. Beef Shank 104
404. Spicy Masala Beef Roast 104
405. Chili Lamb Leg Recipe 105
406. Lamb Kebab Recipe 105
407. Keto Beef Meatballs 105
408. Keto Korean Beef 105
409. Mongolian Style Beef 106
410. Instant Cheddar Beef Hash 106
411. Cheesey Meatballs 106
412. Keto Beef Ragout 107
413. Lamb Neck with Broccoli 107
414. Beef Curry Recipe 107
415. Lamb loin Stew Recipe 108
416. Beef Neck with Fire Roasted Tomatoes 108
417. Easy Beef Chili 108
418. Crispy Lamb Chops 108
419. Lamb Chops with Vegetables 109
420. Easy Beef Bourguignon 109
421. Shredded Beef 109
422. Braised Beef Short Ribs 109
423. Classic Meatloaf 110
424. Korean BBQ Beef 110
425. Bolognese Sauce 110
426. Stewed Beef with Mushrooms 110
427. Beef and Chorizo Chili 111
428. Quick and Easy Taco Meat 111
429. Balsamic Beef Pot Roast 111
430. Zesty Beef Bites 111
431. Cheesy Beef with Tomato Sauce 112
432. Cheesy Garlic Beef Bowls 112
433. Creamy Lime Turkey with Tomato Sauce 112
434. Spicy Garlic Pork and Okra Jumble 112
435. Lamb in Tomato Sauce with Olives 112
436. Chili Lamb And Zucchini In Tomato Sauce 113
437. Balsamic Pork Tenderloin 113
438. Easy Lamb with Gravy 113
439. Spicy Pork Carnitas 113
440. Braised Lamb Chops 114
441. Ginger Soy-Glazed Pork Tenderloin 114
442. Herb-Roasted Lamb Shoulder 114
443. Curried Pork Shoulder 114
444. Curried Lamb Stew 115
445. Nutrition Values: 115
446. Smothered Pork Chops 115
447. Rosemary Garlic Leg of Lamb 115
448. Hungarian Marha Pörkölt 115
449. Creamy and Saucy Beef Delight 116
450. Sunday Hamburger Pilaf 116
451. Italian-Style Steak Pepperonata 116
452. Wine-Braised Beef Shanks 116
453. Holiday Osso Buco 117
454. Tagliatelle with Beef Sausage and Cheese 117
455. Balkan-Style Beef Stew 117
456. Bacon and Blade Roast Sandwiches 117
457. Tuscan-Style Cassoulet 118
458. Barbecued Beef Round with Cheese 118
459. Home-Style Beef Tikka Kebabs 118
460. Favorite Tex-Mex Tacos 118
461. Traditional Beef Pho Noodle Soup 119
462. Ground Beef Taco Bowls 119
463. Barbeque Chuck Roast 119
464. Beef Pad Thai 119
465. Easy Balsamic Beef 120
466. Juicy Round Steak 120
467. Ground Beef Bulgogi 120
468. Classic Beef Stroganoff 120
469. Pepper Jack Beef and Cauliflower Casserole 121
470. Hayashi Rice Stew 121
VEGETABLES 122
Healthy Brussels Sprouts with Mushrooms 122
472. Keto Spinach Pepper Stew 122
473. Easy Portobello Mushrooms in Lime Sauce 122
474. Creamy Broccoli Avocado 122
475. Kale Spinach Muffins 123
476. Button Mushrooms in Tomato Sauce ... 123
477. Keto Vegetarian Pizza 123
478. Cauliflower with Avocado 124
479. Zucchini Eggplant with Cucumber Sauce 124
480. Broccoli Cauliflower Frittata 124
481. Tofu with Mushrooms 124
482. Keto Green Quiche 125
483. Yummy Greens in Cayenne Sauce 125
484. Steamed Broccoli with Basil 125

485. Classic Cauliflower Spread with Thyme 126
486. Chessy Cannelloni Eggplant 126
487. Spinach with Goat's Cheese 126
488. Simple Stuffed Bell Peppers 127
489. Bell Pepper Zucchini Salad 127
490. Tasty Stuffed Bell Peppers 127
491. Sauteed Vegetables 128
492. Zucchini Eggplant Recipe 128
493. Yummy Creamy Spinach Balls 128
494. Braised Kale Recipe 128
495. Corn Pudding 129
496. Pinto Bean Stew 129
497. Collard Greens 129
498. Mushroom Kale Stroganoff 129
499. Tuscan Stew 130
500. Hearts Of Palm Soup 130
501. Asian Coconut Rice and Veggies 130
502. Moo Goo Gai Pan 131
503. Sweet Potato and Black Bean Tacos 131
504. Red Curry Cauliflower 131
505. Vegetable Salad 132
506. Cabbage Rolls 132
507. Black Eyed Peas 132
508. Mucho Burritos 133
509. Barbecue Chickpea Tacos 133
510. Asian Gobi Masala 133
511. Sloppy Janes 134
512. Polenta and Kale 134
513. Corn Chowder 134
514. Vegetable Soup 134
515. Chickpea Kale Korma 135
516. Butternut Mac N Cheese 135
517. Layered Casserole 135
518. Vegetable Stock 136
519. Kimchi Pasta 136
520. Tomato Basil Pasta 136
521. Vegetarian Quinoa Chili 136
522. Kerala Mixed Vegetable Curry 137
523. Creamy Vegan Tomato Soup 137
524. Portobello Pot Roast 137
525. Vegan Green Chile Stew 138
526. Buttery Garlic Mashed Potatoes 138
527. Vegetarian Pasta Rigatoni Bolognese ... 138
528. Lentil Bolognese Sauce 139
529. Vegan Butter Chicken with Soy Curls & Chickpeas 139
530. Maple Bourbon Sweet Potato Chili 140
531. Walnut Lentil Tacos 140
532. Cilantro Lime Quinoa 140
533. Black Bean Chili 140
534. Vegan Lentil Chili 141
535. Spaghetti Squash 141
536. Mushroom Risotto 141
537. Vegan Potato Curry 142
538. Mashed Potatoes with Fried Onions and Bacon 142
539. Vegan Alfredo Sauce 142
540. Carrot Ginger Soup 142

GRAINS & BEANS 144
541. Chicken & Wild Rice Soup 144
542. Quinoa Beef Pot 144
543. Keto Clam Chowder 144
544. Stuffed Cuttlefish 144
545. Saffron Chicken 145
546. Sesame Meatball Stew 145
547. Burrito with Chili Colorado 145
548. Sour Dumplings 145
549. Sausage Radish Cakes 146
550. Seafood Jambalaya 146
551. Shredded Pork Fajitas 146
552. Sausage Gumbo 146
553. Pork Fried Whole Grain Rice 147
554. Bacon Wrapped Jalapenos 147
555. Shredded Beef Tacos 147
556. Beef Stuffed Eggplant 147
557. Spicy Fire Chicken with Rice 147
558. Spiced Apple & Walnut Chicken 148
559. Pulled Chicken in Soft Whole Wheat Tacos 148
560. Pesto Chicken & Whole Wheat Pasta ... 148
561. Pasta & Brown Turkey Sauce 148
562. Orange Chicken Drumsticks & Rice 148
563. Mediterranean Mint & Basil Chicken & Rice 149
564. Mango Citrus Chicken & Rice 149
565. Lemon, Capers, Chicken & Chinese Black Rice 149
566. Jerk Chicken Strips & Wild Rice 149
567. Greek Chicken & Sprouted Rice 149
568. Chicken Fried Wild Rice 150
569. Stuffed Bell Peppers 150
570. Chipotle Tacos 150
571. Breakfast Burritos 150
572. Wild Mushroom Rice 150
573. Spinach Casserole 151
574. Mexican Rice 151
575. Rice Pilaf 151
576. Red Beans Over Sprouted Brown Rice . 151
577. Israeli Couscous 152
578. Wild Rice & Black Beans 152
579. Perfect Brown Rice 152
580. Lentil & Wild Rice Pilaf 152
581. Mung Bean Dahl 152
582. Red Bean & Lentil Chili 152
583. Falafel 153
584. Chickpea Curry 153
585. Lentil Sloppy Joe's 153
586. Lentil and Wild Rice Pilaf 154
587. Instant Pot Hummus 154
588. Stewed Chickpeas 154
589. Rainbow Beans 154
590. Northern White Bean Dip 155
591. Greek-Style Gigantes Beans with Feta . 155
592. Chili Con Carne 155
593. Smokey Sweet Black-Eyed Peas & Greens 155
594. Tex Mex Pinto Beans 156
595. Instant Pot Charros 156
596. Three Bean Salad 156
597. Beans Stew 156
598. Classic Chili Lime Black Beans 157
599. Instant Wheat Berry Salad 157
600. Pasta & Cranberry Beans 157
601. Kidney Beans Dish 157
602. Lentils Tacos 158
603. Couscous with Veggies and Chicken 158
604. Mediterranean Lentils 158
605. Asian Rice 158

606. Black Beans.................................. 159
607. Cilantro Lime Brown Rice 159
608. Black Beans and Chorizo........................ 159
609. Green Chile and Baked Beans................ 159
610. Green Chile Chickpeas 160
611. Red Beans and Rice............................... 160
612. Spicy Lentils 160
613. Butternut Lentils..................................... 160
614. Shrimp and White Beans 161
615. Mushroom and Leek Risotto 161
616. Italian Lentils Dinner 161
617. Veggies Rice Pilaf................................. 161
618. Black Bean Soup.................................... 162
619. Chickpea Basil Salad 162
620. Re-fried Pinto Beans.............................. 162
621. Coconut Jasmine Rice........................... 162
622. Pepper Lemon Quinoa 163
623. Chinese Fried Rice................................. 163
624. Barley and Mushroom Risotto................. 163
625. Barley with Vegetables 163
626. Cracked Wheat and Vegetables 164
627. Cracked Wheat Surprise 164
628. Barley Salad... 164
629. Wheat Berry Salad 164
630. Bulgur Salad... 165
631. Bulgur Pilaf.. 165
632. Israeli Couscous 165
633. Millet with Vegetables 165
634. Buckwheat Porridge.............................. 166
635. Couscous with Chicken and Vegetables 166
636. Creamy Millet.. 166
637. Oats and Vegetables.............................. 167
638. Cranberry Beans and Pasta.................... 167
639. Cranberry Beans Mixture 167
640. Quinoa and Vegetables 167
641. Mexican Cranberry Beans 168
642. Cranberry Bean Chili 168
643. Lentil Tacos 168
644. Indian Lentils 168
645. Lentils Salad 169
646. Italian Lentils 169
647. Lentils and Tomato Sauce..................... 169
648. Chickpeas Curry.................................... 170
SOUPS AND STEWS....................................... 171
649. Creamy Kale Soup................................. 171
650. Broccoli Cheese Soup 171
651. Broccoli Cauliflower Soup 171
652. Clam and Cauliflower Chowder........... 171
653. Turkey Soup 171
654. Buffalo Chicken Soup 172
655. Ham & Asparagus Soup 172
656. Hearty Beef and Bacon Chili 172
657. Chicken Tomato Sausage Stew 173
658. Green Beans Soup................................. 173
659. Bay Leaves Carrots Kale Chicken Soup 173
660. Broccoli and Zucchini Soup.................. 173
661. Healthy Creamy Mushroom Stew 174
662. Beef Soup... 174
663. Creamy Artichoke Spinach Soup........... 174
664. Spinach Soup 174
665. Cilantro Avocado Chicken Soup 174
666. Broccoli Coconut Beef Curry Stew........ 175
667. Cabbage Soup.. 175
668. Mouth Watering Smoked Sausage Stew & Chicken.. 175
669. Pomodoro Soup with Basil.................... 175
670. Fish Stew.. 176
671. Bolognese Soup..................................... 176
672. Keto Chili 176
673. Mexican Chicken Soup.......................... 176
674. Pressure-Cooked Beef Stew.................. 177
675. Lentil Spinach Stew............................... 177
676. Veal Bean Soup..................................... 177
677. Purple Cabbage Stew............................. 177
678. Garbanzo Turkey Soup.......................... 178
679. Green Bean Soup with Beef.................. 178
680. Trout Stew... 178
681. Brisket Broccoli Stew............................ 179
682. Instant Pot Spiced Coconut Fish Stew.. 179
683. Instant Pot Chicken and Vegetable Stew.. 179
684. Ground Beef and Vegetable Stew......... 179
685. Instant Pot Spiced and Creamy Vegetable Stew with Cashews.. 180
686. Coconut Fish Stew with Spinach 180
687. Filling Herbed Turkey Stew.................. 180
688. Low Carb Bouillabaisse Fish Stew....... 180
689. Instant Pot Thai Nut Chicken 181
690. Tasty Instant Pot Greek Fish Stew........ 181
691. Pressure Cooker Vegetable and Fish Stew.. 181
692. Easy Cheesy Turkey Stew..................... 181
693. Instant Pot Beef and Sweet Potato Stew.. 182
694. Instant Pot Coconut Fish Stew.............. 182
695. Instant Pot Loaded Protein Stew 182
696. Instant Pot Low Carb Mussel Stew....... 182
697. Scrumptious Beef Stew......................... 182
698. Turkish Split Pea Stew.......................... 183
699. Delicious Seafood Stew........................ 183
700. Curried Chicken Stew........................... 183
701. Beef Chuck & Green Cabbage Stew 183
702. Madras Lamb Stew................................ 184
703. Curried Goat Stew 184
704. Instant Pot Lemon Chicken Stew.......... 184
705. Hearty Lamb & Cabbage Stew............... 184
706. Rosemary-Garlic Beef Stew.................. 185
707. Instant Pot Oxtail Stew......................... 185
708. Pressure Cooked Lamb-Bacon Stew..... 185
709. Instant Pot Low Carb Vegetable Stew.. 185
710. Best Beef Stew for a King!.................... 186
DESSERTS.. 187
711. Keto Mocha Brownies........................... 187
712. Keto Raspberry Cheesecake 187
713. Choco Cinnamon Cake......................... 187
714. Delicious Raspberry Muffins with Chocolate Topping.. 188
715. Amazing Keto Almond Coffee Cups...... 188
716. Keto Cherry Mousse 188
717. Chocolate Chip Pudding....................... 189
718. Tasty Crumbled Lemon Muffin Parfait 189
719. Sweet Potato & Cinnamon Patties........ 189
720. Keto Coconut Bars................................ 189
721. Chocolate Bounties............................... 190
722. Lemon Cake 190
723. Choco Orange Muffins.......................... 190
724. Rum Cheesecake 191

725. Yummy Vanilla Mint Cake 191
726. Strawberry Pancakes 191
727. Keto Vanilla Cherry Panna Cotta 192
728. Delicious Vanilla Cream with
 Raspberries 192
729. Keto Mocha de Creme 192
730. Keto Mint Brownies 193
731. Creamy Keto Coconut Cake 193
732. Almond Vanilla Brownies 193
733. Special Strawberry Cream Cake 193
734. Yummy Chocolate Cupcakes 194
735. Coconut Flan 194
736. Blueberry Mug Cake 194
737. Ricotta Lemon Cheesecake 195
738. Creamy Lemon Curd 195
739. Chocolate Pudding Cake 195
740. Mini Vanilla Custards 195
741. Coconut Almond Cake 196
742. Maple Almond Cake in a Jar 196
743. Easy Chocolate Cheesecake 196
744. Classic Crème Brulee 196
745. Chili Cauliflower Spread 197
746. Artichokes Spread 197
747. Shrimp and Leeks Appetizer 197
748. Easy Italian Asparagus 197
749. Nutmeg Spiced Endives 198

INTRODUCTION

Going on a ketogenic diet is a lofty idea. It is good for you to know how your body functions and what to expect when you're on a ketogenic diet so as to get the most benefits.

During the adjustment period when your body switches gears on energy sources, there is a likelihood of fatigue, brain fog and sometimes bad breath. These issues will subside on their own once you've fully adjusted to your new lifestyle.

Weight loss is another common occurrence. Research studies have confirmed that much of the weight loss that occurs during the initial stage of going keto is water weight and as such can be regained within a short period of time. Also, the hormones are expected to circulate and they can promote the storage of fats.

In addition, since there is a reduction in your intake of carbohydrates, this also reduces the volume of fiber you consume and may lead to constipation. For the beginners who are just consuming large quantity of fats for the first time, diarrhea is another common occurrence. Again, it takes just a short adjustment period for all these symptoms to subside on their own. To be on the safe side, the amount of carbohydrates you consume should be rich in fiber to prevent constipation.

Instant Pot is basically a type of electric pressure cooker that comes with a bunch of different pre-programmed features. However, before having a lucid knowledge of what an Instant Pot really is, it is salient that you first understand the process of "Pressure Cooking".

Now what is pressure cooking? Well, the process of pressure cooking basically takes an air tight vessel, inside which a large amount of steam is generated and modern pressure cookers take full advantage of these steams produced, in order to cook the meals in a swift manner.

Also, it should be noted that this very process works at the whims of a strong scientific theory that enables it to carryout heating processes without obstruction, which is the reason why when the pressure inside the sealed vessels starts to climb; invariably causes the boiling point of water to also increase.

This very mechanism allows the device to generate a huge amount of heat without the water being actually "boiled" and cook foods at an accelerated rate.

BREAKFAST

01. Beef & Kale Casserole
Cooking Time: 20 minutes
Servings: 4
Ingredients:
2 cups of kale, fresh, chopped
1 lb. ground beef
13 ounces mozzarella cheese, shredded
16 ounces tomato puree
1 celery stalk
1 carrot, chopped
1 yellow onion, chopped
2 tablespoons butter
1 tablespoons red wine
Salt and pepper to taste
Directions:
Set your instant pot on sauté mode, add the butter and melt it. Add the onion, carrot, stir and cook for 5 minutes. Add the beef, salt, pepper and cook for 10 minutes. Add the wine and stir and cook for 1 minute. Add the kale, tomato puree, cover with water and stir set on manual setting for 6 minutes. Release the pressure naturally. Uncover the pot and add the cheese and stir. Divide into serving bowls. Serve.
Nutrition Values:
Calories: 182Fat: 11gFiber: 1.4gCarbs: 31gProtein: 22g

02. Korean Beef
Cooking Time: 25 minutes
Servings: 6
Ingredients:
1 cup beef stock
¼ cup soybean paste
2 lbs. beefsteak, cut into strips
1 yellow onion, sliced thin
1-ounce shiitake mushroom caps, cut into quarters
1 zucchini, cubed
¼ teaspoon red pepper flakes
1 scallion, chopped
1 chili pepper, sliced
12 ounces extra firm tofu, cubed
Salt and pepper to taste
Directions:
Set the instant pot on sauté mode and add the stock and soybean paste, stir and simmer for 2 minutes. Add the beef, pepper flakes, salt and pepper. Cover the instant pot and cook on the meat/stew setting for 15 minutes. Release the pressure naturally. Add the zucchini, onion, tofu, and mushrooms, stir and bring to a boil. Cover the instant pot and cook on manual setting for 4 minutes. Release the pressure naturally again, uncover the instant pot, add more salt and pepper, add the chili pepper and scallion. Stir. Divide into serving bowls. Serve.
Nutrition Values:
Calories: 310Fat: 9.3gFiber: 0.2gCarbs: 18.4gProtein: 35.3g

03. Beef & Broccoli
Cooking Time: 10 minutes
Servings: 4
Ingredients:
3 lbs. beef chuck roast, cut into thin strips
1 tablespoon peanut oil
2 tablespoons almond flour
2 teaspoons toasted sesame oil
1 lb. broccoli florets
1 yellow onion, chopped
½ cup beef stock
For the marinade:
1 tablespoon sesame oil
2 tablespoons fish sauce
1 cup soy sauce
5 garlic cloves, minced
3 red peppers, crushed, dried
½ teaspoon Chinese five spice powder
Toasted sesame seeds for serving
Directions:
Mix the soy sauce, with the fish sauce and 1 tablespoon of sesame oil in a bowl. Add in garlic and five spice powder along with crushed red peppers and stir well. Add the beef strips and toss to coat. Set the instant pot to sauté mode, adding peanut oil and heat it up. Add the onions and cook for 4 minutes. Add the beef and marinade and cook for 2 minutes. Add the stock and stir, cover the instant pot. Cook on the meat/stew setting in 5 minutes. Release the pressure naturally for 10 minutes.
Uncover the instant pot and add the almond flour with ¼ cup liquid from the instant pot, add the broccoli to the steamer basket, cover the instant pot again and cook for 3 minutes on manual mode. Release the pressure and uncover the instant pot and divide the beef into serving bowls add the broccoli on top and drizzle with toasted sesame seeds. Serve.
Nutrition Values:
Calories: 338Fat: 18gFiber: 5gCarbs: 50gProtein: 40g

04. Beef and Cabbage
Cooking Time: 1 hour and 20 minutes
Servings: 6
Ingredients:
2 ½ lbs. beef brisket
6 potatoes, cut into quarters
1 cabbage head, cut into wedges
4 carrots, peeled and chopped
3 cloves garlic, peeled, chopped
2 bay leaves
4 cups water
1 turnip cut into quarters
Horseradish sauce, for serving
Salt and pepper to taste
Directions:
Add the beef brisket and water into your instant pot, add garlic, bay leaves, salt and pepper, cover the instant pot. Set on the meat/stew setting for 1 hour and 15 minutes. Release the pressure with quick-release. Add to instant pot carrots, potatoes, cabbage, and turnip, stir and cover. Cook on the manual setting for 6 minutes. Release the pressure naturally,

and uncover your instant pot. Divide among serving plates. Serve with horseradish sauce on top.
Nutrition Values:
Calories: 340Fat: 24gFiber: 1gCarbs: 14gProtein: 46g

05. Instant Pot Beef Cabbage Rolls
Cooking Time: 38 minutes
Servings: 6
Ingredients:
2 lbs. lean ground beef
½ teaspoon, freshly ground black pepper
4 cloves garlic, minced, finely
1 cup green onion
1 large egg
1 large head of cabbage
1 cup brown rice
1 teaspoon sea salt
For the sauce:
1 cup onion, finely chopped
2 tablespoons butter
3 cloves of garlic, finely minced
Chopped, fresh parsley for garnish
2 tablespoons cold water
1 tablespoon cornstarch
4 dashes Worcestershire sauce
½ teaspoon freshly ground black pepper
1 teaspoon onion powder
½ teaspoon garlic powder
¼ cup white vinegar
2 teaspoons low-sodium instant beef bouillon
1 (8-ounce can tomato sauce
2 (14-ounce cans tomatoes, diced with their juice
Directions:
Cook the brown rice according to package directions. Fluff with fork and set aside. Fill a deep large pot half full of water, and bring to a boil over high heat. Remove the core from the cabbage, and place the cabbage core side down into the pot of water. Cover and allow the head of cabbage to boil for 10 minutes. Keep checking and removing the outer leaves as they soften on the cabbage, removing them to a plate to cool. Once you have removed all the large leaves to make rolls, cook the smaller leaves until they are crisp-tender. When done remove them from heat and coarsely chop them and set aside.
For your sauce take a large saucepan and melt the butter in it, add the onion, and cook over medium heat for 2 minutes, add the garlic and stir for another minute. Add in the tomatoes, bouillon, vinegar, garlic powder, Worcestershire sauce, onion powder, salt and pepper, mix well. Remove from heat and stir in some of the chopped cabbage and set aside.
For your cabbage roll filling add to a large bowl, beaten egg, onion, cooked rice, garlic, salt, pepper, ground beef and mix with your hands until ingredients are well combined.
Take a cabbage leaf and lay it flat on a work surface with the stem end facing you. Take to tablespoonfuls of filling and place it at the bottom of the cabbage leaf. Fold in the sides of the leaf and roll away from you. Repeat this with the remaining cabbage leaves and filling, on average you should get about 15 rolls.
Place a layer of sauce in your instant pot then a layer of cabbage rolls, repeat this, layer, do not fill too much, you might have to do two batches. Secure the lid so that it is sealed and set to the Meat/Stew setting for 20 minutes. When the cooking is completed, release the pressure naturally for 15 minutes, then use quick-release to get rid of any remaining steam. Remove cabbage rolls to a platter. Set instant pot to sauté mode and bring sauce to a boil. In small bowl whisk the cornstarch and cold water, then add into sauce to thicken. Divide rolls into serving bowls, pour sauce over rolls. Serve hot!
Nutrition Values:
Calories: 389Fat: 25gFiber: 1gCarbs: 23gProtein: 37g

06. Beef & Mushroom Soup
Cooking Time: 25 minutes
Servings: 4
Ingredients:
1 ½ lbs. steak, thinly sliced
32 ounces beef stock
10 ounces Cremini mushrooms, thinly sliced
3 tablespoons butter
3 tablespoons garlic, minced
1 medium onion, diced
1 cup heavy cream
1 cup sour cream
2 tablespoons beef bouillon granules
2 tablespoons Dijon mustard
2 tablespoons Italian parsley, chopped
1 ½ teaspoons onion powder
1 ½ teaspoons garlic powder
1 teaspoon Oregano, dried
1 teaspoon sea salt
Black pepper to taste
Directions:
Set your instant pot onto sauté mode and add the butter and heat. Add in the onions and garlic. Add in the beef strips, mushrooms and beef stock. Sauté for a few minutes or until beef is no longer pink. Press the keep warm/cancel button to stop sauté mode. Add in rest of ingredients and press the meat/stew button on instant and set for 20 minutes. Release pressure naturally. Remove lid and divide into serving bowls. Serve.
Nutrition Values:
Calories: 310Fat: 18.4gFiber: 1.3gCarbs: 22.5gProtein: 30.1g

07. Spicy Beef & Cashew Curry
Cooking Time: 20 minutes
Servings: 4
Ingredients:
2lbs chuck roast
6 tablespoons coconut milk
2 tablespoons Thai fish sauce
2 red chilis, fresh, chopped
1 tablespoon onion flakes
1 tablespoon cumin, ground
5 cardamom pods, cracked
3 tablespoons red curry paste
2 cups water
1 tablespoon coriander, ground
1 tablespoon ginger, ground

¼ cup cashews, roughly chopped, for garnish when serving
¼ cup cilantro, fresh, chopped, top when serving
2 tablespoons coconut oil
Directions:
Set your instant pot on sauté mode and add coconut oil and heat. Add in the beef and brown on all sides for a few minutes. Press the keep warm/cancel button to cancel sauté mode once meat is browned. Set instant pot to meat/stew setting for 20 minutes. Add remaining ingredients to instant pot except the cashews and cilantro. Release pressure naturally. Open the lid and divide into serving dishes. Serve.
Nutrition Values:
Calories: 374Fat: 20gFiber: 2.6gCarbs: 14gProtein: 35.5g

08. BBQ Pot Roast with Garlic Sauce
Cooking Time: 1 hour
Servings: 4
Ingredients:
4 lbs. chuck shoulder roast
5 teaspoons garlic, minced
1 yellow onion, chopped
2 tablespoons Worcestershire sauce
3 tablespoons butter
4 tablespoons vinegar
1 tablespoon mustard
1 teaspoon liquid smoke
Salt and pepper to taste
Directions:
Rub the roast with salt and pepper. Set instant pot to sauté and add butter, then add the roast and brown meat on all sides. Press keep warm/cancel button to cancel the sauté mode. Add all other ingredients into the instant pot and set on meat/stew setting for 1 hour. Release the pressure naturally. Open the lid of pot and stir. Divide into serving dishes. Serve with choice of veggies.
Nutrition Values:
Calories: 270Fat: 20gFiber: 1gCarbs: 2gProtein: 23g

09. Cheesesteak Casserole
Cooking Time: 1 hour
Servings: 6
Ingredients:
2 lbs cube steak, cut into strips
1 red pepper, cut into strips
1 green pepper, cut into strips
½ lb. mushroom, sliced
¼ lb. pepperoni, thinly sliced
8 ounces provolone cheese, thinly sliced
1 tablespoon coconut oil
1 onion, thinly sliced
Salt and pepper to taste
Directions:
Set your instant pot to sauté mode, and add in the coconut oil. Add the mushrooms and steak and saute until meat is no longer pink. Add in remaining ingredients except the cheese, and press the keep warm/cancel button to cancel sauté mode. Set your instant pot to the meat/stew setting for 50 minutes. Release pressure naturally. Remove the lid and stir. Divide into serving dishes. Top each dish with cheese, allow cheese to melt and then serve.
Nutrition Values:
Calories: 296Fat: 18.4gFiber: 1.3gCarbs: 20.5gProtein: 30.1g

10. Cabbage Stew and Beef Shank
Cooking Time: 50 minutes
Servings: 4
Ingredients:
2 center-cut beef shanks
4 cloves garlic, minced
½ lb. baby carrots
2 medium onions, chopped
1 small cabbage, cut into wedges
15-ounce can tomato, diced, drained
1 cup beef stock
Salt and pepper to taste
2 tablespoons coconut oil
Directions:
Set your instant pot to sauté mode, and add in coconut oil. Add in the beef shanks and sauté until the meat is no longer pink. Press the keep warm/cancel button to stop sauté mode. Open lid of instant pot and add rest of ingredients. Set on meat/stew setting for 50 minutes. Release pressure naturally. Open lid and stir. Remove the meat and shred with fork. Divide into serving dishes. Serve.
Nutrition Values:
Calories: 310Fat: 22gFiber: 1gCarbs: 14gProtein: 42g

11. Shredded Beef with Avocado Salsa
Cooking Time: 1 hour and 10 minutes
Servings: 6
Ingredients:
2 lbs. beef chuck roast, cut into strips
1 tablespoon taco seasoning
2 tablespoons coconut oil
2 cans diced green chilies with juice
Cabbage Slaw & Dressing Ingredients:
½ a small head of cabbage
1 small green cabbage
½ cup thinly sliced green onion
2 teaspoons green tabasco sauce
6 tablespoons mayo
4 teaspoons lime juice, fresh squeezed
Avocado Salsa Ingredients:
2 large avocados, diced
1 tablespoon lime juice, fresh squeezed
1 medium Poblano pepper, diced very small
1 tablespoon extra-virgin olive oil
1 cup cilantro, freshly chopped
Directions:
Remove all excess fat from the meat and cut into strips. Season the meat strips with taco seasoning. Set your instant pot to sauté mode. Add in coconut oil and meat, sauté until meat is no longer pink and browned on all sides. Press the keep warm/cancel button to stop sauté once the meat is browned. Set to meat/stew setting for 1 hour. Release the pressure naturally. Remove the meat from instant pot and shred on chopping board with a fork. Place shredded meat back into your instant pot and replace the lid

and keep on the keep warm/cancel setting. Slice the cabbage and the green onions to tiny strips using a slicer. Make the dressing by whisking the green Tabasco, mayo, and lime juice together. Mix the strips of cabbage and onions with the dressing. Slice the avocados and mix with lime juice. Chop cilantro and Poblano pepper very finely, and mix with the avocado. Pour in olive oil and mix. Place slaw in serving bowls. Top with beef and avocado salsa. Serve.
Nutrition Values:
Calories: 296Fat: 21gFiber: 1gCarbs: 14gProtein: 33g

12. Cheeseburger Soup
Cooking Time: 25 minutes
Servings: 4
Ingredients:
1 lb lean ground beef
4 cups beef broth low sodium
1 teaspoon Worcestershire sauce
2 teaspoons parsley, fresh chopped
½ red bell pepper
2 tomatoes, chopped
8 ounces tomato paste
½ cup onions, chopped
1 teaspoon garlic powder
½ cup cheese
Salt and pepper to taste
2 tablespoons coconut oil
Directions:
Set your instant pot to sauté mode. Add the coconut oil. Add in the ground beef and sauté until the meat is no longer pink and is browned. Press the keep warm/cancel button to stop sauté mode. Set the instant pot to meat/stew setting for 20 minutes. Add the rest of the ingredients and stir. Close the lid. Once done release pressure naturally. Add to serving dishes. Top with cheese. Serve.
Nutrition Values:
Calories: 187Fat: 5gFiber: 1.4gCarbs: 32gProtein: 38g

13. Beef Sirloin Lettuce Wraps
Cooking Time: 40 minutes
Servings: 6
Ingredients:
2 lbs. sirloin roast, excess fat removed
1 teaspoon smoked paprika
1 tablespoon chili powder
2 cups beef broth
1 onion, chopped
Salt and pepper to taste
Lettuce leaves to use to wrap meat, as needed
Directions:
Add all your ingredients into your instant pot. Set your instant pot on the meat/stew setting for 40 minutes. Once done release the pressure naturally. Remove the lid and stir. Remove the meat to chopping board and shred the meat with a fork. Return the meat to the instant pot. Place lettuce leaves on serving plates then top them with meat. Serve.
Nutrition Values:
Calories: 296Fat: 20gFiber: 1gCarbs: 14gProtein: 37g

14. Ropa Vieja
Cooking Time: 25 minutes
Servings: 4
Ingredients:
2 lbs. flank steak, cut into strips
1 yellow pepper
1 green pepper
1 onion, thinly sliced
4 teaspoons cumin
4 teaspoons oregano
3 teaspoons garlic, minced
3 tablespoons tomato paste
1 tablespoon capers
Sea salt to taste
2 tablespoons olive oil
Directions:
Add the olive oil to your instant pot and set it to sauté mode. Add in meat strips and sauté until browned. Press the keep warm/cancel button to turn off the sauté mode. Add remaining ingredients into the pot and set to meat/stew setting for 20 minutes. Release the pressure with quick-release. Remove the lid and stir ingredients. Divide into serving dishes. Serve.
Nutrition Values:
Calories: 282Fat: 20gFiber: 1gCarbs: 14gProtein: 39g

15. Italian-style Beef
Cooking Time: 45 minutes
Servings: 4
Ingredients:
2 lbs. boneless beef brisket
6 cloves of garlic, minced
1 onion, sliced
1 teaspoon red pepper flakes
½ cup red wine
2 cups fat-free beef broth
Salt and pepper to taste
1 tablespoon Italian seasoning
Directions:
Rub the beef with salt and pepper. Place the beef along with the rest of the ingredients into your instant pot. Set to meat/stew setting for 45 minutes. Once done release the pressure naturally. Remove the lid and stir. Remove the meat and shred with fork then place it back into the instant pot.
Nutrition Values:
Calories: 274Fat: 22gFiber: 1gCarbs: 16gProtein: 42g

16. Asian Shredded Beef
Cooking Time: 50 minutes
Servings: 4
Ingredients:
2 lbs. beef eye of round roast
¼ cup rice wine vinegar
½ cup soy sauce
¼ cup brown sugar
2 tablespoons ketchup
2 tablespoons sesame seeds
1-inch piece of ginger, fresh, grated
2 teaspoons Asian chili sauce
6 cloves of garlic, minced
½ red onion, minced
1 jalapeno, minced

Directions:
In a bowl add the soy sauce, brown sugar, vinegar, sesame seeds, ginger, ketchup, Asian chili sauce. Whisk these ingredients, add in the onion, jalapeno, and garlic. Place the roast into the instant pot. Pour the sauce over the roast. Cook on the meat/stew setting for 50 minutes. When done release naturally. Remove the meat and shred the meat with a fork. Replace the meat back into the instant pot. Allow it to sit for 30 minutes on the keep warm setting.
Nutrition Values:
Calories: 287Fat: 22gFiber: 1gCarbs: 12gProtein: 36g

17. Instant Pot Beef Ragu with Herbs
Cooking Time: 30 minutes
Servings: 4
Ingredients:
2 lbs lean chuck beef
½ onion, diced
1 rib of celery, diced
2 tablespoons oregano, fresh, chopped
2 tablespoons rosemary, fresh, minced
cups beef broth
1-14 ounce can tomatoes, diced
1-14 ounce can tomatoes, crushed
4 garlic cloves, minced
1 carrot, peeled, diced
Directions:
Rub the meat with salt and pepper and place it in the instant pot. Add remaining ingredients to the instant pot. Set to meat/stew setting and cook for 30 minutes. Once done then release the pressure naturally. Remove the lid and stir ingredients. Divide into serving dishes. Serve.
Nutrition Values:
Calories: 292Fat: 19gFiber: 2gCarbs: 14gProtein: 36g

18. Hot Roast Machaca
Cooking Time: 45 minutes
Servings: 4
Ingredients:
2 lbs. rump roast
3 serrano chiles, stemmed, seeded, and minced
3 garlic cloves, minced
1 cup red bell pepper, diced
1 ½ cups onion, diced
4 tablespoons fresh lime juice
2 tablespoons Worcestershire sauce
2 tablespoons of Maggi sauce
Salt and pepper to taste
½ cup beef broth
½ teaspoon oregano, dried
½ 14-ounce can diced tomatoes with juice
Directions:
Rub the meat with salt and pepper and place into your instant pot. In a bowl mix Maggi, beef broth and lime juice. Pour the mixture over the meat. Add all other ingredients into instant pot. Set to meat/stew setting for 45 minutes. Once it is done release pressure naturally. Remove the lid and stir the ingredients, remove meat shred with fork. Return meat to pot. Keep on warm setting for 20 minutes. Divide into serving dishes. Serve.

Nutrition Values:
Calories: 296Fat: 23gFiber: 3gCarbs: 14gProtein: 34g

19. Korean-style Beef Tacos
Cooking Time: 55 minutes
Servings: 6
Ingredients:
2 lbs. beef roast
½ tablespoon Truvia
1/3 soy sauce
4 garlic cloves, minced
1-inch ginger root, fresh, peeled, grated
½ red onion, diced
2 jalapenos, diced
2 tablespoons seasoned rice wine vinegar
2 tablespoons sesame seeds
Serve on flour tortillas
Directions:
In a bowl add Truvia, sesame seeds, jalapenos, ginger and mix well. Add in the rice wine vinegar and soy sauce. Add the beef into instant pot, rub garlic into meat. Pour sauce over the meat and place lid on instant pot. Set to meat/stew setting for 55 minutes. When done release the pressure naturally. Remove the meat and shred, then place back into the instant pot and allow to stay for 20 minutes on keep warm setting. Divide into serving dishes on top of flour tortillas. Serve.
Nutrition Values:
Calories: 302Fat: 23gFiber: 3gCarbs: 14gProtein: 34g

20. Instant Pot Beef Stew
Cooking Time: 40 minutes
Servings: 4
Ingredients:
2 lbs cubed beef
1 tablespoon ghee
2 cups beef broth
1 red onion, sliced
1 carrot, peeled, chopped
2 celery stalks, diced
1 cinnamon stick
5 cloves
¼ teaspoon nutmeg
1-star anise
Salt and pepper to taste
Head of lettuce
Directions:
Set your instant pot to sauté mode, add in the ghee. Place your cubed beef into instant pot and brown on all sides. Also add onion. When you are finished with sautéing the meat and onions press the keep warm/cancel button to stop the sauté mode. Place your other ingredients into instant pot along with meat and onions. Set your instant pot to meat/stew setting for 35 minutes. Once done release pressure naturally. Stir the ingredients. Add lettuce leaves to serving dished then top with meat mixture.
Nutrition Values:
Calories: 292Fat: 21gFiber: 3gCarbs: 14gProtein: 32g

21. Caribbean Ginger Oxtails
Cooking Time: 45 minutes
Servings: 4
Ingredients:

2 lbs. beef oxtails
2 carrots, diced
2 onions, sliced
4 sprigs thyme, fresh
1 teaspoon fish sauce
3 tablespoons tomato paste
2 cups beef stock
1 jalapeno pepper, minced
4 garlic cloves, minced
1-inch piece ginger, peeled, minced
2 tablespoons of ghee
Sea salt and pepper to taste
Directions:
Rub the oxtails with seasonings. Set your instant pot to sauté mode and add in the ghee. Add in the oxtails into instant pot and brown them on all sides. Toss in the garlic, onion, jalapeno, carrot, ginger and continue to sauté for a few minutes. Set the instant pot to keep warm/cancel setting to stop sauté mode. Add remaining ingredients into instant pot and set to meat/stew setting for 40 minutes. Once done release pressure naturally. Stir the ingredients. Divide into serving dishes. Serve.
Nutrition Values:
Calories: 303Fat: 24gFiber: 2gCarbs: 13gProtein: 33g

22. Coconut Yogurt Mix
Preparation time: 5 minutes
Cooking time: 5 minutes
Servings: 2
Ingredients:
1 cup coconut milk
½ cup coconut, unsweetened and flaked
1 cup yogurt
½ teaspoon stevia
¼ teaspoon vanilla extract
½ teaspoon cinnamon powder
Directions:
In your instant pot, combine the coconut milk with the coconut and the rest of the ingredients, toss, put the lid on and cook on High for 5 minutes.
Release the pressure fast for 5 minutes, divide the yogurt mix into bowls and serve.
Nutrition Values: calories 218, fat 18.4, fiber 2.2, carbs 6.7, protein 5.2

23. Artichokes Pudding
Preparation time: 10 minutes
Cooking time: 15 minutes
Servings: 4
Ingredients:
2 cups almond milk
¼ cup coconut cream
1 and ½ cups canned artichokes, drained and chopped
1 teaspoon sweet paprika
A pinch of salt and black pepper
1 tablespoon chives, chopped
Directions:
In your instant pot, mix the almond milk with cream and the rest of the ingredients, put the lid on and cook on High for 15 minutes.
Release the pressure naturally for 10 minutes, divide the mix between plates and serve.
Nutrition Values: calories 312, fat 23.4, fiber 3.2, carbs 7.3, protein 3.2

24. Scotch Eggs and Tomato Passata
Preparation time: 6 minutes
Cooking time: 18 minutes
Servings: 4
Ingredients:
1 pound pork, ground
A pinch of salt and black pepper
1 teaspoon cilantro, chopped
1 teaspoon hot paprika
4 eggs, hard boiled and peeled
1 tablespoon avocado oil
1 cup tomato passata
Directions:
In a bowl, mix the pork with the rest of the ingredients except the eggs, tomato passata and the oil and stir well.
Divide the mix into 4 balls and flatten them on a working surface.
Divide the eggs on each pork ball and wrap them well. Set the instant pot on Sauté mode, add the oil, heat it up, add the scotch eggs and brown them for 2 minutes on each side.
Add the tomato passata, put the lid on and cook on High for 12 minutes.
Release pressure fast for 6 minutes, divide the mix between plates and serve for breakfast.
Nutrition Values: calories 245, fat 8.9, fiber 1.1, carbs 3.9, protein 36

25. Parsley Cauliflower Mix
Preparation time: 10 minutes
Cooking time: 20 minutes
Servings: 4
Ingredients:
2 cups cauliflower florets
2 ounces cheddar cheese, shredded
1 teaspoon garlic powder
1 teaspoon chili powder
2 eggs, whisked
1 tablespoon parsley, chopped
1 tablespoon avocado oil
½ cup heavy cream
A pinch of salt and black pepper
Directions:
Set your instant pot on sauté mode, add the oil, heat it up, add the cauliflower, garlic and chili powder and cook for 5 minutes.
Add the rest of the ingredients, toss, put the lid on and cook on High for 15 minutes.
Release the pressure naturally for 10 minutes, divide the mix into bowls and serve for breakfast.
Nutrition Values: calories 164, fat 13.1, fiber 1.7, carbs 4.6, protein 7.9

26. Pork Pie
Preparation time: 10 minutes
Cooking time: 30 minutes
Servings: 4
Ingredients:
½ cup heavy cream
A pinch of salt and black pepper
4 eggs, whisked

2 cups pork meat, ground and browned
2 green onions, chopped
1 cup cheddar cheese, shredded
1 cup water
Directions:
In a bowl, mix the eggs with the rest of the ingredients except the water, whisk well and spread into a pie pan.
Add the water to your instant pot, add the trivet, add the pan inside, put the lid on and cook on High for 30 minutes.
Release the pressure naturally for 10 minutes, divide the mix between plates and serve hot for breakfast.
Nutrition Values: calories 231, fat 19.3, fiber 0.2, carbs 1.7, protein 13

27. Ginger Cauliflower Rice Pudding
Preparation time: 10 minutes
Cooking time: 15 minutes
Servings: 4
Ingredients:
2 cups almond milk
1 cup cauliflower rice
1 teaspoon cinnamon powder
1 tablespoon ginger, grated
3 tablespoons stevia
1 teaspoon vanilla extract
Directions:
In your instant pot, mix the cauliflower rice with the milk and the other ingredients, toss, put the lid on and cook on High for 15 minutes.
Release the pressure naturally for 10 minutes, stir the pudding, divide it into bowls and serve.
Nutrition Values: calories 284, fat 28.7, fiber 2.8, carbs 7.7, protein 2.9

28. Bok Choy Bowls
Preparation time: 10 minutes
Cooking time: 20 minutes
Servings: 4
Ingredients:
1 and ½ cups veggie stock
2 cups bok choy, roughly torn
2 tablespoons ginger, grated
2 garlic cloves, minced
1 tablespoon coconut aminos
1 tablespoon sweet paprika
2 tomatoes, cubed
A pinch of salt and black pepper
Directions:
In your instant pot, mix the bok choy with the stock and the rest of the ingredients, toss, put the lid on and cook on High for 20 minutes.
Release the pressure naturally for 10 minutes, divide the mix into bowls and serve for breakfast.
Nutrition Values: calories 89, fat 6.8, fiber 2.1, carbs 6.1, protein 1.7

29. Mushroom and Avocado Salad
Preparation time: 10 minutes
Cooking time: 20 minutes
Servings: 4
Ingredients:
2 avocados, pitted, peeled and cubed
1 tablespoon olive oil
1 tablespoon chives, chopped
A pinch of salt and black pepper
½ pound white mushrooms, sliced
1 tablespoon balsamic vinegar
½ cup veggie stock
1 cup baby arugula
Directions:
Set the instant pot on Sauté mode, add the oil, heat it up, add the mushrooms and cook for 4 minutes.
Add the rest of the ingredients except the avocado and the arugula, put the lid on and cook on High for 15 minutes.
Release the pressure naturally for 10 minutes, transfer the mix to a bowl, add the avocado and the arugula, toss and serve for breakfast.
Nutrition Values: calories 250, fat 23.3, fiber 6.4, carbs 7.6, protein 3.8

30. Salmon and Eggs Mix
Preparation time: 10 minutes
Cooking time: 12 minutes
Servings: 4
Ingredients:
4 ounces smoked salmon, skinless, boneless and cut into strips
4 eggs
A pinch of salt and black pepper
½ cup coconut cream
1 tablespoon chives, chopped
1 tablespoon cilantro, chopped
Cooking spray
Directions:
In a bowl, mix the salmon with the eggs and the rest of the ingredients except the cooking spray and whisk well.
Grease the instant pot with the cooking spray, pour the salmon mix, spread, put the lid on and cook on High for 12 minutes.
Release the pressure naturally for 10 minutes, divide the mix between plates and serve.
Nutrition Values: calories 167, fat 12.9, fiber 0.7, carbs 2.1, protein 11.4

31. Italian Beef and Green Beans Mix
Preparation time: 10 minutes
Cooking time: 30 minutes
Servings: 6
Ingredients:
2 spring onions chopped
1 red bell pepper, chopped
1 pound beef, ground
½ cup veggie stock
A pinch of salt and black pepper
1 tablespoon Italian seasoning
1 tablespoon cilantro, chopped
1 teaspoon olive oil
½ pound green beans, trimmed and halved
Directions:
Set your instant pot on sauté mode, add the oil, heat it up, add the meat, Italian seasoning, salt and pepper and brown for 5 minutes.
Add the rest of the ingredients, toss, put the lid on and cook on High for 25 minutes.

Release the pressure naturally for 10 minutes, divide everything between plates and serve for breakfast.
Nutrition Values: calories 259, fat 9.4, fiber 2.4, carbs 6.7, protein 35.8

32. Herbed Mushroom Mix
Preparation time: 10 minutes
Cooking time: 20 minutes
Servings: 4
Ingredients:
1 and ½ pounds brown mushrooms, chopped
2 tablespoons chicken stock
A pinch of salt and black pepper
1 tablespoon olive oil
½ teaspoon garlic powder
½ teaspoon basil, dried
1 teaspoon rosemary, chopped
1 red bell pepper, cut into strips
Directions:
Set your instant pot on sauté mode, add the oil, heat it up, add the mushrooms, stir and sauté for 5 minutes.
Add the rest of the ingredients, put the lid on and cook on High for 15 minutes.
Release the pressure naturally for 10 minutes, divide the mix between plates and serve for breakfast.
Nutrition Values: calories 42, fat 3.7, fiber 0.6, carbs 2.7, protein 0.4

33. Creamy Zucchini Pan
Preparation time: 10 minutes
Cooking time: 20 minutes
Servings: 4
Ingredients:
4 zucchinis, sliced
1 tablespoon avocado oil
1 shallot, minced
¼ cup heavy cream
2 tablespoons parsley, chopped
6 eggs, whisked
2 tablespoons cheddar, grated
A pinch of salt and black pepper
Directions:
Set the instant pot on Sauté mode, add the oil, heat it up, add the shallot and sauté for 2-3 minutes.
Add the zucchinis and the rest of the ingredients, toss, put the lid on and cook on High for 15 minutes.
Release the pressure naturally for 10 minutes, divide the mix between plates and serve for breakfast.
Nutrition Values: calories 163, fat 10.4, fiber 2.4, carbs 7.7, protein 11.8

34. Leeks and Pork Mix
Preparation time: 10 minutes
Cooking time: 30 minutes
Servings: 4
Ingredients:
1 pound pork meat, ground
¼ cup coconut cream
2 leeks, chopped
4 eggs, whisked
1 tablespoon sweet paprika
1 tablespoon chives, chopped
A pinch of salt and black pepper
¼ teaspoon garlic powder
1 tablespoon olive oil
Directions:
Set your instant pot on sauté mode, add the oil, heat it up, add the leeks and sauté for 5 minutes.
Add the meat and brown for 4-5 minutes more.
Add the eggs and the rest of the ingredients, toss, put the lid on and cook on High for 20 minutes.
Release the pressure naturally for 10 minutes, divide the mix between plates and serve for breakfast.
Nutrition Values: calories 160, fat 11.8, fiber 1.8, carbs 7.1, protein 6.9

35. Cardamom Walnuts Pudding
Preparation time: 5 minutes
Cooking time: 10 minutes
Servings: 2
Ingredients:
1 teaspoon cardamom, ground
½ cup walnuts, chopped
1 teaspoon swerve
1 and ½ cups coconut cream
2 tablespoons almond meal
Directions:
In your instant pot, mix the cream with the cardamom and the rest of the ingredients, toss, put the lid on and cook on High for 10 minutes.
Release the pressure fast for 5 minutes, divide everything into bowls and serve.
Nutrition Values: calories 231, fat 21.9, fiber 3.2, carbs 5.1, protein 8.9

36. Basil Eggs Mix
Preparation time: 5 minutes
Cooking time: 15 minutes
Servings: 4
Ingredients:
2 tablespoons basil, chopped
Cooking spray
A pinch of salt and black pepper
4 eggs, whisked
1 cup cheddar cheese, shredded
1 teaspoon chili powder
Directions:
Grease the instant pot with the cooking spray, add the eggs and the rest of the ingredients, toss, put the lid on and cook on High for 15 minutes.
Release the pressure fast for 5 minutes, divide the mix between plates and serve for breakfast.
Nutrition Values: calories 180, fat 14, fiber 0.3, carbs 1.1, protein 12.7

37. Creamy Blueberries and Nuts
Preparation time: 5 minutes
Cooking time: 8 minutes
Servings: 6
Ingredients:
½ cup walnuts, chopped
½ cups almonds, chopped
2 teaspoons swerve
1 cup blueberries
1 teaspoon vanilla extract
1 cup coconut cream
Directions:

In your instant pot, combine the walnuts with the almonds and the rest of the ingredients, toss, put the lid on and cook on High for 8 minutes.
Release the pressure fast for 5 minutes, divide the mix into bowls and serve for breakfast.
Nutrition Values: calories 218, fat 19.7, fiber 3.2, carbs 5.8, protein 5.3

38. Kale and Bok Choy Muffins
Preparation time: 10 minutes
Cooking time: 20 minutes
Servings: 4
Ingredients:
½ cup almond milk
4 eggs, whisked
1 tablespoon avocado oil
A pinch of salt and black pepper
½ cup bok choy, chopped
½ cup kale, chopped
1 tablespoon chives, chopped
1 and ½ cups water
Directions:
In a bowl, mix the almond milk with the eggs and the rest of the ingredients except the water and the oil and stir well.
Grease a muffin tray with the oil and pour the muffin mix inside.
Add the water to your instant pot, add the trivet, add muffin tray inside, put the lid on and cook on High for 20 minutes.
Release the pressure naturally for 10 minutes, cool the muffins down and serve for breakfast.
Nutrition Values: calories 142, fat 12, fiber 1.1, carbs 3.3, protein 6.7

39. Spinach and Artichokes Muffins
Preparation time: 10 minutes
Cooking time: 20 minutes
Servings: 12
Ingredients:
1 cup baby spinach, chopped
1 cup canned artichoke hearts, drained and chopped
A pinch of salt and black pepper
1 and ½ cups water
Cooking spray
3 cups almond flour
1 teaspoon baking soda
4 eggs
Directions:
In a bowl, mix the spinach with the artichokes and the rest of the ingredients except the water and the cooking spray and stir well.
Grease a muffin tray with the cooking spray and pour the muffin mix inside.
Add the water to your instant pot, add the trivet, add the muffin tray inside, put the lid on and cook on High for 20 minutes.
Release the pressure naturally for 10 minutes, cool the muffins down and serve for breakfast.
Nutrition Values: calories 66, fat 4.5, fiber 0.2, carbs 0.6, protein 5.8

40. Mozzarella and Kale Muffins
Preparation time: 10 minutes
Cooking time: 20 minutes
Servings: 4
Ingredients:
Cooking spray
2 cups water
1 cup mozzarella cheese, grated
4 eggs, whisked
½ teaspoon basil, dried
¼ teaspoon baking soda
1 cup almond flour
¼ cup kale, chopped
A pinch of salt and black pepper
½ cup almond milk
Directions:
In a bowl, mix the mozzarella with the eggs and the rest of the ingredients except the water and the cooking spray and whisk well.
Grease a muffin tray with the cooking spray and pour the muffins mix inside.
Add the water to your instant pot, add the trivet, add the muffin tray inside, put the lid on and cook on High for 20 minutes.
Release the pressure naturally for 10 minutes, divide the muffins between plates and serve for breakfast.
Nutrition Values: calories 155, fat 12.9, fiber 0.7, carbs 2.7, protein 8.4

41. Chicken Bowls
Preparation time: 10 minutes
Cooking time: 15 minutes
Servings: 4
Ingredients:
1 avocado, peeled and cut into wedges
2 tomatoes, cubed
1 and ½ cups baby spinach
A pinch of salt and black pepper
2 chicken breasts, skinless, boneless and cubed
2 tablespoons olive oil
2 tablespoons chicken stock
¼ cup tomato passata
1 shallot, chopped
Directions:
Set your instant pot on sauté mode, add the oil, heat it up, add the shallot and sauté for 2 minutes.
Add the chicken, stock and tomato passata, put the lid on and cook on High for 13 minutes.
Release the pressure naturally for 10 minutes, transfer the chicken mix to a bowl, add the remaining ingredients, toss and serve for breakfast.
Nutrition Values: calories 1, fa78t 17, fiber 4.6, carbs 7.6, protein 1.7

42. Coconut Pudding
Preparation time: 5 minutes
Cooking time: 5 minutes
Servings: 6
Ingredients:
2 cups coconut milk
1 cup coconut cream
¼ cup walnuts, chopped
½ cup coconut, unsweetened and shredded
4 teaspoons swerve
Directions:

In your instant pot, combine the coconut milk with the rest of the ingredients, toss, put the lid on and cook on High for 5 minutes.
Release the pressure fast for 5 minutes, divide the pudding into bowls and serve.
Nutrition Values: calories 332, fat 33.8, fiber 3.6, carbs 7.8, protein 4.2

43. Zucchini Spread
Preparation time: 10 minutes
Cooking time: 12 minutes
Servings: 4
Ingredients:
4 zucchinis, sliced
A pinch of salt and black pepper
½ cup heavy cream
½ cup cream cheese, soft
2 garlic cloves, minced
½ cup veggie stock
1 tablespoon avocado oil
1 tablespoon dill, chopped
Directions:
In your instant pot, mix the zucchinis with the stock, salt and pepper, put the lid on and cook on High for 12 minutes.
Release the pressure naturally for 10 minutes, drain the zucchinis, transfer them to a blender, add the rest of the ingredients, pulse, divide into bowls and serve as a morning spread.
Nutrition Values: calories 193, fat 16.5, fiber 2.5, carbs 7.8, protein 5.2

44. Blackberries Jam
Cooking Time: 30 minutes
Servings: 4
Ingredients:
5 cups sugar
4 pints' blackberries
3 tbsp. pectin powder
Juice of 1 small lemon
Directions:
Put the blackberries in your instant pot.
Add the sugar; then stir well and select sauté mode and cook for 3 minutes.
Transfer the jam to clean jars, close them and place them in the steamer basket of your instant pot.
Add water to cover the jars halfway, select Canning mode on your pot, close the lid and leave them for 20 minutes
Remove jars after 20 minutes, leave them to cool down and keep your jam in the fridge until you serve it in the morning with some toasted bread and some butter.

45. Delicious Poached Eggs
Cooking Time: 20 minutes
Servings: 2
Ingredients:
2 bell peppers; ends cut off
2 slices mozzarella cheese
2 eggs
1 bunch rucola leaves
1 cup water
2 slices whole wheat bread; toasted
For the sauce:
1 ½ tsp. mustard
3 tbsp. orange juice
1 tsp. turmeric powder
1 tsp. lemon juice
1 tbsp. white wine vinegar
2/3 cup homemade mayonnaise
Salt to the taste
Directions:
In a bowl; mix mayo with salt, turmeric, mustard, lemon juice, orange juice and vinegar, stir well, cover the bowl and keep in the fridge for now
Break an egg in each bell pepper, place them in the steamer basket of your instant pot, cover the basket with tin foil, add the water to the pot and cook on Low for 5 minutes.
Release the pressure naturally and open the instant pot lid.
Divide toasted bread into 2 plates, add cheese on each, some rucola leaves and top with pepper cups.
Drizzle the sauce all over and serve

46. Spinach & Tomato Breakfast
Cooking Time: 30 minutes
Servings: 6
Ingredients:
3 cups baby spinach; chopped.
12 eggs
1/2 cup milk
3 green onions; sliced
4 tomatoes sliced
1/4 cup parmesan; grated
1 ½ cups water
1 cup tomato; diced
Salt and black pepper to the taste
Directions:
Pour the water in your instant pot
In a bowl; mix the eggs with salt, pepper and milk and stir well.
Put diced tomato, spinach and green onions in a baking dish and stir them.
Pour the eggs mix over veggies, spread tomato slices on top and sprinkle parmesan at the end.
Arrange this in the steamer basket of your instant pot, seal the instant pot lid and cook everything at High for 20 minutes
Quick release the pressure; open the pot and introduce the baking dish in preheated broiler until the mixture is brown on top.
Divide among plates and serve

47. Banana Cake
Cooking Time: 1 hour
Servings: 5
Ingredients:
3 bananas, peeled and mashed
2 tsp. baking powder
1 cup water
2 eggs
1 stick butter; soft
1 tsp. nutmeg
1 ½ cups sugar
1 tsp. cinnamon
2 cups flour
A pinch of salt

Directions:
In a bowl, mix eggs with butter and sugar and stir very well
Add salt, baking powder, cinnamon and nutmeg and stir well again.
Add bananas and flour and stir again
Grease a spring form pan with some butter, pour the batter in it and cover the pan with a paper towel and tin foil
Add 1 cup water to your instant pot, place the pan in the pot, close the instant pot lid and cook at High for 55 minutes
Quick release the pressure, remove the pot, leave banana breakfast cake to cool down, cut and serve it

48. Breakfast Hash
Cooking Time:18 minutes
Servings:4
Ingredients:
8 oz. sausage, ground.
1 package hash browns; frozen
1/3 cup water
1 yellow onion; chopped.
1 green bell pepper; chopped.
4 eggs; whisked
1 cup cheddar cheese; grated
Salt and black pepper to the taste
Salsa for serving
Directions:
Set your instant pot on Sauté mode; add sausage, stir and cook for 2 minutes.
Drain excess fat; add bell pepper and onion, stir and cook for 2 more minutes
Add hash browns, water, eggs, salt and cheese; then stir well and close the instant pot lid and cook on Low for 4 minutes
Quick release the pressure, divide hash among plates and serve with salsa

49. Blueberry Bliss Bowls
Cooking Time: 22 minutes
Servings: 5
Ingredients:
1 cup nondairy milk, plus more as needed
1 cup fresh blueberries
1 cup millet; rinsed
1/2 cup sliced toasted almonds
2 ¼ cups water
1 tbsp. freshly squeezed lemon juice
2 tbsp. maple syrup
1/4 tsp. ground cinnamon
1/4 tsp. ground nutmeg
1/2 tsp. salt or as your liking
Zest of ½ lemon
Directions:
In the Instant Pot, stir together the millet, water, maple syrup, lemon juice, nutmeg, cinnamon and salt.
Lock the lid and turn the steam release handle to Sealing. Using the Manual function, set the cooker to High Pressure for 10 minutes
After completing the cooking time, let the pressure release naturally for 10 minutes; quick release any remaining pressure
Remove the lid carefully and stir in the milk, adding more if you like a creamier texture. Top with the blueberries, almonds and lemon zest before serving.

50. Quinoa and Granola Bowls
Cooking Time: 20 minutes
Servings: 4
Ingredients:
1/2 to 1 cup nondairy milk
1 cup quinoa; rinsed
2 cups granola (any variety
2 cups Fresh Fruit Compote
1 ½ cups water
2 tbsp. maple syrup
1 tsp. vanilla extract
1/2 tsp. ground cinnamon
Pinch salt
Sliced bananas; for topping (If you like
Toasted walnuts; for topping (If you like
1. Directions:
In the Instant Pot, combine the quinoa, water, maple syrup, vanilla, cinnamon and salt.
Lock the lid and turn the steam release handle to Sealing. Using the Manual function, set the cooker to High Pressure for 8 minutes
After completing the cooking time, let the pressure release naturally for 10 minutes; quick release any remaining pressure
Remove the lid carefully and stir the quinoa. Add enough milk to get the desired consistency.
Spoon the quinoa mix into bowls and top with granola, compote and any additional toppings, as desired.

51. Tofu and Potato Casserole
Cooking Time: 2 hours
Servings: 5
Ingredients:
2 cups frozen hash browns, thawed
1 (14-ouncepackage firm tofu, pressed for 30 to 60 minutes
⅓ cup nutritional yeast
1/4 cup nondairy milk
1 batch Tempeh "Sausage"
1 cup water
1/4 tsp. freshly ground black pepper, plus more for seasoning
1 tsp. garlic powder
1 tsp. ground cumin
1 tsp. sea salt
1 tsp. onion powder
1/2 tsp. dried oregano
Sliced scallion, green and light green parts; for serving
Garden Salsa; for serving
Nonstick cooking spray; for preparing the pan
Hot sauce; for serving
Cashew Sour Cream; for serving
Directions:
Lightly coat the bottom of a 7-inch springform pan with nonstick spray and set aside. In a large bowl, toss the hash browns with salt to taste and pepper and set aside.

In a food processor, combine the tofu, yeast, milk, sea salt, onion powder, garlic powder, cumin and oregano. Blend until smooth
Add the tempeh sausage to the hash browns along with one-fourth of the tofu mixture. Stir to combine. Layer this mixture on the bottom of the prepared pan. Top with the remaining tofu mixture. Cover the pan with a paper towel and wrap it tightly in aluminum foil.
Pour the water into your Instant Pot and place a trivet inside the inner pot. Put the springform pan on the trivet.
Lock the lid and turn the steam release handle to Sealing. Using the Manual function, set the cooker to High Pressure for 52 minutes.
After completing the cooking time, quick release the pressure
Remove the lid carefully and remove the pan from the Instant Pot. Take off the foil and paper towel. Let cool before releasing the sides of the pan. Serve topped as desired

52. French Toast Casserole
Cooking Time: 30 minutes
Servings: 5
Ingredients:
6 cups cubed, stale French bread
1/4 cup maple syrup, Or more for serving
1/4 cup Bailey's Almande Almond Milk Liqueur
1 cup water
Nonstick cooking spray; for preparing the bowl
1/4 tsp. kala namak; or sea salt
1 tsp. vanilla extract
1 large banana, plus more for topping; optional
Vegan butter; for topping
Directions:
Spray a 7-cup oven-safe glass bowl with nonstick spray and set aside. Pour the water into your Instant Pot and place a trivet inside the inner pot
In a large bowl, mash the banana with a fork. Stir in the maple syrup, Bailey's, vanilla and kala namak, making sure the banana is completely mixed in
Quickly toss the bread in the banana mixture, making sure to get even coverage.
Transfer to the prepared bowl, cover tightly with aluminum foil and place the bowl on top of the trivet in the Instant Pot
Lock the lid and turn the steam release handle to Sealing. Using the Manual function, set the cooker to High Pressure for 25 minutes
After completing the cooking time, quick release the pressure. Remove the lid carefully. Serve with toppings as desired and enjoy!

53. Tomato Spinach Quiche.
Cooking Time:30 minutes
Servings:6
- **Ingredients:**
12 large eggs
1/4 tsp. fresh ground black pepper
3 large green onions, sliced
1/2 tsp. salt
4 tomato slices, for topping the quiche
1/2 cup. milk
1 cup. tomato, seeded, diced
1 ½ cup. water, for the pot
3 cups. fresh baby spinach, roughly chopped
1/4 cup. Parmesan cheese, shredded.
Directions:
Pour the water into the Instant Pot container. In a large-sized bowl, whisk the eggs with the milk, pepper, and salt
Add the tomato, spinach, and the green onions into a 1 ½ quart-sized baking dish; mix well to combine
Pour the egg mix over the vegetables; stir until combined. Put the tomato slices gently on top
Sprinkle with the shredded parmesan cheese. Put the baking dish into the rack with a handle
Put the rack into the Instant Pot and then lock the lid. Set the pressure to "High" and the timer to 20 minutes.
When the timer beeps, wait for 1o minutes, then turn the steamer valve to "Venting" to release remaining pressure. Open the pot lid carefully
Hold the rack handles and lift the dish out from the pot
Broil till the top of the quiche is light brown, if desired
TIP: You can cover the baking dish with foil to prevent moisture from gathering on the quiche top. You can cook uncovered; just soak the moisture using a paper towel

54. Mushroom Oatmeal.
Cooking Time:25 minutes
Servings:4
Ingredients:
8 oz. mushroom; sliced
1 small yellow onion; chopped.
3 thyme springs; chopped.
1 cup steel cut oats
2 garlic cloves; minced.
2 tbsp. butter
2 tbsp. extra virgin olive oil
1/2 cup water
1/2 cup gouda; grated
14 oz. canned chicken stock
Salt and black pepper to the taste
Directions:
Select Sauté mode on your instant pot; add butter and melt it.
Add onions, stir and cook for 3 minutes.
Add garlic, stir and cook for 1 minute more
Add oats, stir and cook for 1 minute.
Add water, salt, pepper, stock, and thyme, seal the instant pot lid and cook at High for 10 minutes.
Release the pressure and leave the pot aside
Meanwhile; heat up a pan with the olive oil over medium heat, add mushrooms and cook them for 3 minutes.
Add them to the instant pot; also add more salt and pepper to the taste and the gouda, stir and divide among plates.

55. Healthy Oats
Cooking Time: 24 minutes
Servings: 5
Ingredients:

2 cups steel cut oats
1/2 cup chia seeds
1 cup chopped walnuts
1 cup fresh blueberries
4 ½ cups water
1 cup nondairy milk
2 tbsp. agave; or maple syrup; optional
1/4 tsp. salt; optional
Directions:
In the Instant Pot, stir together the oats and water.
Lock the lid and turn the steam release handle to Sealing. Using the Manual function, set the cooker to High Pressure for 12 minutes
After completing the cooking time, turn off the Instant Pot. Let the pressure release naturally for 10 minutes; quick release any remaining pressure
Remove the lid carefully and add the milk. Stir in the agave and salt and top with the chia seeds, walnuts and blueberries.

56. Lemon Marmalade Recipe
Cooking Time:25 minutes
Servings:8
Ingredients:
2 lb. lemons; washed and sliced with a mandolin
1 tbsp. vinegar
4 lb. sugar
Directions:
Put lemon slices in your instant pot.
Close the instant pot lid and cook the marmalade at High for 10 minutes.
Quick release the pressure; add the sugar, seal the instant pot lid again and cook at High for 4 more minutes
Release the pressure again, stir your marmalade, pour it into jars and refrigerate until your serve it.

57. Tasty Sausage
Cooking Time: 23 minutes
Servings: 5
Ingredients:
1 (8-ouncepackage unflavored tempeh
1 cup water
1 tbsp. olive oil
1 tsp. garlic powder
1 tsp. dried sage
1/2 tsp. dried oregano
2 tsp. vegan Worcestershire sauce
1 ½ tsp. smoked paprika
1 tsp. onion powder
1/2 tsp. salt or as your liking
1/4 tsp. freshly ground black pepper
Pinch chili powder
Directions:
Select the "Sauté" Low mode on your instant pot.
When the display reads "Hot," add the oil and heat until it begins to shimmer.
With your hands, crumble the tempeh into the hot oil and stir to coat
Add the Worcestershire sauce, paprika, onion powder, garlic powder, sage, oregano, salt, pepper and chili powder. Continue to sauté, stirring as needed, for 6 to 7 minutes more

Turn off the Instant Pot and add the water. Use your spoon to scrape up any bits of flavor that have stuck to the bottom of the pot. Stir well.
Lock the lid and turn the steam release handle to Sealing. Using the Manual function, set the cooker to High Pressure for 3 minutes
After completing the cooking time, quick release the pressure.
Remove the lid carefully. Select Sauté Low again and let the remaining liquid cook off. Taste and season with more salt, as needed.

58. Pecan Sweet Potatoes
Cooking Time:20 minutes
Servings:8
Ingredients:
1 cup pecans chopped
1 cup water
1/4 cup butter
1/4 cup maple syrup
1 tbsp. lemon peel
1/2 cup brown sugar
1 tbsp. cornstarch
1/4 tsp. salt
3 sweet potatoes peeled and sliced
Whole pecans for garnish
Directions:
Pour the water in your instant pot; add lemon peel, brown sugar and salt and stir.
Add potatoes, seal the instant pot lid and cook at High for 15 minutes
Release the pressure and transfer the potatoes to a serving plate.
Select sauté mode on your instant pot; add the butter and melt it.
Add pecans, maple syrup, cornstarch and stir very well.
Pour this over the potatoes, garnish with whole pecans and serve!

59. Mixed Mushroom Pate
Cooking Time:25 minutes
Servings:6
Ingredients:
1 oz. dry porcini mushrooms
1 tbsp. extra-virgin olive oil
1 shallot finely chopped
1/4 cup white wine
1 lb. button mushrooms sliced
1 cup boiled water
1 bay leaf
1 tbsp. truffle oil
3 tbsp. grated parmesan cheese
1 tbsp. butter
Salt and pepper to the taste
Directions:
Put dry mushrooms in a bowl, add 1 cup boiling water over them and leave them aside for now.
Set your instant pot on sauté mode; add butter and the olive oil and heat them up.
Add the shallot; stir and cook for 2 minutes.
Add dry mushrooms and their liquid, fresh mushrooms, wine, salt, pepper, and bay leaf

Stir; seal the instant pot lid and cook at High for 16 minutes.
Quick release the pressure, discard bay leaf and some of the liquid, transfer everything to your blender and pulse until you obtain a creamy spread
Add truffle oil and grated parmesan cheese; blend again, transfer to a bowl and serve.

60. Chocolate Steel Cut Oats
Cooking Time: 25 minutes
Servings: 5
Ingredients:
2 cups steel cut oats
2 ½ cups nondairy milk; divided; or more as needed
1/4 cup chocolate chips
1/4 cup peanut butter
2 ½ cups water
2 tbsp. agave; or maple syrup
1/4 tsp. salt or as your liking
Directions:
In Your Instant Pot, combine the oats, water, 2 cups of milk, the salt and chocolate chips. Stir to mix.
Lock the lid and turn the steam release handle to Sealing. Using the Manual function, set the cooker to High Pressure for 12 minutes.
After completing the cooking time, turn off the pressure cooker
Let the pressure release naturally for 10 minutes; quick release any remaining pressure
Add the remaining ½ cup of milk "more if you want the oats thinner". Stir in the peanut butter and agave and enjoy.
Note: Inner pot of your pressure cooker is never filled more than halfway when cooking oats or the foam may clog the pressure release valve.

61. Breakfast Quiche
Cooking Time:40 minutes
Servings:4
Ingredients:
1/2 cup ham, diced
1 cup sausage; already cooked and ground.
1 cup cheese; shredded.
4 bacon slices; cooked and crumbled.
1 ½ cups water
2 green onions; chopped.
1/2 cup milk
6 eggs, whisked
Salt and black pepper to taste
Directions:
Put the water in your instant pot and leave it aside for now.
In a bowl; mix eggs with salt, pepper, milk, sausage, ham, bacon, onions and cheese and stir everything well.
Pour this into a baking dish, cover with some tin foil, place the dish in the steamer basket of your instant pot, cover and cook at High for 30 minutes.
Release the pressure naturally for 10 minutes, then release remaining pressure by turning the valve to 'Venting', and carefully open the lid, take the quiche out and leave it aside for a few minutes to cool down.
Cut the quiche, arrange it on plates and serve.

62. Eggs Breakfast
Cooking Time:30 minutes
Servings:6
Ingredients:
1 cup ham; cooked and crumbled.
1 cup kale leaves; chopped.
1 cup water
1 yellow onion; finely chopped
1/2 cup heavy cream
6 eggs
1 tsp. herbs de Provence
1 cup cheddar cheese; grated
Salt and black pepper to taste
Directions:
In a bowl; mix eggs with salt, pepper, heavy cream, onion, kale, cheese and herbs, whisk very well and pour into a heat proof dish.
Put 1 cup water in your instant pot; place dish in the steamer basket, close the instant pot lid and cook at High for 20 minutes
Release the pressure, open the instant pot lid, remove the dish, divide eggs between plates and serve.

63. Chickpeas Spread
Cooking Time:25 minutes
Servings:8
Ingredients:
1 cup chickpeas soaked and drained
6 cups water
1 bay leaf
4 garlic cloves crushed.
2 tbsp. tahini paste
Juice of 1 lemon
1/4 tsp. cumin
1/4 cup chopped parsley
A pinch of paprika
Extra virgin olive oil
Salt to the taste
Directions:
Put chickpeas and water in your instant pot.
Add bay leaf, 2 garlic cloves, seal the instant pot lid and cook at High for 18 minutes
Quick release the pressure, discard excess liquid and bay leaf and reserve some of the cooking liquid.
Add tahini paste, the cooking liquid you've reserved, lemon juice, cumin, the rest of the garlic and salt to the taste
Transfer everything to your food processor and pulse well
Transfer your chickpeas spread in a serving bowl, sprinkle olive oil and paprika on top and enjoy!

64. Maple Millet
Cooking Time: 22 minutes
Servings: 5
Ingredients:
1/4 cup maple syrup
1 cup millet
1/2 to 1 cup nondairy milk
2 cups water
1/2 tsp. ground cinnamon
1/2 tsp. salt or as your liking
Fresh berries; for topping
Directions:

In the Instant Pot, stir together the millet, water, cinnamon and salt.
Lock the lid and turn the steam release handle to Sealing. Using the Manual function, set the cooker to High Pressure for 10 minutes
After completing the cooking time, let the pressure release naturally for 10 minutes; quick release any remaining pressure
Remove the lid carefully and stir in the maple syrup and as much milk as you need to get the consistency you prefer "more milk makes it creamier"
You can add an extra sprinkle of salt, too. Top with the berries and serve.

65. Barbeque Tofu
Cooking Time:20 minutes
Servings:6
Ingredients:
28 oz. firm tofu; cubed
12 oz. BBQ sauce
1 red bell pepper; chopped.
1 yellow onion; chopped.
1 celery stalk; chopped.
1 green bell pepper; chopped.
2 tbsp. extra virgin olive oil
4 garlic cloves; minced.
Salt to the taste
A pinch of curry powder
Directions:
Set your instant pot on Sauté mode; add the oil and heat it up.
Add bell peppers, garlic, onion and celery and stir
Add salt and curry powder, stir and cook for 2 minutes.
Add tofu, stir and cook 4 minutes more
Add BBQ sauce; then stir well and seal the instant pot lid and cook at High for 5 minutes
Quick release the pressure, open the instant pot lid, transfer to plates and serve.

66. Apple Porridge
Cooking Time: 24 minutes
Servings: 4
Ingredients:
1 apple, chopped
1/2 to 1 cup nondairy milk
1 cup quinoa; rinsed
1 ½ cups water
2 tbsp. ground cinnamon
2 tbsp. maple syrup
1/2 tsp. vanilla extract
1/2 tsp. salt or as your liking
Directions:
In the Instant Pot, stir together the quinoa, water, maple syrup, cinnamon, vanilla, salt and apple.
Lock the lid and turn the steam release handle to Sealing. Using the Manual function, set the cooker to High Pressure for 8 minutes
After completing the cooking time, let the pressure release naturally for 10 minutes; quick release any remaining pressure
Remove the lid carefully and stir in as much milk as needed to make it creamy.
If you didn't cook the apples, add them now and put the cover back on for 1 to 2 minutes to warm them.

67. Feta Spinach Egg Cups.
Cooking Time:22 minutes
Servings:4
Ingredients:
6 eggs
1/2 cup. mozzarella cheese
1/4 cup. feta cheese
1 cup. water
1 tsp. black pepper
1/2 tsp. salt
1 cup. chopped baby spinach
1 chopped tomato
Directions:
Pour water into the Instant Pot and lower in trivet
Layer silicone ramekins with spinach.
In a bowl, mix the rest of the ingredients and pour into cups, leaving 1/4-inch of head room
Put in the instant pot pressure cooker [you may have to cook in batchesand adjust time to 8 minutes on "High" pressure
When time is up, turn off the instant pot and quick-release.

68. Cheesy Chili Eggs
Preparation Time: 20 minutes,
servings: 4
Ingredients:
1 cup Shredded cheddar cheese
4 Whisked eggs
2 tbsp Chopped basil .
A pinch of salt and black pepper
Cooking spray
1 tsp Chili powder .
Directions:
Coat the instant pot with the cooking spray and mix in the basil, chili powder, cheddar cheese, eggs, salt, and pepper then seal the lid to cook for 15 minutes at high pressure.
Quick-release the pressure for 5 minutes, share into plates and serve.
Nutrition Values:
Calories 180, fat 14, carbs 1.1, protein 12.7, fiber 0.3

69. Nutty Blueberries Mix
Preparation Time: 13 minutes,
servings: 6
Ingredients:
½ cup Chopped walnuts
½ cup Chopped almonds
1 cup Blueberries
2 tsp Swerve .
1 cup Coconut cream
1 tsp Vanilla extract .
Directions:
Mix all the ingredients in the instant pot and seal the lid to cook for 8 minutes on high pressure.
Quick-release the pressure for 5 minutes, share into bowls and serve.
Nutrition Values:
Calories 218, fat 19.7, carbs 5.8, protein 5.3, fiber 3.2

70. Veggie Pastry

Preparation Time: 30 minutes,
servings: 4
Ingredients:
1 tbsp Chopped chives .
½ cup Chopped kale
½ cup Chopped Bok Choy
½ cup Almond milk
4 Whisked eggs
1 tbsp Avocado oil .
A pinch of salt and pepper
Directions:
Mix the chives, kale, Bok Choy, almond milk, eggs, salt, and pepper in a bowl.
Coat the muffin pastry tray with oil and pour the mix into it.
Pour the 1 and 1/2 cup of water into the instant pot, put in the inner pot and place the pastry tray inside it.
Seal the lid to cook for 20 minutes at high pressure.
Natural release the pressure for 10 minutes and let the pastry cool down and serve.
Nutrition Values:
Calories 142, fat 12, carbs 3.3, protein 6.7, fiber 1.1

71. Artichoke And Spinach Scones
Preparation Time: 30 minutes,
servings: 12
Ingredients:
4 Eggs
1 cup Baby spinach; chopped
2 cup Canned artichoke hearts; drained and chopped
3 cups Almond flour
1 tsp Baking soda .
A pinch of salt and black pepper
Cooking spray
Directions:
Combine the eggs, spinach, baking soda, artichoke hearts, almond flour, salt, and pepper in a bowl and set aside.
Coat the muffin tray with cooking spray and pour the spinach mix in the tray.
Pour the 1 ½ cups water into the instant pot and place the inner pot inside it. Put the muffin tray inside the pot and seal the lid to cook for 20 minutes at high pressure.
Natural release the pressure for 10 minutes and let the scones cool and serve.
Nutrition Values:
Calories 66, fat 4.5, carbs 0.6, protein 5.8, fiber 0.2

72. Nutty Coconut Mousse
Preparation Time: 10 minutes,
servings: 6
Ingredients:
2 cups Coconut milk
4 tsp Swerve .
½ cup Unsweetened and shredded coconut
¼ cup Chopped walnuts
1 cup Coconut cream
Directions:
Mix all the ingredients in the instant pot and seal the lid to cook for 5 minutes at high pressure.
Quick-release the pressure for 5 minutes, share into bowls and serve.
Nutrition Values:
Calories 332, fat 33.8, carbs 7.8, protein 4.2, fiber 3.6

73. Creamy Zucchini
Preparation Time: 22 minutes,
servings: 4
Ingredients:
4 Sliced zucchini
1 tbsp Chopped dill .
½ cup Veggie stock
½ cup Softened cream cheese
½ cup Heavy cream
A pinch of salt and black pepper
1 tbsp Avocado oil .
2 cloves Minced garlic
Directions:
Put the zucchini in the instant pot and mix in the stock, salt, and pepper then seal the lid to cook for 12 minutes at high pressure.
Natural release the pressure for 10 minutes, strain the zucchini and put it in a food processor. Mix in the rest of the ingredients and blend well. Share into bowls and serve as a spread.
Nutrition Values:
Calories 193, fat 16.5, carbs 7.8, protein 5.2, fiber 2.5

74. Cheesy Radish And Tomatoes Jumble
Preparation Time: 20 minutes,
servings: 4
Ingredients:
¼ cup Sliced radishes
½ cup Shredded mozzarella
1 tbsp Chopped chives .
1 lb. Halved cherry tomatoes .
1 tbsp Chopped basil .
A pinch of salt and black pepper
1 tbsp Olive oil .
Directions:
Put the chives, radishes, basil, tomatoes, olive oil, salt, and pepper inside the instant pot and mix it well.
Drizzle the mozzarella cheese over the spread and seal the lid to cook for 10 minutes at high pressure.
Natural release the pressure for 10 minutes, share into plates and serve.
Nutrition Values:
Calories 62, fat 4.4, carbs 4.9, protein 2.1, fiber 1.5

75. Garlic Pork Meat With Kale
Preparation Time: 25 minutes,
servings: 4
Ingredients:
1 Lb. Torn kale .
1 Chopped spring onion
½ cup Beef stock
2 cups Ground pork meat
A pinch of salt and black pepper
1 tbsp Avocado oil .
2 cloves Minced garlic
Directions:
Press 'Sauté' on the instant pot and pour in the oil. When hot, add the garlic, onion, and pork meat to brown for 5 minutes.

Mix in the kale, spring onion, beef stock, salt, and pepper and seal the lid to cook for 10 minutes on high pressure.
Natural release the pressure for 10 minutes, share into plates and serve.
Nutrition Values:
Calories 66, fat 5.3, carbs 6.5, protein 3.8, fiber 2

76. Creamy Zucchini With Walnuts
Preparation Time: 20 minutes,
servings: 4
Ingredients:
¼ cup Chopped walnuts
2 tbsp Swerve .
1 tsp Ground nutmeg .
4 Sliced zucchinis
1 ½ cups Coconut cream
Directions:
Mix all the ingredients in the instant pot and seal the lid to cook for 10 minutes on high pressure.
Natural release the pressure for 10 minutes, share into bowls and serve.
Nutrition Values:
Calories 83, fat 8.2, carbs 7.8, protein 4.3, fiber 2.8

77. Bacon And Turkey Frittata With Avocado And Tomatoes
Preparation Time: 25 minutes,
servings: 4
Ingredients:
2 Bacon slices: cooked and crumbled
1 cup Skinless and boneless turkey breast; cut into strips
1 Chopped tomato
1 Small avocado; peeled and chopped
4 Whisked eggs
A pinch of salt and black pepper
2 tbsp Olive oil .
Directions:
Press 'Sauté' on the instant pot and add 1 tablespoon of olive oil to the pot. When hot, add the turkey to brown for 5 minutes.
Mix in the remaining ingredients and seal the lid to cook for 10 minutes at high pressure.
Natural release the pressure for 10 minutes, share the frittata and serve.
Nutrition Values:
Calories 228, fat 21.2, carbs 5.3, protein 6.6, fiber 3.6

78. Creamy Nuts And Strawberries
Preparation Time: 20 minutes,
servings: 4
Ingredients:
½ cup Chopped almonds
½ tsp Ground nutmeg .
2 cups Strawberries; halved
½ cup Chopped walnuts
1 cup Coconut cream
1 tbsp Stevia .
Directions:
Mix the cream, almonds, nutmeg, strawberries, walnuts, and stevia in the instant pot and seal the lid to cook for 10 minutes on low pressure.

Natural release the pressure for 10 minutes, share into bowls and serve.
Nutrition Values:
Calories 328, fat 29.8, carbs 7.6, protein 8.1, fiber 5.4

79. Garlic Turkey With Leeks And Egg
Preparation Time: 25 minutes,
servings: 4
Ingredients:
1 Skinless and boneless turkey breasts; cut into strips
2 Chopped leeks
8 Whisked eggs
½ cup Chicken stock
2 tbsp Olive oil .
2 cloves Minced garlic
Directions:
Press 'Sauté' on the instant pot and add the oil. When it is hot, mix in the turkey, garlic, and leeks to cook for 5 minutes.
Mix in the eggs and chicken stock then seal the lid to cook on high pressure for 10 minutes.
Natural release the pressure for 10 minutes, share into plates and serve.
Nutrition Values:
Calories 216, fat 16, carbs 7.6, protein 11.9, fiber 0.8

80. Coconut and Berries Mix
Preparation Time: 22 minutes,
servings: 6
Ingredients:
1 tsp Swerve .
3 tbsp Unsweetened coconut flakes .
2 cups Almond milk
1 cup Blackberries
1 cup Strawberries
1 tsp Vanilla extract .
Directions:
Combine all the ingredients in the instant pot and seal the lid to cook for 12 minutes at high pressure.
Natural release the pressure for 10 minutes, share into bowls and serve.
Nutrition Values:
Calories 213, fat 20.1, carbs 6.7, protein 2.4, fiber 3.7

81. Chili Mushrooms with Okra Egg Dish
Preparation Time: 25 minutes,
servings: 2
Ingredients:
4 Whisked eggs
½ cup Chopped cilantro
1 Lb. Sliced white mushrooms-.
1 cup Okra
2 Chopped spring onions-
2 Minced chili peppers
1 tbsp Avocado oil .
2 Minced garlic cloves
Directions:
Press 'Sauté' on the instant pot and add the oil. When hot, mix in the garlic and onions to reduce for 2 minutes.
Add in the mushrooms to cook for 2 minutes.

Mix the eggs, cilantro, okra, and chili peppers with the mushrooms in the pot and seal the lid to cook for 10 minutes at high pressure.
Natural release the pressure for 10 minutes, share the egg dish and serve.
Nutrition Values:
Calories 108, fat 5.2, carbs 4.7, protein 9.9, fiber 2.4

82. Creamy Cocoa Vanilla Coconut Meal
Preparation Time: 20 minutes,
servings: 6
Ingredients:
1 cup Almond milk
1 cup Unsweetened coconut flakes
1 tsp Cocoa powder .
1 cup Coconut cream
2 tsp Vanilla extract .
2 tbsp Stevia .
Directions:
Combine all the ingredients in the instant pot and seal the lid to cook for 10 minutes at high pressure.
Natural release the pressure for 10 minutes then share into bowls and serve.
Nutrition Values:
Calories 236, fat 23.6, carbs 6.5, protein 2.3, fiber 3.1

83. Creamy Almonds And Broccoli With Coconut
Preparation Time: 20 minutes,
servings: 4
Ingredients:
1 cup Broccoli florets
2 Whisked eggs
½ cup Coconut flakes
½ cup Toasted and chopped almonds
1 cup Heavy cream
Cooking spray
Directions:
Coat the instant pot with the cooking spray and mix in the almonds and the broccoli florets then pour in the heavy cream mixed with the eggs over the broccoli and nuts.
Drizzle the coconut flakes over the mix then seal the lid to cook for 15 minutes at high pressure.
Natural release the pressure for 10 minutes, share into plates and serve.
Nutrition Values:
Calories 248, fat 22.8, carbs 6.6, protein 6.9, fiber 3

84. Creamy Cinnamon And Coconut With Strawberries
Preparation Time: 15 minutes,
servings: 6
Ingredients:
1 cup Halved strawberries
2 cups Almond milk
1 cup Coconut flakes
1 tbsp Cinnamon powder .
½ cup Coconut cream
Directions:
Mix all the ingredients together in the instant pot and seal the lid to cook for 10 minutes at high pressure.
Quick-release the pressure for 5 minutes, share into bowls and serve.
Nutrition Values:
Calories 285, fat 28.4, carbs 7.5, protein 2.9, fiber 3.9

85. Creamy Coconut Frittata
Preparation Time: 20 minutes,
servings: 4
Ingredients:
4 Whisked eggs
½ cup Coconut milk
1 cup Coconut flakes
A pinch of salt and black pepper
Cooking spray
1 tbsp Sweet paprika .
Directions:
Whisk the paprika, eggs, coconut milk, salt, pepper, and coconut flakes in a bowl.
Spray the instant pot with the cooking spray and pour in the egg mix then seal the lid to cook for 10 minutes at high pressure.
Natural release the pressure for 10 minutes, share the frittata and serve.
Nutrition Values:
Calories 209, fat 18.6, carbs 6, protein 7.2, fiber 3.1

86. Spicy Leek And Veggie Egg Dish
Preparation Time: 25 minutes,
servings: 4
Ingredients:
1 Chopped red bell pepper
4 Whisked eggs
2 Sliced leeks
1 Chopped shallot
A pinch of salt and black pepper
Cooking spray
1 tbsp Sweet paprika .
Directions:
Coat the instant pot with the cooking spray then mix in all the ingredients and seal the lid to cook for 15 minutes at high pressure.
Natural release the pressure for 10 minutes, share into bowls and serve.
Nutrition Values:
Calories 106, fat 9.4, carbs 6.6, protein 6.8, fiber 1.9

87. Cauliflower Rice With Broccoli And Tomatoes
Preparation Time: 22 minutes,
servings: 6
Ingredients:
1 tsp Chili flakes .
1 Broccoli head with florets separated
4 Cubed tomatoes
1 cup Veggie stock
1 cup Cauliflower rice
2 tsp Curry powder .
1 tbsp Grated ginger .
Directions:
Mix all the ingredients in the instant pot and seal the lid to cook at high pressure for 12 minutes.
Natural release the pressure for 10 minutes, share into bowls and serve.
Nutrition Values:
Calories 30, fat 5, carbs 4.5, protein 1.3, fiber 1.3

MAINS

88. Stuffed Bell Peppers
Preparation Time: 35 MIN
Servings: 4
Ingredients:
5 bell peppers, seeds removed
1 medium-sized onion, peeled and finely chopped
7oz button mushrooms, sliced
4 garlic cloves, peeled and crushed
4 tbsp of extra-virgin olive oil
1 tsp of salt
¼ tsp of freshly ground black pepper
¼ cup of rice
½ tbsp. of Cayenne pepper
2 cups vegetable stock
Directions:
With the cooker's lid off, heat up two tablespoons of olive oil on the "Sautee" mode. Add onions and garlic and stir-fry until translucent. Press the "Cancel" button and set aside.
Rinse well each bell pepper and pat dry with some kitchen paper. Remove the stem along with seeds. In a small bowl, combine rice with the mixture from your pot. Add mushrooms and stir all well. Season with salt, pepper, and cayenne pepper. Stuff each bell pepper with this mixture. Gently place them in your instant pot, filled side up, and pour in the broth.
Seal the lid and set the steam release handle. Press the "Manual" mode and set the timer for 15 minutes. When done, press "Cancel" button and release the pressure naturally.
Enjoy!

89. Ginger Stew
Preparation Time: 35 MIN
Servings: 4
Ingredients:
2 cups green peas
1 large onion, chopped
4 cloves of garlic, finely chopped
3 ½ oz of olives, pitted
1 tbsp of ginger, ground
1 tbsp of turmeric, ground
1 tbsp of salt
4 cups of vegetable stock
3 tbsp olive oil
Directions:
Rinse well the green peas using a large colander. Drain and set aside.
Plug in your instant pot and press "Sautee" button. Heat up the olive oil in the stainless steel insert and add onions and garlic. Stir-fry for 2-3 minutes, or until translucent.
Now, add the remaining ingredients and close the lid. Set the steam release handle and press "Stew" button. When you hear the cooker's end signal, perform a quick release.
Open the pot and serve immediately.

90. Chickpeas with Onions
Preparation Time: 35 MIN
Servings: 5
Ingredients:
1 lb chickpeas, soaked
3 large purple onions, peeled and sliced
2 large tomatoes, roughly chopped
3 oz parsley, chopped
2 cups vegetable broth
1 tbsp cayenne pepper
3 tbsp almond butter
2 tbsp olive oil
1 tsp salt
½ tsp freshly ground black pepper
Directions:
Plug in your instant pot and heat up the oil in the stainless steel insert. Press the "Sautee" button and add onions. Stir-fry for five minutes. Now, add soaked chickpeas, chopped tomatoes, chopped parsley, and vegetable broth. Stir in the cayenne pepper, salt, and freshly ground black pepper. Close the lid and set the steam release handle. Press the "Stew" button and cook for 30 minutes.
When done, press "Cancel" button and turn off the pot. Perform a quick release and open the pot. Serve chickpeas warm.

91. Portobello Mushrooms with Green Peas
Preparation Time: 65 MIN
Servings: 4
Ingredients:
8 oz Portobello mushrooms, sliced
1 cup green peas
1 cup pearl onions, minced
2 large carrots
½ cup celery stalks, chopped
2 garlic cloves, crushed
2 large potatoes, chopped
1 tbsp apple cider vinegar
1 tsp rosemary
1 tbsp cayenne pepper
1 tsp salt
½ tsp pepper, freshly ground
2 tbsp almond butter
3 cups vegetable stock
Directions:
Set your instant pot to "Sautee" mode. Add onions, carrots, celery stalks, and garlic. Sprinkle with some salt, pepper, rosemary, and cayenne pepper. Stir-fry for a few minutes.
Now, add the remaining ingredients and seal the lid. Set the steam release handle and press the "Manual" mode. Set the timer for 30 minutes.
When done, press "Cancel" button and release the pressure naturally.
Open the lid and serve immediately.

92. Lentil Stew
Preparation Time: 35 MIN
Servings: 4
Ingredients:
1 cup red lentils, soaked
1 medium-sized onion, peeled and finely chopped
½ cup sweet carrot puree
1 tbsp all-purpose flour
½ tsp freshly ground black pepper

½ tsp cumin, ground
½ tsp salt
2 tbsp olive oil
Directions:
Soak the lentils overnight.
Rinse well the lentils under cold running water using a large colander. Drain well and set aside.
Plug in your instant pot and grease the stainless steel insert with olive oil. Press "Sautee" button and heat it up. Add onions and flour. Cook for 10 minutes, stirring constantly.
Now, add the remaining ingredients and pour in about 4 cups of water. Close the lid and set the release steam handle. Press "Manual" button and cook for 30 minutes on high pressure.
Press "Cancel" button and release the steam handle. Turn off the pot and set aside to chill for a while before serving.
Optionally, sprinkle with cayenne pepper and parsley.

93. One Pot Quinoa
Preparation Time: 20 MIN
Servings: 2
Ingredients:
4 cups water
2 cups quinoa
3 garlic cloves, minced
2 tbsp rice vinegar
2 tbsp soy sauce
1tsp grated ginger
2 tbsp sugar
8 oz bag of frozen vegetables (Asian-style
Directions:
Combine all the ingredients (except for frozen vegetablesin Instant Pot. Cover the pot with lid. Set steam release handle to 'sealing' and set Instant Pot to manual to 1 minute over high pressure.
Once done, allow it to naturally release pressure for 10 minutes. Change steam release handle to 'venting' to release any remaining steam. Open the lid. Then add thawed frozen veggies and mix well.

94. Instant Pot Hot Dogs
Preparation Time: 35 MIN
Servings: 4
Ingredients:
For Marinade:
¼ cup soy sauce
¼ cup water
1 tbsp rice vinegar
½ tsp liquid smoke
½ tsp garlic powder
½ tsp onion powder
For Topping:
Ketchup, mustard, etc
For Hot Dog:
4 large carrots
4 oil-free vegan hot dog buns
Directions:
Place trivet in the inner pot. Pour in 1½ cups water. Place 4 carrots on a trivet and cover the pot with lid. Switch the manual button for 3 minutes over high pressure. Set steam release handle to 'sealing'.
When the timer beeps, change the steam release handle to 'venting' to release the steam immediately. Mix the marinade ingredients together in a container. Add carrots along with the marinade. Let it marinade for 24 hours.
Take them from marinade and transfer them to Instant Pot. Pour in marinade and switch on sauté button. Switch adjust button to get 'high' temperature setting. Sauté it for 10 minutes.
Serve carrot dogs over desired oil-free hot dog buns topped with favorite sauces.

95. Curried Potato and Cauliflower (Indian Aloo Gobi
Preparation Time: 40 MIN
Servings: 2
Ingredients:
1 head cauliflower
1½ lbs potatoes, peeled and then chopped
2 cups water
1 red onion, chopped finely
1 tsp salt
3 garlic cloves, minced
1 tsp ground coriander
1 tsp garam masala
1 tsp chili powder
1/2 tsp turmeric
1 tsp grated ginger
Directions:
Steam the cauliflower head in Instant Pot for 2 minutes on a trivet with 1½ cups water. Immediately release pressure and take out trivet out from Instant Pot. Allow it to cool. Empty the pot of water.
Sauté onions, ginger and garlic for 5 minutes along with ½ cup water (using the sauté function. Once timer beeps, switch on 'Keep Warm/Cancel' button. Add 1½ cups water to the inner pot. Add potatoes and all spices. Mix everything around using a spoon. Cover the pot with lid and switch on manual button for 8 minutes over high pressure. Set steam release handle to 'sealing'. Once finished cooking, allow pressure to release naturally for about 5-10 minutes. In the meanwhile, chop cauliflower into bite-size bits. Using the steam release handle to release remaining steam after 5-10 minutes. Add cauliflower pieces and stir around using a spoon.

96. Sloppy Joe in Instant Pot
Preparation Time: 35 MIN
Servings: 6-8 sloppy joes
Ingredients:
1 cup of red lentils
1 rib of celery, chopped
1 yellow onion, chopped
1/2 of a yellow pepper, chopped
1/2 can (1/2 of an 8 oz canof tomato paste
2 1/2 cups of water
1/4 cup of red wine vinegar
2 tbsp of brown sugar
1 tsp of salt
1 tsp of liquid smoke
3 garlic cloves, minced
2 tbsp of sriracha (optional
1/4 cup of oil-free breadcrumbs

6 or 8 oil-free hamburger buns
Directions:
Except for breadcrumbs and buns, combine all ingredients in Instant Pot. Set steam release handle to 'sealing' and switch on manual button. Cover the pot with lid and set to 15 minutes over high pressure. Allow the pressure to release naturally for 10-15 minutes. Change steam release handle to 'venting' to release extra steam. Open the lid. Add breadcrumbs and give it a stir.
Serve this sloppy Joe mix over hamburger buns topped with fresh mixed greens, if desired.

97. Pizza Alla Puttanesca.
Preparation Time: 15 MIN
Servings: 6
Ingredients:
Dough:
1½ cups unbleached all-purpose flour
½ cup warm water, or as needed
1 tablespoon olive oil
1½ teaspoons instant yeast
½ teaspoon salt
½ teaspoon Italian seasoning
Sauce:
½ cup crushed tomatoes
½ cup shredded vegan mozzarella cheese
¼ cup pitted green olives, sliced
¼ cup pitted kalamata olives, sliced
1 tablespoon chopped fresh flat-leaf parsley
1 tablespoon capers, rinsed and drained
¼ teaspoon garlic powder
¼ teaspoon sugar
¼ teaspoon dried basil
¼ teaspoon dried oregano
¼ teaspoon hot red pepper flakes
Salt and freshly ground black pepper
Directions:
Get a bowl to mix your dough. Whisk together the flour, yeast, salt, and seasoning.
Add the oil slowly whilst stirring, then add water little by little until the dough ball is formed.
Knead the dough on a floured surface for 2 minutes. Shape it and put it in a warm bowl to rise for an hour.
Whilst the dough rises, mix the sauce. Combine tomatoes, olives, capers, parsley, basil, oregano, garlic powder, sugar, red pepper, salt and pepper.
Oil a tray that will fit in your instant pot and stretch the dough to fit it.
Spread the sauce over the dough.
Insert the tray into your instant pot and cook for 10 minutes on steam.
Release the pressure quickly and sprinkle the mozzarella on top at the end.

98. Seitan Fajitas.
Preparation Time: 40 MIN
Servings: 6
Ingredients:
1lb seitan, cut into strips
2 tablespoons tomato paste
1½ cups tomato salsa
1 tablespoon chili powder
1 tablespoon soy sauce
2 large bell peppers (any color, seeded and cut into ¼-inch-thick strips
1 large yellow onion, thinly sliced
1 garlic clove, minced
Salt and freshly ground black pepper
2 tablespoons freshly squeezed lime juice
1 ripe Hass avocado, peeled, pitted, and diced, for garnish
1 large ripe tomato, diced, for garnish
Directions:
Mix the tomato paste, salsa, chili powder, and soy sauce until combined well.
Put the bell peppers, onion, and garlic in your instant pot.
Put your seitan strips on top. Try and avoid them touching.
Pour the tomato mix over everything.
Seal and cook on Poultry for 30 minutes.
Depressurize naturally, stir in the lime to taste.
Serve and top with avocado and tomato.

99. Zesty Stuffed Bell Peppers.
Preparation Time: 30 MIN
Servings: 4
Ingredients:
4 large bell peppers (any color or a combination
1 (14-ouncecan tomato sauce
2 cups cooked brown or white rice
1½ cups cooked pinto beans or black beans or 1 (15-ouncecan beans, rinsed and drained
1 cup fresh or thawed frozen corn kernels
1 cup diced fresh tomatoes or 1 (14-ouncecan diced tomatoes, drained
2 teaspoons olive oil (optional
4 garlic cloves, minced
4 scallions, chopped
1 tablespoon chili powder
2 teaspoons minced chipotle chiles in adobo
1½ teaspoon ground cumin
1¼ teaspoon dried oregano
½ teaspoon sugar
Salt and freshly ground black pepper
Directions:
Warm the oil in your instant pot, leaving the lid open. When the oil is hot, add the garlic and scallions and soften for 3 minutes.
Add the chili powder, and a teaspoon of both the cumin and the oregano.
Put the garlic mixture in a bowl to one side. Add the rice, beans, corn, tomatoes, and chiles with a little salt and pepper. Mix well.
Top and hollow your bell peppers.
Fill the peppers evenly with the mix and set them in the steamer basket of your instant pot.
Mix the tomato sauce, remaining cumin, remaining oregano, sugar, and salt in the base of your instant pot.
Lower the steamer basket, seal, and cook on Steam for 24 minutes.
Depressurize fast and serve immediately.

100. Moroccan Stuffed Peppers
Preparation Time: 30 MIN
Servings: 4

Ingredients:
4 large bell peppers (assorted colors look great
2 cups boiling water or vegetable broth
2 cups couscous
1 cup cooked chickpeas or 1 (15-ouncecan chickpeas
1 medium-size yellow onion, minced
2 carrots, peeled and minced
1 large zucchini, minced
3 garlic cloves, minced
3 tablespoons tomato paste
2 teaspoons olive oil
2 teaspoons harissa or hot chili paste
2 teaspoons ground coriander
1 teaspoon paprika
1 teaspoon ground cinnamon
½ tablespoon ground cumin
1 teaspoon salt
¼ teaspoon freshly ground black pepper
1 tablespoon minced fresh flat-leaf parsley leaves, for garnish

Directions:
Top and hollow our the peppers. Remove the stems, then chop the tops and keep the diced pepper.
Warm the oil in your instant pot.
When hot, add the onion and soften for 4 minutes.
Add the carrots, pepper tops, zucchini, garlic, and cook for 2 more minutes.
Add the harissa, tomato paste, coriander, cinnamon, cumin, paprika, salt and pepper.
Add the couscous and water, stir well.
Add the chickpeas and stir again.
Pack the stuffing into the peppers and put them in the steamer basket of your instant pot.
Put a cup of water in your instant pot. Lower the steamer basket.
Seal and cook on Steam for 24 minutes.
Depressurize naturally and serve immediately, topped with parsley.

101. Corn Chorizo pie
Preparation Time: 6 Min
Servings: 6
Ingredients:
12 soft corn tortillas
1 crumbled vegan chorizo
1 onion, minced
1 teaspoon olive oil
2 canned chipotle chilies in adobo, minced
1½ cups corn kernels
1½ cups shredded vegan cheddar cheese
2 tablespoons chili powder
1 tablespoon tomato paste
1 tablespoon grated unsweetened dark chocolate
1 (15-ouncecan vegan refried beans, stirred
1 teaspoon ground cumin
¼ teaspoon black pepper
1 teaspoon smoked paprika
1 teaspoon dark brown sugar
1 teaspoon dried oregano
8 ounces steamed diced tempeh, chopped seitan
½ teaspoon salt
1 (14.5-ouncecan crushed tomatoes
4 garlic cloves, minced
1½ cups cooked pinto beans

Directions:
Add the onion, garlic and oil in the instant pot.
Cook for 30 seconds and then add the tomato paste, cumin, chipotle chiles, chocolate, oregano, chili powder, paprika, brown sugar, and seasoning.
Add some water and cover with lid.
Cook for 2 minutes and then add the tomatoes.
Cover and cook for 1 minute.
Add the tempeh, beans, corn and mix well.
Cover and cook for another 5 minutes.
Serve hot.

102. Cheesy Tomato Gratin
Preparation Time: 10 Min
Servings: 6
Ingredients:
1(14.5-ouncecan petite diced tomatoes
1 cup shredded vegan mozzarella cheese
3 large potatoes, peeled and sliced
½ teaspoon smoked paprika
¼ cup vegetable broth
1 onion, minced
2 tablespoons chili powder
½ teaspoon ground cumin
¼ teaspoon cayenne pepper
3 garlic cloves, minced
1 teaspoon dried oregano
3 tablespoons tomato paste
Salt and black pepper

Directions:
Add the onion, garlic in your instant pot.
Cover and cook for 30 seconds.
Add the broth, oregano, cumin, tomato paste, cayenne, paprika and chili powder.
Add the tomatoes, and mix well.
Cook for 2 minutes.
Add the potato slices and cook for 4 minutes.
Add the cheese and cook for another minute.
Serve warm.

103. Sweet Potatoes and Onions with Jerk Sauce
Preparation Time: 6 Min
Servings: 6
Ingredients:
2 sweet potatoes, peeled and diced
1 pound tempeh, diced
½ sweet onion, diced
¼ teaspoon cayenne pepper
1 garlic clove, crushed
¼ teaspoon paprika
2 scallions, coarsely chopped
2 teaspoons soy sauce
1 tablespoon ginger
2 tablespoons lime
1 teaspoon dried thyme
1 teaspoon dark brown sugar
1 hot green chile, seeded and chopped
½ teaspoon ground allspice
¼ teaspoon ground cinnamon
½ teaspoon salt
1 tablespoon rice vinegar
¼ teaspoon black pepper
⅓ cup water

½ large or 1 small Vidalia or other sweet onion, cut into ½-inch dice
Directions:
In a blender add the chile, scallions, ginger, garlic and onion.
Blend for 30 seconds and add the soy sauce, cinnamon, cayenne, seasoning, vinegar, marmalade, allspice, sugar and thyme.
Add some water and blend again.
Add the tempeh, onion and potatoes in the instant pot.
Add the jerk sauce you made.
Mix well and cook for 5 minutes.
Serve warm.

104. Ziti Mushroom Stew
Preparation Time: 6 Min
Servings: 4
Ingredients:
1 bell pepper, seeded and minced
1 onion, minced
1 (14-ounce can crushed tomatoes
4 garlic cloves, minced
2 tablespoons tomato paste
½ cup dry red wine
8 ounces white mushrooms, coarsely chopped
1 cup hot water
8 ounces uncooked ziti
1 teaspoon dried basil
Salt and black pepper
2 teaspoons minced fresh oregano
1 teaspoon natural sugar
2 tablespoons chopped parsley
Directions:
Add the ziti, mushroom, red wine, tomato paste in an instant pot.
Add the sugar, herbs, spices, hot water and the rest of the ingredients.
Mix well and cook for 5 minutes with the lid on.
Serve hot.

105. Tofu Cheesecake
Preparation Time: 15 MIN
Servings: 8-12
Ingredients:
8 ounces silken tofu
¼ cup dried bread crumbs
3 garlic cloves, crushed
1 teaspoon salt
1 cup raw cashews, soaked
2 tablespoons sun-dried tomatoes, chopped
1 cup vegan cream cheese
2 tablespoons parsley, minced
2 tablespoons pitted olives, chopped
¼ teaspoon cayenne pepper
2 tablespoons minced fresh basil
1 tablespoon cornstarch
1 teaspoon minced oregano
Directions:
Combine the parsley, basil, and tomatoes in a bowl. Mix well and set aside for now.
Add the breadcrumbs onto a baking pan and use hands to make the top even.
Add the cashew, salt and garlic in a blender. Blend until smooth.
Add the tofu, cream cheese and blend again.
Add tomatoes, oregano, olives, cayenne, basil, cornstarch, and blend again.
Add on top of the crust.
Use aluminum foil to cover the top. Make some holes.
Add to your instant pot and cook for about 8 minutes.
Serve cold with the cherry tomato mix on top.

106. Garlic Pimento Fondue
Preparation Time: 15 MIN
Servings: 4
Ingredients:
1 can white beans, drained and rinsed
2 cups shredded vegan cheddar cheese
1 jar diced pimentos, drained
1/2 teaspoon Dijon mustard
1 clove garlic, minced
2 tablespoons vegan chicken-flavored bouillon
2 tablespoons olive oil
1/4 teaspoon salt
1/4 teaspoon pepper
3/4 cup water
Directions:
Process the beans and water in a food processor until pureed.
Spray the instant pot with nonstick spray and the pureed beans and everything but the cheese. Seal the lid and cook on high 4 minutes, then let the pressure release naturally. Remove the lid and stir in the cheese. Serve in a fondue pot to keep warm.

107. Sweet and Nutty Fondue
Preparation Time: 15 MIN
Servings: 4
Ingredients:
1/2 cup almond butter
1/2 tablespoons grated ginger
1 can coconut milk
1 teaspoon soy sauce
1 clove garlic, minced
1/4 teaspoon chili powder
1/4 teaspoon cayenne pepper
1/2 teaspoon garam masala
1 tablespoon cornstarch, if needed
Directions:
Spray the instant pot with nonstick spray.
Stir together all the ingredients except for the cornstarch and add them to the instant pot. Seal the lid and cook on high 4 minutes. Quick release the pressure.
Remove the lid and check the consistency. If it needs to be thickened, switch to the sauté setting of the instant pot, add the cornstarch, and cook for 15 minutes.

108. Beefy Cajun Po Boy
Preparation Time: 35 MIN
Servings: 4
Ingredients:
3 cups cubed beef-flavored seitan, thinly sliced
2 cloves garlic, minced
1 tablespoon vegan Worcestershire sauce
2 tablespoons vegan beef-flavored bouillon

1/2 teaspoon Cajun seasoning
1/4 teaspoon pepper
1 bay leaf
1 tablespoons cornstarch
1 1/2 cups water
French bread, for serving
Lettuce, for serving
Tomato, for serving
Vegan Mayonnaise, for serving.
Directions:
Mix together the garlic, water, Worcestershire sauce, Cajun seasoning, bouillon, water, and bay leaf in the instant pot.
Add the sliced seitan. Seal the lid and cook on high 4 minutes. Let pressure release naturally, then remove the lid and the bay leaf.
Return to sauté setting and add the cornstarch. Cook an additional 20 minutes, adding additional cornstarch if needed.
Serve on French bread, topped with lettuce, tomato, and vegan mayonnaise.

109. Meatless Philly Cheesesteak Hoagie
Preparation Time: 30 MIN
Servings: 6
Ingredients:
4 large Portobello mushrooms, sliced
2 large bell peppers, cut into strips
1 onion, halved and sliced
2 tablespoons vegan beef-flavored bouillon
1 tablespoon vegan Worcestershire sauce
1 tablespoon cornstarch
1/2 cup water
6 hoagie rolls, for serving
Shredded vegan cheddar cheese, for serving
Directions:
Combine all the ingredients in the instant pot. Seal the lid and cook on high 3 minutes, then let the pressure release naturally.
Switch to sauté setting and add the cornstarch. Simmer for 20 minutes, until gravy is thickened.
Serve on a toasted hoagie roll topped with shredded cheese.

110. Sloppy Tempeh Sandwich
Preparation Time: 25 MIN
Servings: 6
Ingredients:
16 ounces tempeh, cubed
1 tablespoon tomato paste
1 onion, diced
3 cloves garlic
1/2 bell pepper, chopped
1 can diced tomatoes
1/4 cup water
1 tablespoon maple syrup
1 teaspoon vegan Worcestershire sauce
1 tablespoon apple cider vinegar
1/2 teaspoon smoked paprika
1/2 teaspoon chipotle chili powder
1/2 teaspoon cumin
1/2 teaspoon chili powder
1/4 teaspoon hot sauce
1/2 teaspoon salt
1 teaspoon Dijon
12 buns, for serving
Directions:
Use a steamer basket to steam the tempeh for 10 minutes.
Heat the oil in the instant pot on the sauté setting and cook the onion for 5 minutes. Add the garlic and peppers and cook an additional 5 minutes.
Add the rest of the ingredients to the instant pot, seal the lid, and cook on high 4 minutes. Let the pressure release naturally, then remove the lid and serve on buns.

111. Tex Mex Tofu Taco 'Meat'
Preparation Time: 20 MIN
Servings: 6
Ingredients:
15 ounces firm tofu, cubed
1 clove garlic, minced
1/2 teaspoon chili powder
3 tablespoons salsa
1/4 teaspoon cumin
1/8 teaspoon cayenne pepper
1/2 teaspoon fresh ground pepper
1/4 teaspoon smoked paprika
1/4 teaspoon salt
Zest of 1 lime
Juice of 1 lime
Taco shells, for serving
Directions:
Spray the instant pot with nonstick spray. Combine all the ingredients and cook on high 4 minutes. Let the pressure release naturally, then remove the lid. If the sauce is too thin, switch to sauté setting and cook for 5 to 10 minutes to reduce the sauce.
Serve on taco shells with your favorite toppings, or use as a taco salad topping.

112. Black Bean and Potato Burrito Filling
Preparation Time: 20 MIN
Servings: 6
Ingredients:
4 large russet potatoes, peeled and chopped
8 ounces corn
1/2 bell pepper, chopped
8 ounces black beans
1 cup water
1 1/2 cups salsa
1/4 teaspoon chili powder
1/4 teaspoon salt
Tortillas, for serving
Directions:
Spray the instant pot with nonstick spray.
Add all the ingredients. Seal the lid and cook on high 4 minutes. Let the pressure release naturally.
Use an immersion blender to puree the mixture. Add additional salt if needed and serve wrapped in warm tortillas.

113. Pesto Butternut Grilled Sandwiches
Preparation Time: 25 MIN

Servings: 6
Ingredients:
1 butternut squash, halved
1 teaspoon ground sage
4 fresh rosemary leaves
1/2 teaspoon ground thyme
5 fresh basil leaves
1/2 cup walnuts
2 tablespoons olive oil
1/4 cup nutritional yeast
12 slices bread, for serving
Directions:
Combine seasonings, herbs, walnuts, and olive oil in a food processor and blend to make the pesto. Set aside.
Find a butternut squash that will fit into your instant pot and cut it in half. Remove the seeds and place squash in an oiled instant pot.
Seal the lid and cook on high for 6 minutes, then let pressure release naturally.
Remove the lid and allow the squash to cool.
Scoop out the flesh from the squash. You will use about 2 cups.
Mix the squash with the pesto and the yeast.
To serve, spread the mixture on bread. Top with another piece of bread and grill in a hot, oiled skillet.

114. Soy Ginger Lettuce Wraps
Preparation Time: 25 MIN
Servings: 6
Ingredients:
8 ounces tempeh cubed
1 large stalk celery
2 carrots, chopped
1 can water chestnuts, drained
1 jalapeno, diced
2 cloves garlic, minced
1 tablespoon grated ginger
1 1/4 cups water
1/4 cup soy sauce
1/4 cup rice vinegar
1 teaspoon sugar
1/4 teaspoon red pepper flakes
1/2 teaspoon sesame seeds
Whole butter lettuce leaves, for serving
Cooked rice, for serving
Directions:
Use a steamer basket to steam the tempeh for 10 minutes.
Mix together the rest of the ingredients in a medium-sized bowl to make the ginger sauce.
Add all the ingredients to the instant pot and cook on high 4 minutes. Let the pressure release naturally before removing the lid.
Place a small scoop of rice into each lettuce leaf, then add tempeh mixture to each leaf and serve.

115. Quinoa Pecan Stuffed Squash
Preparation Time: 20 MIN
Servings: 2
Ingredients:
1 small acorn squash, halved and seeded
1 tablespoon chopped dried cranberries
1 can kidney beans, drained and rinsed
1 tablespoon chopped pecans
1 cup cooked quinoa
1 clove garlic, minced
1 teaspoon thyme, minced
Salt and pepper, to taste
1/4 cup white wine
Water
Directions:
Mix together the rice, pecans, garlic, thyme, kidney beans, cranberries, salt, and pepper. Add white wine to moisten the mixture.
Fill each squash half with the stuffing mixture.
Spray the instant pot with nonstick spray. Place the squash halves into the instant pot. If they do not both fit in the bottom, place foil on top of one and place the other on top, making sure they stay below the fill line. You may need to cook each half separately if the halves are too large.
Seal the lid and cook on high 6 minutes, then release pressure naturally and serve.

116. Chicken Noodles Soup
Preparation Time: 10 minutes
Cooking time: 25 minutes
Servings: 4
Ingredients:
4 oz egg noodles
8 oz chicken breast, skinless, boneless
1 carrot, grated
1 onion, diced
1 teaspoon salt
1 teaspoon peppercorns
1 teaspoon dried oregano
1 teaspoon olive oil
4 cups of water
Directions:
Heat up the instant pot on Saute mode.
When it is hot, add diced onion and grated carrot.
Cook the vegetables on Saute mode for 5 minutes. Stir them occasionally.
Then add chicken breast, salt, peppercorns, and oregano.
Add water and close the lid.
Cook the soup for 10 minutes on Manual mode (High pressure. Then make quick pressure release.
Open the lid and add egg noodles.
Cook the soup on Saute mode for 7 minutes more or until noodles are cooked.
Nutrition Values:calories 134, fat 3.3, fiber 1.6, carbs 11.8, protein 13.8

117. Taco Soup
Preparation Time: 15 minutes
Cooking time: 20 minutes
Servings: 3
Ingredients:
1 cup ground beef
1 teaspoon taco seasoning
1 teaspoon garlic powder
½ teaspoon onion powder
1 teaspoon salt
¼ cup fresh cilantro, chopped
3 oz Garbanzo beans, canned
1 tablespoon sesame oil

1 chili pepper, chopped
2 cups of water
1 teaspoon chili flakes
2 oz Cheddar cheese, shredded
1 corn tortilla, chopped
1. Directions:
Put the ground beef in the instant pot and set Saute mode.
Add Taco seasoning, garlic powder, onion powder, and salt.
Then add sesame oil and cook the ground beef on Saute mode for 10 minutes.
After this, add Garbanzo beans, chopped chili pepper, chili flakes, and water.
Stir the soup well and close the lid.
Set Manual mode (High pressureand cook soup for 10 minutes.
Then allow natural pressure release for 10 minutes more.
Open the lid and add fresh cilantro.
Ladle the soup in the serving bowls and garnish it with Cheddar cheese and chopped tortilla.
Nutrition Values:calories 311, fat 16.8, fiber 5.6, carbs 22.9, protein 17.9

118. Chicken Transparent Soup
Preparation Time: 20 minutes
Cooking time: 25 minutes
Servings: 4
Ingredients:
1-pound chicken breast
4 cups of water
1 onion, diced
1 teaspoon salt
1 teaspoon ground black pepper
1 carrot, chopped
1 teaspoon coconut oil
Directions:
Put coconut oil in the instant pot and heat it up on Saute mode.
Then add onion and carrot.
Saute the vegetables for 5 minutes.
After this, add salt, ground black pepper, chicken breast, and water.
Close the lid and set Manual mode (High pressure.
Cook the soup for 20 minutes.
Then allow natural pressure release for 10 minutes.
After this, open the lid and remove the chicken breast.
Chop it into serving pieces and put in the serving bowls.
Add hot soup in every bowl.
Nutrition Values:calories 158, fat 4, fiber 1.1, carbs 4.4, protein 24.5

119. Egg Loaf
Preparation Time: 10 minutes
Cooking time: 10 minutes
Servings: 3
Ingredients:
6 eggs
1 teaspoon salt
1 teaspoon ground black pepper
Cooking spray
1 cup water, for cooking
Directions:
Pour water in the instant pot and insert the rack.
Then take the round baking pan and spray it with cooking spray from inside.
Crack the eggs in the baking pan and sprinkle them with salt and ground black pepper.
After this, insert the baking pan on the rack and close the lid.
Set manual mode (High pressure and cook the egg loaf for 6 minutes.
Then allow natural pressure release for 3 minutes more.
Carefully remove the pan from the instant pot and them remove egg loaf from the pan.
Slice it into servings.
Nutrition Values:calories 128, fat 8.8, fiber 0.2, carbs 1.1, protein 11.2

120. Lentil Soup
Preparation Time: 10 minutes
Cooking time: 30 minutes
Servings: 2
Ingredients:
½ cup red lentils
1 tablespoon coconut oil
1 teaspoon salt
1 teaspoon chili flakes
1 bell pepper, chopped
½ red onion, chopped
1 teaspoon ground turmeric
1 teaspoon tomato paste
½ cup corn kernels, frozen
4 cups of water
Directions:
Put coconut oil in the instant pot and heat it up on Saute mode.
When the coconut oil is melted, add red onion and bell pepper.
Saute the vegetables for 5 minutes. Stir them occasionally.
After this, add salt, chili flakes, ground turmeric, tomato paste, and 1 cup of water.
Mix up the mixture well and add lentils.
Then add the remaining water and close the lid.
Set Manual mode (High pressureand cook soup for 20 minutes.
Then make quick pressure release and open the lid.
Ladle the soup into the serving bowls.
Nutrition Values:calories 297, fat 8.1, fiber 17.4, carbs 44.4, protein 14.8

121. Chicken Pilaf
Preparation Time: 15 minutes
Cooking time: 20 minutes
Servings: 4
Ingredients:
1 cup of rice
cups chicken stock
1 teaspoon butter
½ onion, diced
½ carrot, grated
1 teaspoon salt
½ teaspoon chili powder
½ teaspoon ground black pepper

½ teaspoon dried cilantro
½ teaspoon ground coriander
1 teaspoon tomato sauce
7 oz chicken fillet, chopped
Directions:
Set the Saute mode and heat up the instant pot.
Then add butter and melt it.
Add chopped chicken fillet and sprinkle it with salt, chili powder, ground black pepper, dried cilantro, and ground coriander.
Add diced onion and carrot and mix up the ingredients well.
Saute them for 7 minutes.
Then add tomato sauce, rice, and chicken stock.
Don't stir the pilaf anymore.
Close the lid and set Manual mode (High pressure.
Cook the pilaf for 13 minutes.
Then allow natural pressure release for 10 minutes more.
Open the lid and carefully stir the pilaf.
Transfer it in the serving plates.
Nutrition Values:calories 288, fat 5.4, fiber 1.3, carbs 39.9, protein 18.4

122. Creamy Pappardelle
Preparation Time: 10 minutes
Cooking time: 10 minutes
Servings: 4
Ingredients:
8 oz pappardelle pasta
1 cup cream
1 cup chicken stock
1 teaspoon dried oregano
1 teaspoon salt
6 oz tuna, canned, shredded
Directions:
Pour cream and chicken stock in the instant pot.
Add pappardelle pasta, salt, and dried oregano.
Close and seal the lid and set Manual mode (High pressure.
Cook pasta for 7 minutes. Then make quick pressure release for 3 minutes more.
Open the lid and add tuna.
Mix up the pappardelle well and transfer in the serving plates.
Nutrition Values:calories 338, fat 7.5, fiber 3.3, carbs 42.5, protein 23.3

123. Parmesan Mac&Cheese
Preparation Time: 15 minutes
Cooking time: 4 minutes
Servings: 3
Ingredients:
4 oz elbow macaroni
1 cup Parmesan, grated
½ cup milk, hot
1 teaspoon chives, chopped
½ teaspoon mustard
½ teaspoon ground paprika
1 teaspoon cream cheese
1 cup of water
Directions:
Put macaroni and water in the instant pot.
Add mustard, ground paprika, and cream cheese. Stir the ingredients and close the lid.
Set Manual mode (High pressureand cook macaroni for 4 minutes.
Then make quick pressure release and open the lid.
Stir the macaroni with the help of a spatula and add chives, hot milk, and Parmesan.
Mix up the macaroni until the cheese is melted.
Nutrition Values:calories 288, fat 10, fiber 1.3, carbs 32, protein 18.5

124. Garlic Pasta
Preparation Time: 10 minutes
Cooking time: 15 minutes
Servings: 2
Ingredients:
6 oz linguine
2 tablespoons lemon juice
1 teaspoon garlic powder
1 garlic clove, diced
1 oz Parmesan, grated
1 cup cream
½ cup of water
1 tablespoon fresh parsley, chopped
Directions:
Pour cream and water in the instant pot.
Add diced garlic, garlic powder, and lemon juice.
Set Saute mode and heat up the liquid until hot.
Meanwhile, break the linguine into halves.
Add linguine in the hot cream mixture and stir. Close the lid.
Cook the pasta on Manual mode (High pressurefor 10 minutes.
Make quick pressure release and open the lid.
Add Parmesan and fresh parsley. Stir the pasta well until homogenous and cheese is melted.
Nutrition Values:calories 379, fat 11.8, fiber 0.3, carbs 52.8, protein 15.7

125. Ramen Noodles
Preparation Time: 10 minutes
Cooking time: 25 minutes
Servings: 3
Ingredients:
4 oz ramen noodles
1 tablespoon soy sauce
½ oz scallions, chopped
2 cups chicken stock
5 oz chicken fillet, chopped
1 teaspoon salt
1 teaspoon ground black pepper
1 teaspoon olive oil
1 teaspoon sesame seeds
4 oz bok choy, chopped
Directions:
Place chicken and olive oil in the instant pot.
Add ground black pepper and salt and mix up.
Set Saute mode and cook chicken for 10 minutes.
Then add chicken stock and soy sauce.
Close the lid and cook the liquid for 8 minutes on Manual mode (High pressure.
Then make quick pressure release and open the lid.
Shred the chicken with the help of 2 forks.
Add ramen noodles, bok choy, and scallions.

Set Saute mode and bring the ramen to boil.
Then carefully mix up the ramen and cook it for 3 minutes.
Add sesame seeds and ladle the cooked ramen into the bowls.
Nutrition Values:calories 295, fat 12.3, fiber 1.8, carbs 25, protein 19.8

126. Carrot Chicken Soup
Preparation Time: 10 minutes
Cooking time: 30 minutes
Servings: 4
Ingredients:
7 oz chicken breast
4 carrots, peeled, chopped
4 cups chicken stock
1 teaspoon salt
1 teaspoon sour cream
1 tablespoon fresh dill
½ teaspoon ground coriander
¾ teaspoon ground nutmeg
¼ cup chickpeas, canned
Directions:
Pour chicken stock in the instant pot.
Add chicken breast, carrot, salt, ground coriander, nutmeg and close the lid.
Set Manual mode (High pressureand cook the soup for 18 minutes.
Then make quick pressure release and open the lid.
Remove the chicken breast from the instant pot and shred it.
Then blend the soup until it is smooth.
Add shredded chicken and cook the soup for 5 minutes more on Saute mode.
Add chickpeas and dill.
Top the soup with sour cream.
Nutrition Values:calories 143, fat 3, fiber 3.9, carbs 15, protein 14.3

127. Cabbage Casserole
Preparation Time: 10 minutes
Cooking time: 25 minutes
Servings: 6
Ingredients:
1 cup of rice
1 ½ cup ground beef
½ cup spaghetti sauce
1 teaspoon salt
1 teaspoon chili flakes
1 teaspoon ground paprika
1 teaspoon dried oregano
3 cups chicken stock
1 tablespoon olive oil
5 oz cabbage, chopped
1 onion, diced
Directions:
Place ground beef in the instant pot.
Add salt, olive oil, and diced onion.
Cook the ingredients on Saute mode for 5 minutes.
After this, add spaghetti sauce, chili flakes, ground paprika, dried oregano, chicken stock, rice, and cabbage.
Stir the mixture gently and close the lid.

Set manual mode (high pressureand cook the casserole for 15 minutes.
Make a quick pressure release.
Carefully stir the casserole with the help of the spatula.
Nutrition Values:calories 245, fat 6.4, fiber 2.2, carbs 31.1, protein 14.7

128. Lunch Fritatta
Preparation Time: 10 minutes
Cooking time: 10 minutes
Servings: 2
Ingredients:
¼ cup green peas, frozen
¼ cup corn kernels, frozen
¼ cup fresh spinach, chopped
½ cup ground chicken
3 eggs, beaten
1 teaspoon salt
½ teaspoon white pepper
Cooking spray
Directions:
Spray the instant pot bowl with cooking spray and add ground chicken.
Sprinkle it with salt and white pepper and saute on Saute mode for 5 minutes. Stir it from time to time.
Then add chopped spinach, corn kernels, and green peas.
Mix up well and pour the beaten eggs over the mixture.
Close the lid and cook the frittata for 5 minutes on Manual mode (high pressure.
Then make quick pressure release and remove the cooked frittata from the instant pot.
Nutrition Values:calories 194, fat 9.5, fiber 1.7 carbs 7.2, protein 20.2

129. Chili Black Rice
Preparation Time: 15 minutes
Cooking time: 20 minutes
Servings: 2
Ingredients:
½ cup black rice
½ cup ground pork
1 tablespoon scallions, chopped
½ teaspoon salt
1 ½ cup chicken stock
1 teaspoon chili flakes
1 teaspoon butter
Directions:
Put black rice in the instant pot bowl and add ground pork.
Mix up the ingredients well and add salt, chicken stock, chili flakes, and butter.
Add scallions and close the lid.
Set Manual mode (high pressureand cook rice for 20 minutes.
Then allow natural pressure release for 10 minutes and open the lid.
Mix up the cooked meal well before serving.
Nutrition Values:calories 186, fat 5.4, fiber 0.8, carbs 9.6, protein 24

130. Fettuccine Alfredo
Preparation Time: 10 minutes

Cooking time: 15 minutes
Servings: 3
Ingredients:
1 teaspoon butter
1 garlic clove, diced
1 cup chicken stock
5 oz Fettuccine
1 teaspoon salt
5 oz chicken breast, chopped
½ cup heavy cream
1 oz Parmesan, grated
Directions:
Put butter in the instant pot and melt it on Saute mode.
Add diced garlic and chicken stock.
Then add heavy cream and chopped chicken.
Add salt and bring the liquid to boil.
After this, add Fettuccine and close the lid.
Set the Manual mode (High pressureand cook the meal for 8 minutes.
Use quick pressure release and open the lid.
Add cheese and shake the mixture very well.
Transfer the meal in the serving plates.
Nutrition Values:calories 305, fat 13.2, fiber 0, carbs 27.3, protein 19.1

131. Baked Sweet Potato Soup

Preparation Time: 11 minutes
Cooking time: 20 minutes
Servings: 3
Ingredients:
4 sweet potatoes, peeled, chopped
1 teaspoon minced ginger
½ teaspoon salt
1 carrot, chopped
3 cups beef broth
1 cup cream
1 teaspoon lemon juice
1 teaspoon smoked paprika
Directions:
Put all ingredients in the instant pot and close the lid.
Set Manual mode (High pressureand cook the soup mixture for 20 minutes.
Then allow natural pressure release for 10 minutes and open the lid.
Blend the soup until smooth and ladle in the serving bowls.
Nutrition Values:calories 104, fat 6, fiber 0.9, carbs 6.6, protein 5.8

132. Hawaiian Rice

Preparation Time: 15 minutes
Cooking time: 30 minutes
Servings: 2
Ingredients:
½ cup of rice
1 cup chicken stock
1 teaspoon coconut oil
1 bell pepper, chopped
2 oz pineapple, chopped
1 teaspoon soy sauce
3 oz ham, chopped
½ cup of water
½ onion, diced
1 teaspoon salt
1 teaspoon chili flakes
Directions:
Heat up coconut oil in the instant pot on Saute mode and add chopped bell pepper and diced onion. Saute the vegetables for 5 minutes. Stir them from time to time.
After this, add salt, chili flakes, ham, and pineapple. Saute the ingredients for 5 minutes more.
Then add water, soy sauce, chicken stock, and rice. Stir well.
Close the lid and set Manual mode (high pressure. Cook the rice for 20 minutes.
Then allow natural pressure release for 10 minutes. Mix up the cooked meal well before serving.
Nutrition Values:calories 308, fat 6.7, fiber 3, carbs 50, protein 11.8

133. Butternut Squash and Coconut Soup

Preparation Time: 10 minutes
Cooking time: 25 minutes
Servings: 4
Ingredients:
½ cup coconut cream
3 cups chicken stock
1 cup butternut squash, chopped
1 tablespoon sour cream
½ teaspoon ground ginger
1 teaspoon minced garlic
1 teaspoon olive oil
1 tablespoon fresh cilantro
¼ cup celery stalk, chopped
Directions:
Pour olive oil in the instant pot.
Add minced garlic and ground ginger.
Hen add celery stalk and saute the vegetables for 2-3 minutes on Saute mode.
Then add butternut squash and mix up well.
Add coconut cream, chicken stock, and fresh cilantro.
Close the lid and cook the soup on High (manual modefor 20 minutes.
Then make quick pressure release and open the lid.
Blend the soup until smooth with the help of the hand mixer.
Then ladle it in the serving bowls and garnish with sour cream.
Nutrition Values:calories 111, fat 9.4, fiber 1.5, carbs 7, protein 1.8

134. Spanish Rice

Preparation Time: 10 minutes
Cooking time: 25 minutes
Servings: 4
Ingredients:
1 ½ cup of rice
1 cup spaghetti sauce
1 onion, diced
1 teaspoon dried oregano
1 teaspoon salt
1 tablespoon butter
½ cup tomatoes, canned
cup chicken stock
Directions:

Place butter and onion in the instant pot and heat up on saute mode.
Then keep cooking the onion on Saute mode until it is light brown.
After this, add rice, spaghetti sauce, dried oregano, salt canned tomatoes, and chicken stock.
Mix up the rice carefully with the help of the spatula and close the lid.
Cook the rice on Manual mode (high pressurefor 17 minutes. Use quick pressure release.
Nutrition Values:calories 314, fat 3.9, fiber 2.7, carbs 62.2, protein 6

135. Tuscan Chicken Pasta
Preparation Time: 10 minutes
Cooking time: 15 minutes
Servings: 6
Ingredients:
11 oz penne pasta
8 oz chicken thighs, skinless, boneless
1 tablespoon coconut oil
1 teaspoon Italian seasoning
1/3 cup cremini mushrooms, sliced
1 teaspoon soy sauce
2 cups chicken stock
1 cup cream
2 oz Parmesan, grated
Directions:
Chop the chicken thighs and place them in the instant pot.
Set saute mode and start to cook the,
Add coconut oil, Italian seasonings, and saute them for 5 minutes.
After this, add mushrooms and mix up.
Saute the ingredients for 5 minutes more and add chicken stock, cream, Parmesan, and penne pasta.
Mix up well and close the lid.
Set Manual mode (high pressureand cook pasta for 5 minutes.
Then make quick pressure release and open the lid.
Mix up the cooked pasta well and transfer in the serving plates.
Nutrition Values:calories 304, fat 10.9, fiber 0, carbs 30.6, protein 20.6

136. Egg&Bacon Salad
Preparation Time: 10 minutes
Cooking time: 11 minutes
Servings: 2
Ingredients:
4 eggs
4 bacon slices
1 tablespoon mayonnaise
1 teaspoon chives, chopped
1/3 teaspoon chili pepper
1 cup water, for cooking
Directions:
Pour water in the instant pot and insert rack.
Crack eggs in the baking pan and insert it in the instant pot.
Close the lid and cook the eggs on Manual mode (High pressurefor 7 minutes. Make quick pressure release and remove the eggs from the instant pot.
Chop the eggs and place in the salad bowl.
After this, clean the instant pot and remove the rack.
Chop the bacon slices and put them in the instant pot bowl.
Close the lid and cook on High for 4 minutes. Make quick pressure release and transfer the bacon in the chopped eggs.
Add chili pepper, chives, and mayonnaise.
Mix up the salad well.
Nutrition Values:calories 361, fat 27.1, fiber 0.1, carbs 3.1, protein 25.3

137. Caesar Wrap
Preparation Time: 10 minutes
Cooking time: 10 minutes
Servings: 2
Ingredients:
2 corn tortillas
1/3 cup Cheddar cheese, shredded
2 lettuce leaves
½ teaspoon ground black pepper
½ teaspoon salt
8 oz chicken fillet
1 teaspoon olive oil
1 teaspoon lemon juice
2 tablespoons Caesar dressing
Directions:
Sprinkle the chicken fillet with lemon juice, olive oil, salt, and ground black pepper.
Place the chicken fillets in the instant pot and cook them on Manual mode (high pressurefor 10 minutes.
Meanwhile, sprinkle the corn tortillas with cheese from one side.
Add lettuce leaves.
When the chicken fillet is cooked, make a quick pressure release and chop the chicken roughly.
Add it over the lettuce leaves and top with Caesar dressing.
Wrap the tortillas.
Nutrition Values:calories 397, fat 19.7, fiber 1.9, carbs 14.8, protein 39.1

138. Frito Pie Bowl
Preparation Time: 10 minutes
Cooking time:25 minutes
Servings: 6
Ingredients:
1 cup Cheddar cheese, shredded
½ cup fresh cilantro, chopped
2 cups ground beef
1 cup Taco sauce
5 oz Rotel tomatoes, canned
1 teaspoon dried oregano
1 teaspoon salt
¼ cup tomato sauce
3 tablespoons masa harina
3 tablespoons water
5 oz red kidney beans, canned
1 tablespoon olive oil
1 onion, diced
Directions:
Heat up olive oil in Saute mode and add the onion.
Cook the onion until light brown and add ground beef.
Mix up well and saute for 5 minutes.

After this, add taco sauce, cilantro, Rotel tomatoes, salt, dried oregano, tomato sauce, and red kidney beans.
Saute the mixture for 15 minutes.
Meanwhile, mix up together masa harina and water.
Add the masa harina mixture in the instant pot and mix up well.
Close the lid and saute the meal for 5 minutes.
Then transfer the cooked Frito pie in the bowls and top it with shredded cheese.
Nutrition Values:calories 307, fat 14.7, fiber 4.9 carbs 24.3, protein 20.2

139. Cheddar Soup
Preparation Time: 10 minutes
Cooking time: 15 minutes
Servings: 4
Ingredients:
3 onions, diced
1 cup Cheddar cheese, shredded
1 cup cream
3 cups chicken stock
1 oz bacon, chopped, cooked
1 teaspoon butter
1 teaspoon salt
1 tablespoon dried dill
1 potato, grated
Directions:
Heta up butter on Saute mode and add diced onion.
Cook it until the onion is light brown.
Then add bacon, grated potato, dried dill, salt, cream, and chicken stock.
Close the lid and cook soup on Manual mode for 5 minutes (High pressure.
Use the quick pressure release and open the lid.
Add Cheddar cheese and stir the soup with the help of the spoon until the cheese is melted.
Nutrition Values:calories 274, fat 17.2, fiber 2.8, carbs 18.5, protein 12.6

140. Lasagna
Preparation Time: 10 minutes
Cooking time: 40 minutes
Servings: 6
Ingredients:
cup ground beef
1 onion, diced
1 cup marinara sauce
1 teaspoon olive oil
1 teaspoon Italian seasoning
1 teaspoon salt
4 oz ricotta cheese
5 oz Parmesan, grated
1 tablespoon fresh parsley
4 oz lasagna noodles
Cooking spray
1 cup water, for cooking
Directions:
Pour olive oil in the instant pot and heat it up on Saute mode.
Add diced onion and ground beef.
Then add salt and mix up well.
Saute the ground beef for 10 minutes.
After this, add marinara sauce and parsley. Mix up well and saute the ground beef for 5 minutes more.
Then remove the ground beef from the pot.
Pour water in the instant pot and insert rack.
Spray the baking pan with cooking spray and arrange ½ part of lasagna noodles.
Spread the noodles with ½ part of ground beef mixture.
In the separated bowl combine together ricotta cheese and Parmesan.
Top the ground beef with ½ part of Parmesan mixture.
Cover the cheese layer with lasagna noodles and repeat the same steps.
Then cover the surface of lasagna with foil and transfer om the rack.
Close the lid and cook the meal on Manual mode (High pressurefor 25 minutes.
Make quick pressure release and open the lid.
Remove the foil from lasagna.
Nutrition Values:calories 237, fat 13.1, fiber 1.5, carbs 19.8, protein 19.4

141. Fish Casserole
Preparation Time: 20 minutes
Cooking time: 8 minutes
Servings: 4
Ingredients:
8 oz salmon, chopped
1 cup potatoes, chopped
1 cup chicken stock
1 teaspoon ground coriander
½ teaspoon ground nutmeg
1 teaspoon dried oregano
¼ cup marinara sauce
½ cup chickpeas, canned
Directions:
Mix up together ground coriander, nutmeg, oregano, and salmon.
Then pour the marinara sauce in the instant pot.
Add potatoes.
Place salmon over potatoes.
Then add chickpeas and chicken stock. Close the lid.
Cook the casserole for 8 minutes in Manual mode (high pressure.
Then allow natural pressure release for 10 minutes.
Mix up the casserole well before serving.
Nutrition Values:calories 211, fat 5.8, fiber 5.9, carbs 23.8, protein 17

142. Bacon Chowder
Preparation Time: 10 minutes
Cooking time: 30 minutes
Servings: 4
Ingredients:
3 cups chicken stock
1 cup of water
1 tablespoon butter
1-pound chicken breast, skinless, boneless, chopped
½ cup corn kernels
3 oz bacon, chopped, roasted
1 teaspoon salt
1 tablespoon cream cheese
1 tablespoon chives

Directions:
Melt butter in the instant pot on Saute mode.
Then add chopped chicken, chives, salt, bacon, and corn kernels.
Saute the ingredients for 5 minutes.
Add cream cheese, water, and chicken stock. Close the lid.
Saute the chowder for 25 minutes.
Nutrition Values:calories 303, fat 16.1, fiber 0.6, carbs 4.6, protein 33.3

143. Stuffed Pepper Rings
Preparation Time: 10 minutes
Cooking time: 25 minutes
Servings: 4
Ingredients:
4 bell peppers
½ cup of rice
1 cup ground chicken
1 cup tomato sauce
1 teaspoon salt
1 teaspoon minced garlic
1 teaspoon olive oil
½ cup of water
Directions:
Pour olive oil in the instant pot.
Heat it up on Saute mode.
Then add minced garlic and ground chicken.
Saute the chicken for 5 minutes.
Then add rice and water.
Saute the ingredients for 10 minutes.
After this, trim the bell peppers.
Fill them with the rice-chicken mixture and slice into the rings.
Arrange the pepper rings in the instant pot.
Add tomato sauce and close the lid.
Cook the meal on High-pressure mode for 9 minutes.
Use quick pressure release.
Nutrition Values:calories 215, fat 4.3, fiber 2.8, carbs 31, protein 13.8

144. Zucchini Meat Cakes
Preparation Time: 10 minutes
Cooking time: 20 minutes
Servings: 4
Ingredients:
2 zucchini, grated
1 egg, beaten
1 teaspoon salt
1 onion, minced
1 teaspoon ground black pepper
1 cup ground chicken
1 teaspoon olive oil
Directions:
Heat up olive oil in the instant pot.
Add ground chicken and sprinkle it with ground black pepper.
Saute the chicken for 5 minutes.
After this, transfer the cooked ground chicken in the bowl.
Add egg, salt, minced onion, and mix up well.
With the help of the spoon place small cakes from the zucchini mixture in the instant pot bowl.

Saute them for 5 minutes from each side or until they are light brown.
If the cakes are too liquid – add wheat flour to make the batter thicker.
Nutrition Values:calories 120, fat 5.1, fiber 1.8, carbs 6.3, protein 13.1

145. Fragrant Tomato Soup
Preparation Time: 15 minutes
Cooking time: 20 minutes
Servings: 4
Ingredients:
2 cups tomatoes, chopped
4 oz fennel bulb, chopped
1 tablespoon coconut oil
1 teaspoon salt
½ teaspoon ground black pepper
1 teaspoon fresh basil, chopped
1 bell pepper, chopped
½ teaspoon cayenne pepper
½ cup cream
2 cups chicken stock
1 oz Parmesan, grated
Directions:
Tosso coconut oil in the instant pot and heat it up on Saute mode.
When the coconut oil is melted, add bell pepper and fennel bulb.
Mix up well and saute the vegetables for 3 minutes.
After this, add salt, ground black pepper, basil, cayenne pepper, cream, and chicken stock.
Add tomatoes and close the lid.
Set manual mode (High pressureand cook the soup for 15 minutes.
Then allow natural pressure release for 10 minutes.
With the help of the hand blender, blend the soup until smooth.
Ladle the soup in the serving bowls and top with grated cheese.
Nutrition Values:calories 112, fat 7.2, fiber 2.5, carbs 9.7, protein 4.4

146. Oregano Soup
Preparation Time: 15 minutes
Cooking time: 18 minutes
Servings: 4
Ingredients:
1 potato, chopped
½ carrot, chopped
¼ cup of rice
3 cups chicken stock
1 tablespoon dried oregano
1 teaspoon butter
4 chicken drumsticks, skinless
1 teaspoon salt
1 teaspoon cayenne pepper
Directions:
Heat up butte on Saute mode and add carrot and potato.
Sprinkle the vegetables with salt and cayenne pepper and mix up.
Saute the vegetables for 5 minutes.
After this, add rice and chicken drumsticks. Mix up well.

Add chicken stock and close the lid.
Set Manual mode (High pressureand cook soup for 18 minutes.
Then allow natural pressure release for 15 minutes.
Open the lid, add dried oregano and mix up the soup well.
Let it cook for 10 minutes before serving.
Nutrition Values:calories 176, fat 4.3, fiber 1.9, carbs 18.9, protein 15.1

147. Filipino Sinigang
Preparation Time: 10 minutes
Cooking time: 40 minutes
Servings: 4
Ingredients:
1-pound beef sirloin, chopped
½ cup tamarind soup
3 cups of water
1 teaspoon salt
1 chayote, chopped
1 eggplant, chopped
3 oz bok choy, chopped
1 teaspoon ground black pepper
2 tomatoes, chopped
Directions:
Put beef sirloin in the instant pot bowl.
Add water, salt, and ground black pepper. Close the lid.
Cook the beef on Manual mode (High pressurefor 30 minutes.
Then make quick pressure release and open the lid.
Add eggplant, chayote, and bok choy.
Close the lid and cook on High Pressure for 5 minutes more. Make a quick pressure release.
Add tomatoes and mix up well. Add tamarind soup.
Close the lid and cook the meal for 5 minutes more on High pressure.
When the time is over, make a quick pressure release and open the lid.
Nutrition Values:calories 265, fat 7.5, fiber 6.1, carbs 12.3, protein 36.9

148. Taco Pie
Preparation Time: 15 minutes
Cooking time: 17 minutes
Servings: 4
Ingredients:
4 corn tortillas
1 teaspoon taco seasoning
½ cup Cheddar cheese, shredded
½ cup red kidney beans, canned, mashed
1 teaspoon olive oil
1 teaspoon minced garlic
1 cup ground beef
1 cup water, for cooking
Directions:
Pour olive oil in the instant pot.
Add minced garlic and ground beef.
Saute the mixture for 10 minutes on Saute mode.
Then line the baking pan with baking paper.
Place 1 corn tortilla inside and spread it with red kidney mixture.
After this, place the ground beef mixture over the beans and top it with Cheddar cheese.

Cover the mixture with second corn tortilla.
Repeat the same steps till you use all the ingredients.
Top the last tortilla with shredded cheese.
Clean the instant pot and pour water inside.
Insert the rack and place the baking pan on it.
Close the lid and cook the pie on High (Manual modefor 7 minutes.
Then allow natural pressure release for 10 minutes.
Cool the cooked pie little before serving.
Nutrition Values:calories 265, fat 10.9, fiber 5, carbs 25.7, protein 16.6

149. Nutritious Rice Bowl
Preparation Time: 10 minutes
Cooking time: 35 minutes
Servings: 2
Ingredients:
½ cup of rice
2 cups chicken stock
4 oz tofu, cubed
1 teaspoon soy sauce
¼ teaspoon sugar
1 teaspoon apple cider vinegar
1 teaspoon salt
1 teaspoon sunflower oil
Directions:
Pour chicken stock in the instant pot.
Add rice and salt.
Close the lid and cook the rice on Rice mode for 20 minutes.
When the rice is cooked, transfer it into the serving bowls.
Pour the oil in the instant pot.
Heat it up on Saute mode.
Then mix up together tofu, soy sauce, sugar, and apple cider vinegar.
Put the tofu mixture in the instant pot and saute for 10 minutes. Stir it occasionally.
Top the cooked rice with tofu.
Nutrition Values:calories 222, fat 3.2, fiber 1.1, carbs 39.4, protein 8.8

150. Lentils&Rice Mix
Preparation Time: 8 minutes
Cooking time: 20 minutes
Servings: 2
Ingredients:
¼ cup red lentils
¼ cup of rice
½ cup tomato sauce
½ cup chicken stock
1 teaspoon cayenne pepper
1 teaspoon butter
½ teaspoon salt
Directions:
Preheat butter in the instant pot on Saute mode.
Add rice and red lentils.
Then sprinkle the mixture with cayenne pepper and salt.
Mix up well.
Add tomato sauce and saute the mixture for 10 minutes.
Then add chicken stock.
Close the lid and set Manual mode (high pressure.

Cook the mixture for 10 minutes. Then make quick pressure release.
Mix up the cooked meal well before serving.
Nutrition Values:calories 206, fat 2.7, fiber 8.8, carbs 36.9, protein 9

151. Chicken Mole
Preparation Time: 10 minutes
Cooking time: 15 minutes
Servings: 2
Ingredients:
1 teaspoon olive oil
½ onion, diced
1 garlic clove, diced
3 oz tomatoes, canned
1 chipotle pepper, chopped
1 teaspoon Adobo sauce
1 teaspoon ground cinnamon
½ teaspoon ground cumin
5 oz chicken breast, skinless, boneless, chopped
2 oz Parmesan, grated
2 corn tortillas
Directions:
Pour olive oil in the instant pot.
Add diced onion and garlic clove. Saute the vegetables for 5 minutes.
After this, add tomatoes, chipotle pepper, Adobo sauce, ground cinnamon, cumin, and mix up well.
Bring the mixture to boil on Saute mode.
Then blend it with the help of the hand blender.
When the mixture is smooth, add chopped chicken and mix up well.
Close the lid and set Manual mode (High pressure.
Cook the chicken for 10 minutes. Make a quick pressure release.
Open the lid.
Fill the tortillas with cooked chicken mixture and top with Parmesan.
Nutrition Values:calories 282, fat 11.2, fiber 3.7, carbs 20.6, protein 26.9

152. Mushroom Risotto
Preparation Time: 10 minutes
Cooking time: 17 minutes
Servings: 3
Ingredients:
½ cup arborio rice
¼ cup green peas, frozen
¼ teaspoon minced garlic
½ teaspoon salt
¾ teaspoon dried thyme
½ cup cremini mushrooms, sliced
2 cups beef broth
¼ cup Mozzarella, shredded
1 tablespoon butter
Directions:
Melt butter in the instant pot on Saute mode.
Add minced garlic, salt, dried thyme, green peas, cremini mushrooms, and mix up well.
Saute the vegetables for 10 minutes.
After this, add arborio rice and beef broth.
Close the lid and cook risotto for 7 minutes on Manual mode (High pressure.
Then make a quick pressure release and open the lid.
Add Mozzarella and mix up risotto.
Nutrition Values:calories 194, fat 5.4, fiber 1.6, carbs 28.4, protein 7

153. Lunch Saute
Preparation Time: 10 minutes
Cooking time: 25 minutes
Servings: 2
Ingredients:
4 oz chicken fillet, chopped
½ teaspoon salt
½ teaspoon ground black pepper
2 oz celery stalk
1 carrot, chopped
1 potato, chopped
¼ cup broccoli florets
1 tablespoon cream cheese
1 teaspoon olive oil
½ teaspoon ground cumin
1/3 cup chicken stock
Directions:
Put all ingredients in the instant pot and shake well.
Close the lid and set Saute mode.
Cook the meal for 25 minutes.
When the saute is cooked, gently shake it and transfer in the serving plates.
Nutrition Values:calories 237, fat 8.7, fiber 3.6, carbs 20.3, protein 19.5

154. Chickpeas&Noodles Soup
Preparation Time: 5 minutes
Cooking time: 8 minutes
Servings: 4
Ingredients:
3 oz spaghetti
½ cup chickpeas, cooked
1 teaspoon cream cheese
4 cups chicken stock
1 onion, diced
1 teaspoon cayenne pepper
½ teaspoon salt
1 teaspoon olive oil
Directions:
Heat up olive oil on Saute mode.
Add onion and cook it until light brown.
Add cayenne pepper, cream cheese, salt, chickpeas, and spaghetti.
Close the lid and set Manual mode (High pressure.
Cook the soup for 4 minutes.
Then make quick pressure release.
Nutrition Values:calories 187, fat 4.1, fiber 5.1, carbs 30.4, protein 8.3

155. Lo Mein
Preparation Time: 10 minutes
Cooking time: 8 minutes
Servings: 2
Ingredients:
½ cup mushroom, sliced
1 carrot, spiralized
1 teaspoon minced garlic
1 teaspoon hot sauce
½ cup chicken stock
1 teaspoon corn starch
4 tablespoons water

1 teaspoon cumin seeds
1 teaspoon soy sauce
4 oz spaghetti
4 oz chicken fillet, chopped
Directions:
Place mushrooms in the instant pot.
Add carrot, minced garlic, hot sauce, chicken stock, soy sauce, chicken fillet, and spaghetti.
Close the lid and cook the ingredients on High pressure (Manual modefor 6 minutes.
Then make quick pressure release.
Whisk together corn starch and water.
Pour the mixture over the spaghetti and stir well.
Cook Lo Mein on High for 2 minutes more. Make a quick pressure release.
Sprinkle the cooked meal with cumin seeds.
Nutrition Values:calories 303, fat 5.9, fiber 1.1, carbs 37.5, protein 24.2

156. Cajun Rice Bowl
Preparation Time: 15 minutes
Cooking time: 12 minutes
Servings: 3
Ingredients:
5 oz Andouille sausages, sliced
½ cup of rice
1 teaspoon Cajun seasonings
½ teaspoon ground turmeric
½ teaspoon chili flakes
2 chicken thighs, skinless, boneless
½ teaspoon smoked paprika
1 ½ cup water
1 teaspoon salt
Directions:
Chop the chicken thighs roughly and place in the instant pot.
Add rice and sprinkle the ingredients with Cajun seasonings.
After this, add sausages, ground turmeric, chili flakes, smoked paprika, and salt.
Add water and mix up the rice mixture with the help of the spoon.
Close and seal the lid.
Set the manual mode (high pressureand cook the rice mixture for 12 minutes.
Then allow natural pressure release for 10 minutes.
Open the lid and transfer hot chicken-rice mixture directly in the serving bowls.
Nutrition Values:calories 329, fat 16, fiber 0.7, carbs 27.1, protein 18.9

157. American Goulash
Preparation Time: 10 minutes
Cooking time: 35 minutes
Servings: 4
Ingredients:
4 oz elbow macaroni
½ cup ground chicken
½ cup tomato sauce
1 teaspoon minced garlic
2 oz celery stalk, chopped
1 teaspoon Italian seasoning
2 cups of water
½ cup green beans, chopped

1 teaspoon salt
1 onion, chopped
1 tablespoon cream cheese
Directions:
Put all ingredients from the list above in the instant pot bowl and stir carefully with the help of the wooden spatula.
After this, close the lid and set Saute mode.
Cook the goulash for 35 minutes.
Cool the cooked goulash to the room temperature.
Nutrition Values:calories 177, fat 3.1, fiber 2.7, carbs 27.2, protein 10

158. Rice Casserole
Preparation Time: 10 minutes
Cooking time: 10 minutes
Servings: 4
Ingredients:
1/3 cup long-grain rice
1 cup broccoli florets
1 cup cream
½ cup Mozzarella, shredded
1 teaspoon chili pepper
½ teaspoon ground nutmeg
1 teaspoon butter
1 teaspoon salt
1 garlic clove, chopped
½ cup chicken stock
1 tablespoon fresh cilantro, chopped
Directions:
Heta up butter in the instant pot on Saute mode.
When the butter is melted, add chopped garlic and broccoli florets.
Saute the vegetables for 3 minutes.
Then mix up well with the help of the spatula and ad cream, Mozzarella, chili pepper, ground nutmeg, salt, and rice.
Add chicken stock and close the lid.
Cook casserole on Manual mode (High pressurefor 7 minutes.
Then allow natural pressure release for 5 minutes more.
Nutrition Values:calories 126, fat 5.3, fiber 0.9, carbs 16.5, protein 3.4

159. Ham Casserole
Preparation Time: 25 minutes
Cooking time: 8 minutes
Servings: 6
Ingredients:
7 oz ham, sliced
4 tablespoons cream cheese
1 teaspoon minced garlic
2 tomatoes, sliced
1 cup cream
1 tablespoon cornstarch
1 cup corn kernels, frozen
½ teaspoon ground black pepper
1 oz pineapple, chopped
1 teaspoon avocado oil
Directions:
Brush the instant pot bowl and avocado oil.
Then place the layer of ham.

In the separated bowl, mix up together cream cheese with minced garlic.
Spread the ham layer with cream cheese mixture gently.
After this, top it with sliced tomatoes and chopped pineapple.
Then make the layer od ham again and repeat all the steps.
Spread the last layer with cream cheese mixture.
After this, whisk together corn starch and cream.
Pour the liquid over the casserole and close the lid.
Cook the ham casserole on Manual mode (High pressurefor 8 minutes.
Then allow natural pressure release for 15 minutes.
Nutrition Values:calories 142, fat 7.9, fiber 1.8, carbs 11.3, protein 7.6

160. Ham Rotini
Preparation Time: 10 minutes
Cooking time: 5 minutes
Servings: 4
Ingredients:
7 oz rotini
1 cup chicken stock
1 teaspoon salt
1 teaspoon dried cilantro
1 tablespoon spaghetti sauce
4 oz ham, chopped
¼ cup Cheddar cheese, shredded
1 tablespoon sour cream
Directions:
Pour chicken stock in the instant pot.
Add rotini, salt, and dried cilantro.
Then close the lid and cook the pasta on Manual (High pressurefor 5 minutes. Make a quick pressure release.
After this, open the lid and add spaghetti sauce, ham, Cheddar cheese, and sour cream.
Mix up the ham rotini well.
Nutrition Values:calories 261, fat 6.2, fiber 2.2, carbs 38.6, protein 13.2

161. Tortilla Soup
Preparation Time: 15 minutes
Cooking time: 15 minutes
Servings: 6
Ingredients:
1 cup corn kernels
1 cup red kidney beans, cooked
1 cup bell pepper, chopped
1 tablespoon olive oil
1 onion, diced
½ cup tomatoes, canned
1 tablespoon taco seasoning
1 teaspoon salt
3 corn tortillas, chopped
½ cup fresh cilantro
7 oz chicken fillet
5 cups of water
Directions:
Pour olive oil in the instant pot. Set Saute mode.
Add bell peppers, onion, and corn kernels.
Saute the vegetables for 5 minutes.
After this, add red kidney beans, tomatoes, taco seasoning, salt, and chicken fillet.
Then add water and close the lid.
Cook the soup on Manual mode (High pressurefor 10 minutes.
Then allow natural pressure release for 10 minutes.
After this, open the lid and remove the chicken fillet.
Shred the chicken fillet and return it back in the soup.
Add fresh cilantro and chopped tortillas.
Nutrition Values:calories 256, fat 5.9, fiber 7, carbs 33.8, protein 18.6

162. Jacket Potato
Preparation Time: 15 minutes
Cooking time: 15 minutes
Servings: 2
Ingredients:
2 russet potatoes
1 tablespoon cream cheese
½ teaspoon chives
1 oz Cheddar cheese, shredded
½ teaspoon salt
½ teaspoon chili flakes
1 cup water, for cooking
Directions:
Pour water in the instant pot and insert rack.
Place the potatoes on the rack and close the lid.
Cook the potatoes on Manual (High pressurefor 15 minutes.
Then make quick pressure release and open the lid.
Make the lengthwise cut in every potato and mash the potato pulp gently with the help of the fork.
After this, in the mixing bowl combine together chives, cream cheese, salt, Cheddar cheese, and chili flakes.
Top every jacket potato with cream cheese mixture.
Serve the potatoes hot.
Nutrition Values:calories 222, fat 6.7, fiber 5.1, carbs 33.8, protein 7.5

163. Tomato Kielbasa
Preparation Time: 10 minutes
Cooking time: 10 minutes
Servings: 2
Ingredients:
7 oz kielbasa, sliced
1/3 cup tomato sauce
1 garlic clove, chopped
½ onion, chopped
1 bay leaf
¼ cup of water
1 teaspoon butter
Directions:
Heat up butter on Saute mode.
Then add chopped onion and garlic.
Saute the ingredients for 2 minutes and add bay leaf, water, tomato sauce, and sliced kielbasa.
Close the lid and cook the meal on Manual (High pressurefor 7 minutes.
Then allow natural pressure release for 10 minutes.
Serve kielbasa with tomato gravy.
Nutrition Values:calories 266, fat 19.5, fiber 1.4, carbs 9.5, protein 14

164. Cauliflower and Mushroom Soup
Preparation Time: 10 minutes
Cooking time: 25 minutes
Servings: 6
Ingredients:
1 teaspoon ground coriander
1 cup mushrooms, chopped
1 cup cauliflower, chopped
5 cups chicken stock
½ cup cream
1 teaspoon smoked paprika
1 teaspoon salt
1 onion, diced
1 teaspoon dried dill
Directions:
Place all ingredients in the instant pot.
Close the lid and cook soup on Manual mode (High pressurefor 25 minutes.
When the time is over, make natural pressure release and open the lid.
With the help of the hand blender make the soup smooth.
Add more salt if desired and ladle into the soup bowls.
Nutrition Values:calories 36, fat 1.7, fiber 1.1, carbs 4.5, protein 1.7

165. Onion Cheesy Soup
Preparation Time: 10 minutes
Cooking time: 20 minutes
Servings: 2
Ingredients:
1 cup onion, chopped
1/3 cup butter
1 teaspoon salt
1 cup Mozzarella cheese
½ cup milk
2 cups of water
1 teaspoon chili flakes
Directions:
Put onion and butter in the instant pot bowl.
Close the lid and cook them in Saute mode for 10 minutes.
Then open the lid, add chili flakes, salt, cheese, and milk.
Saute the mixture for 5 minutes more or until cheese is melted.
After this, add water and close the lid.
Cook onion soup on High (Manual modefor 4 minutes.
Then make quick pressure release.
Mix up the soup well before serving.
Nutrition Values:calories 365, fat 34.5, fiber 1.2, carbs 8.9, protein 7

166. Green Soup
Preparation Time: 15 minutes
Cooking time: 16 minutes
Servings: 2
Ingredients:
2 cups chicken stock
5 oz salmon, chopped
1 cup spinach, chopped
½ cup kale, chopped
¼ cup fresh parsley, chopped
1 teaspoon salt
½ teaspoon ground cumin
1 garlic clove, diced
1 teaspoon olive oil
Directions:
Heat up olive oil in saute mode and add diced garlic.
Saute it for 2 minutes.
Then add ground cumin, salt, parsley, kale, spinach, and salmon.
Mix up the ingredients well and saute them for 3 minutes.
After this, add chicken stock and close the lid.
Cook soup on Manual mode (High pressurefor 6 minutes.
Then allow natural pressure release for 10 minutes.
Nutrition Values:calories 142, fat 7.5, fiber 0.9, carbs 4.2, protein 15.8

167. Vegan Soup
Preparation Time: 15 minutes
Cooking time: 20 minutes
Servings: 4
Ingredients:
1 russet potato, chopped
1 carrot, grated
½ yellow onion, diced
¼ teaspoon minced garlic
2 oz celery stalk, chopped
¼ cup fresh dill, chopped
1 teaspoon salt
1 teaspoon ground black pepper
1 bay leaf
4 cups of water
¼ cup long-grain rice
Directions:
Put all ingredients from the list above in the instant pot bowl.
Close the lid and set Manual mode (High pressure.
Cook the vegan soup for 20 minutes. Then make quick pressure release.
Let the cooked soup rest for 15-20 minutes before serving.
Nutrition Values:calories 99, fat 0.3, fiber 2.6, carbs 22.1, protein 2.8

168. Lentil Curry
Preparation Time: 15 minutes
Cooking time: 20 minutes
Servings: 2
Ingredients:
½ cup red lentils
½ cup of water
½ cup organic almond milk
1 shallot, chopped
1 garlic clove, diced
½ teaspoon salt
1 teaspoon curry paste
1 tablespoon coconut oil
½ teaspoon dried cilantro
¼ teaspoon cayenne pepper
¼ teaspoon minced ginger
Directions:
Put coconut oil in the instant pot.

Set saute mode and heat it up.
When the coconut oil is melted, add shallot, garlic clove, and minced ginger.
Saute the ingredients for 3 minutes. Stir them occasionally.
After this, add cayenne pepper, dried cilantro, curry paste, salt, and almond milk.
Stir the mixture until curry paste is dissolved.
Then add lentils and water.
Mix up the ingredients with the help of the spoon and close the lid.
Set Manual mode (High pressureand cook lentil curry for 16 minutes.
Then allow natural pressure release for 10 minutes.
Mix up the cooked meal well before transfer it into the bowls.
Nutrition Values:calories 264, fat 9.2, fiber 15, carbs 30.9, protein 15.2

169. Lazy Penne
Preparation Time: 10 minutes
Cooking time: 10 minutes
Servings: 2
Ingredients:
5 oz penne pasta
½ cup ground pork
½ white onion, diced
½ teaspoon cayenne pepper
1 cup chicken stock
½ teaspoon salt
1 teaspoon coconut oil
1 teaspoon tomato paste
Directions:
Heat up coconut oil in the instant pot bowl on Saute mode.
When the oil is melted, add diced onion and saute it for 4 minutes or until light brown.
After this, add ground pork, cayenne pepper, and salt. Mix up well.
Saute the meat for 3 minutes more or until it is browned.
Then add tomato paste and mix up well.
Add chicken stock and penne pasta. Stir gently and close the lid.
Cook the meal for 3 minutes on Manual mode (High pressure.
Then make quick pressure release.
Open the lid and mix up the meal well.
Nutrition Values:calories 476, fat 20.6, fiber 0.8, carbs 42.5, protein 28.9

170. Chicken Alfredo Pasta
Preparation Time: 10 minutes
Cooking time: 7 minutes
Servings: 4
Ingredients:
1 cup of water
½ cup heavy cream
4 oz Parmesan, grated
6 oz spaghetti
1/3 teaspoon minced garlic
¼ teaspoon white pepper
Directions:
Put spaghetti in the instant pot.
Add water, heavy cream, minced garlic, and white pepper.
Close the lid and cook spaghetti on High pressure (manual modefor 7 minutes.
Make a quick pressure release.
After this, open the lid and add Parmesan. Stir the meal until cheese is melted.
Nutrition Values:calories 266, fat 12.6, fiber 0, carbs 24.9, protein 14.3

171. Chicken Chili Soup
Preparation Time: 15 minutes
Cooking time: 10 minutes
Servings: 2
Ingredients:
6 oz chicken breast, chopped
¼ cup red kidney beans, canned
1 teaspoon turmeric
½ teaspoon ground black pepper
½ teaspoon salt
½ cup tomatoes, crushed, canned
½ teaspoon chili pepper
½ cup corn kernels
1 tablespoon Ranch dip
2 cups of water
1 teaspoon cream cheese
Directions:
Put all ingredients from the list above in the instant pot bowl and carefully mix.
Then close the lid and set Manual mode (High pressure.
Cook chili soup for 10 minutes and then make quick pressure release.
Open the lid and mix up the soup well with the help of the spoon.
Then cool the cooked soup for 10 minutes and ladle it into the serving bowls.
Nutrition Values:calories 257, fat 6.6, fiber 5.5, carbs 25.3, protein 25.7

SIDES

172. Cantonese Winter Squash.
Preparation Time: 45 MIN
Servings: 4
Ingredients:
1 large butternut squash, peeled, seeded, and diced
4 garlic cloves, thinly sliced
2 tablespoons water
1 tablespoon soy sauce
1 tablespoon light brown sugar
2 teaspoons olive oil
1½ teaspoons grated fresh ginger
Salt and freshly ground black pepper
Directions:
Warm the oil in your instant pot.
Add the garlic and ginger and soften a minute.
Add the water, soy sauce, squash, sugar, salt, and pepper.
Seal and cook on Stew for 40 minutes.
Depressurize naturally.

173. Italian Tomatoes and Zucchini.
Preparation Time: 45 MIN
Servings: 6
Ingredients:
2 pounds zucchini, diced
2 pounds ripe plum tomatoes, diced
1 medium-size yellow onion, minced
3 garlic cloves, minced
2 teaspoons olive oil (optional
1 teaspoon dried basil
¾ teaspoon salt
⅛ teaspoon freshly ground black pepper
2 tablespoons minced fresh flat-leaf parsley or basil, for garnish
Directions:
Warm the oil in your instant pot.
Add the onion and garlic and soften 4 minutes.
Add the remaining ingredients except for the parsley.
Seal and cook on Stew for 35 minutes.
Depressurize naturally and serve topped with parsley.

174. Vegan Braciole.
Preparation Time: 45 MIN
Servings: 6
Ingredients:
1 large eggplant
1 cup marinara sauce
1 cup dry breadcrumbs
⅓ cup nutritional yeast
⅓ cup golden raisins
¼ cup minced fresh flat-leaf parsley leaves
5 garlic cloves, minced
6 ounces white mushrooms, finely chopped
2 tablespoons vegan Parmesan cheese (optional
2 teaspoons olive oil (optional
Salt and freshly ground black pepper
Directions:
Halve your eggplant lengthwise and scoop out the flesh leaving a ¼ inch shell.
Chop the scooped eggplant.
Warm the oil in your instant pot and add the eggplant, garlic, mushrooms, salt, and pepper. Cook 5 minutes with the lid off.
Remove from the heat and mix in bread crumbs, nutritional yeast, raisins, and parsley.
Fill the eggplant shells with the stuffing and put in the slow cooker.
Pour the marinara over them and top with cheese.
Seal and cook for 35 minutes on Stew.

175. Marmalade Beets
Preparation Time: 45 MIN
Servings: 9
Ingredients:
8 to 10 small beets, trimmed and halved, or 4 large beets, trimmed and cubed
3 tablespoons Orange Marmalade
2 teaspoons olive oil
juice of 1 lemon
juice of 1 lime
Salt and freshly ground black pepper
Directions:
Mix the marmalade and juices in a bowl.
Put your beets in your instant pot and stir in the marmalade mixture with some salt and pepper.
Seal and cook on Meat for 35 minutes.
Depressurize naturally.
Skin the beets and discard the skins.
Toss the beets in the marmalade again before serving.

176. Creamy Wild Asparagus
Preparation Time: 35 MIN
Servings: 4
Ingredients:
2 lbs fresh wild asparagus, trimmed
2 small onions, peeled and finely chopped
1 cup of vegan sour cream
4 cups of vegetable broth
2 tbsp of vegetable oil
½ tsp of salt
½ tsp of dried oregano
½ tsp of cayenne pepper
Directions:
Rinse and drain asparagus. Trim off the woody ends and cut into thick pieces. Set aside.
Plug in the instant pot and press "Sautee" button.
Heat up the oil in the stainless steel insert and add finely chopped onions. Stir-fry until translucent.
Add chopped asparagus, oregano, salt, and cayenne pepper. Stir well and continue to cook until asparagus soften.
Add the vegetable broth and mix well to combine.
Stop the "Sautee" mode and close the cooker's lid.
Open the steam release handle on top and press the "Soup" button, or set the cooking time to 20 minutes.
When you hear the cooker's end signal, press "Cancel" button.
Allow the cooker to release the pressure naturally and open the lid. Whisk in the vegan sour cream and serve immediately.

177. Smashed Potatoes
Preparation Time: 35 MIN

Servings: 2
Ingredients:
For Smashed Potatoes:
2 cups water
2 ½ lbs potatoes, peeled and then chopped
1 tsp salt
½ tsp garlic powder
½ tsp onion powder
1 tsp Italian seasoning
For Garnishing:
½ cup corn
1 green onion stalk, sliced
½ cup green beans
Directions:
Add potatoes, salt, garlic powder, onion powder, and Italian seasoning to Instant Pot. Sprinkle seasonings over top for getting even coating. Add water and using a spoon mix the potatoes.
Cover with lid. Switch on manual button and set the timer to 10 minutes over high pressure. Set steam release handle to 'sealing'.
Once done, allow pressure to release naturally for 10 minutes. Use steam release handle to release any remaining steam. Using an immersion blender, blend potatoes until desired consistency is achieved.
Serve it topped with some corn, green onions and green beans.

178. Easy Green Peas
Preparation Time: 45 MIN
Servings: 4
Ingredients:
1 lb green peas, rinsed and drained
1 medium-sized tomato, roughly chopped
1 medium-sized onion, peeled and sliced
2 large carrots, peeled and sliced
2 small potatoes, peeled and chopped
1 celery stalk
A handful of parsley, finely chopped
2 garlic cloves, crushed
2 bay leaves
4 tbsp of fresh tomato sauce
Olive oil
Directions:
Grease the stainless steel insert of your instant pot with some oil. Press "Sautee" button and add onion and garlic. Stir-fry for several minutes and add the sliced carrot, fresh tomato paste, and finely chopped celery.
Cook for 10 minutes, stirring constantly.
Add the remaining ingredients and pour in 4 cups of water. Securely lock the lid and press "Manual" button. Adjust the steam release handle and set the timer for 35 minutes. Cook on low pressure.
When done, press "Cancel" button and release the steam naturally.
Serve warm.

179. Quick Mushrooms
Preparation Time: 45 MIN
Servings: 4
Ingredients:
8 minced garlic cloves
1 teaspoon garlic powder
2 tablespoons olive oil
1 tablespoon cumin
3 tablespoons chili powder
2 cups sliced mushrooms
1 pound cubed potatoes
1 chopped medium zucchini
1 minced medium onion
2 cups tomato sauce
½ cup pureed carrots
2 cups vegetable broth
Directions:
Plug in your instant pot and press "Sautee" button. Heat up the oil in the stainless steel insert and add carrots, cumin, chili powder, tomato sauce, and garlic. Stir properly to mix the ingredients in.
Add mushrooms and zucchini. Stir-fry for 5 minutes and then add all remaining ingredients.
Securely lock the lid and adjust the steam release handle. Press "Manual " button and set the timer for 7 minutes. Cook on high pressure.
When done, press "Cancel" button and turn off the pot. Perform a quick release of the pressure.
Open the pot and serve immediately.

180. Perfect Stuffing
Preparation Time: 25 MIN
Servings: 8
Ingredients:
1 loaf Italian bread, cut into ½-inch dice (about 10 cups
1½ cups vegetable broth, or as needed
¼ cup minced fresh flat-leaf parsley
1 large yellow onion, minced
2 celery ribs, minced
2 teaspoons olive oil (optional
1½ teaspoons dried thyme
1 teaspoon dried marjoram
1 teaspoon ground sage
1 teaspoon salt
½ teaspoon freshly ground black pepper
Directions:
Warm the oil in your instant pot with the lid off.
Add the onion and celery and soften for 5 minutes.
Add the thyme, marjoram, and sage.
Add the bread cubes, onion mix, parsley, salt, and pepper.
Add broth, a little at a time, to soak into the bread. Seal and cook on low for 20 minutes.
Depressurize naturally and either roll into balls to refrigerate or freeze, or use immediately.

181. Instant Pot Refried Beans
Preparation Time: 1 HR 15 MIN
Servings: 6
Ingredients:
1 1/2 cups of dry pinto beans
1 tbsp of cumin
1 tbsp of chili powder
1 tsp of salt
3/4 cups (180mLof salsa
4 oz (80mLof jalapeños, diced
For garnishing (optional
Corn tortillas, sliced and baked with salt and lime juice on top

Directions:
Rinse beans and then place in instant pot. Cover them with enough water (about 2 inches (5cm of water covering the top of beans.
Switch on manual button for 45 minutes over high pressure. Set steam release handle to 'sealing'. After the timer goes off, hit 'Cancel' button and allow pressure to release naturally for 10 minutes.
Drain cooked beans and transfer them to a bowl. Add cumin, chili powder and salt.
Using a potato masher or immersion blender, mash the beans to desired consistency.
Add in diced jalapeños and salsa to beans, stir with a spoon and serve.

182. Autumn Stuffed Squash
Preparation Time: 40 MIN
Servings: 6
Ingredients:
1 large buttercup squash
4 cups cubed bread, dried
1 large Granny Smith apple, peeled, cored, and chopped
1 cup coarsely chopped cooked chestnuts
1 cup vegetable broth, or as needed
1 large yellow onion, minced
1 celery rib, minced
3 tablespoons minced fresh flat-leaf parsley
2 teaspoons olive oil (optional
1 teaspoon salt
1 teaspoon ground sage
½ teaspoon dried thyme
¼ teaspoon freshly ground black pepper
Directions:
Chop the top off your squash so it will fit in your instant pot and scoop out the seeds. Chop the bottom so it sits nicely.
Heat the oil in your instant pot with the lid off.
Add the onion and celery and soften for 5 minutes.
Stir in the sage and thyme, then remove and put in a bowl.
Add the bread, apple, chestnuts, parsley, salt and pepper.
Mix well and add enough water to soak into the bread.
Pack the stuffing into your squash and put the squash in the instant pot.
Pour hot water in so it comes up an inch of the way up your squash.
Seal and cook on Meat for 35 minutes.
Release the pressure quickly and serve.

183. Sweet and Sour Cabbage Rolls.
Preparation Time: MIN
Servings: 6
Ingredients:
1 large head green cabbage, cored
2½ cups cooked brown rice or barley
1 medium-size yellow onion, minced
8 ounces steamed tempeh, finely chopped
1 (14.5-ouncecan crushed tomatoes
⅓ cup dark brown sugar
¼ cup cider vinegar
¼ cup golden raisins
2 tablespoons minced fresh flat-leaf parsley leaves
2 teaspoons freshly squeezed lemon juice
2 teaspoons olive oil (optional
1 teaspoon natural sugar
½ teaspoon ground coriander
½ teaspoon dried thyme
¼ teaspoon ground allspice
¼ teaspoon ground cinnamon
Salt and freshly ground black pepper
Directions:
Steam the cabbage in your instant pot for 3 minutes to soften, then set aside to cool.
Remove the water and warm some oil in your instant pot, with the lid open.
When the oil is hot, soften the onion for 5 minutes.
Add the tempeh, coriander, allspice, thyme, cinnamon, sugar, salt, and pepper and mix well.
Remove from the heat and add rice, raisins, parsley, and lemon.
Lay out each cabbage leaf and make mini burritos out of them using the rice mix.
Place your cabbage rolls back in the instant pot.
In a bowl combine tomatoes, brown sugar, and vinegar. Pour over the cabbage rolls.
Seal and cook on Stew for 10 minutes.
Depressurize quickly and serve.

184. Collard Rolls.
Preparation Time: 40 MIN
Servings: 6
Ingredients:
1 large bunch collard greens, stems removed (about 8 large leaves
1½ cups cooked brown rice
1½ cups cooked black-eyed peas or 1 (15-ouncecan black-eyed peas, rinsed and drained
1 cup vegetable broth
1 large yellow onion, minced
3 garlic cloves, minced
1 chipotle chile in adobo, minced
2 teaspoons olive oil
1 teaspoon dried thyme
1 teaspoon liquid smoke
Salt and freshly ground black pepper
Vegan sour cream, purchased or homemade, for serving
Tabasco sauce, for serving
Directions:
Steam the collard leaves in your instant pot for 3 minutes to soften. Set aside to cool. Clean your instant pot.
Put some oil in the base of your instant pot. Add the onion and soften 5 minutes.
Add the garlic, chile, and thyme and cook another minute.
Mix the onions in a bowl with rice, black-eyed peas, liquid smoke, salt, and pepper.
Make small burritos using the collard leaves and the stuffing.
Arrange in your instant pot and pour the broth over them.
Seal and cook on Stew 10 minutes.
Depressurize quickly and serve.

185. St Patrick's Cabbage Rolls
Preparation Time: 50 MIN
Servings: 6
Ingredients:
1 large head green cabbage, cored
1 medium-size yellow onion, minced
1 small carrot, peeled and grated
3 large Yukon Gold potatoes; 1 peeled and grated, 2 peeled and cut into ½-inch dice
8 ounces seitan (purchased or homemade, chopped
1 cup vegetable broth
¼ cup cider vinegar
3 tablespoons brown mustard
2 tablespoons light brown sugar
2 teaspoons olive oil
1½ teaspoons pickling spices
1 teaspoon ground coriander
¼ teaspoon ground allspice
Salt and freshly ground black pepper
Directions:
Steam the cabbage in your instant pot for 3 minutes. Clean the pot.
Warm the oil in your instant pot with the lid open.
Add the onion and carrot and soften for 5 minutes.
Stir in the grated potato and seitan and cook another 2 minutes.
Remove from the heat and mix in coriander, salt, pepper, allspice, 1 teaspoon of vinegar and 1 of mustard.
In a bowl or cup combine the remaining mustard and vinegar with the brown sugar and the pickling spices. Add the vegetable broth and make a smooth sauce.
Make burritos with the cabbage leaves and stuffing.
Put the diced potatoes in the base of your instant pot.
Arrange the cabbage rolls in your instant pot on top of the potatoes.
Seal. Cook for 35 minutes on Stew.

186. Steamed Artichokes
Preparation Time: 45 MIN
Servings: 8
Ingredients:
4 artichokes
3 cups hot water
Juice of 1 lemon
Directions:
Slice the ends and tops of the artichokes, and snip off the tips of the leaves.
Arrange them in the steamer basket of your instant pot.
Pour the water into the instant pot and lower the basket.
Cook on Steam for 45 minutes.

187. Sprouts and Chestnuts
Preparation Time: 30 MIN
Servings: 8
Ingredients:
1½ pounds Brussels sprouts, trimmed and halved lengthwise, if large
1 cup roasted shelled chestnuts
3 shallots, thinly sliced lengthwise
3 slices vegan bacon, sautéed and chopped
3 tablespoons vegetable broth
2 tablespoons pure maple syrup
1 tablespoon cider vinegar
2 teaspoons olive oil
Salt and freshly ground black pepper
Directions:
Warm 1tsp of the oil in your instant pot with the lid open.
Add the shallots and soften 3 minutes.
Add more oil and put all your ingredients except the chestnuts in.
Seal the instant pot and cook for 15 minutes on Stew. Depressurize quickly, add the chestnuts, seal, and cook another 5 minutes on Stew.
Depressurize naturally. Serve.

188. Sweet and Sour Cabbage
Preparation Time: 45 MIN
Servings: 6
Ingredients:
1 (2-poundhead green cabbage, cored and shredded
1 yellow onion, minced
¼ cup water
3 tablespoons cider vinegar
3 tablespoons light brown sugar or granulated natural sugar
2 tablespoons unbleached all-purpose flour
2 teaspoons olive oil
½ teaspoon caraway seeds
Salt and freshly ground black pepper
Directions:
Warm the oil in your instant pot.
Soften the onion in the oil for 5 minutes.
Add the caraway seeds and flour and cook another minute.
Add the water slowly, stirring to make a smooth sauce.
Add the vinegar and sugar and mix well.
Add the cabbage and stir until coated.
Seal and cook on Stew for 35 minutes.
Depressurize naturally.

189. Mediterranean Cauliflower
Preparation Time: 20 MIN
Servings: 6
Ingredients:
1 large head cauliflower, trimmed, cored, and cut into small florets
1 medium-size yellow onion, minced
3 garlic cloves, minced
1 (14.5-ouncecan diced tomatoes, drained
⅓ cup golden raisins
⅓ cup white wine or vegetable broth
3 tablespoons toasted pine nuts, for garnish
2 tablespoons minced fresh flat-leaf parsley or basil, for garnish
1 tablespoon capers
2 teaspoons olive oil
Salt and freshly ground black pepper
Directions:
Warm the oil in the base of your instant pot with the lid off.
Soften the onion in it for 5 minutes.
Add the garlic and cook another minute.

Add the cauliflower, tomatoes, raisins, wine, capers, salt and pepper.
Seal and cook on Meat for 12 minutes.
Depressurize naturally.

190. Gobi Manchurian
Preparation Time: 30 MIN
Servings: 6
Ingredients:
1 head cauliflower, trimmed, cored, and cut into small florets
½ cup ketchup
½ cup vegetable broth
¼ cup minced scallions, for garnish
¼ cup minced fresh cilantro, for garnish
1 small yellow onion, chopped
4 garlic cloves, minced
3 tablespoons crushed dry-roasted peanuts
2 tablespoons soy sauce
1 tablespoon tapioca starch or cornstarch
2 teaspoons rice vinegar
2 teaspoons vegetable oil
1 teaspoon grated fresh ginger
1 teaspoon ground coriander
½ teaspoon cayenne pepper
¼ teaspoon red pepper flakes
Salt
Directions:
Warm the oil in your instant pot.
Add the onion and soften for 5 minutes.
Add the garlic and ginger and cook another minute.
Add the coriander and a pinch of the cayenne and coat the vegetables.
Mix the remaining cayenne, the ketchup, the tapioca, the soy sauce, 1 teaspoon of the vinegar, the red pepper flakes and the broth in a bowl.
Add the onions to the ketchup.
Put your cauliflower in your instant pot and pour the sauce back over it.
Seal and cook on Steam for 20 minutes.

191. Zucchini Puttanesca
Preparation Time: 30 MIN
Servings: 4
Ingredients:
2 large or 4 small zucchini
1½ cups cooked orzo
1 cup marinara sauce
⅓ cup pitted green olives, chopped
⅓ cup pitted kalamata olives, chopped
6 garlic cloves, minced
3 ripe plum tomatoes, chopped
2 tablespoons capers
2 tablespoons minced fresh flat-leaf parsley leaves
2 tablespoons minced fresh basil leaves
2 teaspoons olive oil (optional
½ teaspoon red pepper flakes
Salt and freshly ground black pepper
Directions:
Slice the zucchini lengthwise and hollow out the flesh, leaving a ¼ inch of skin.
Chop up the scooped zucchini.
Warm the oil in your instant pot with the lid off.
Add the garlic and chopped zucchini and cook 5 minutes.
Add the tomatoes, pepper flakes, olives, capers, parsley, orzo, basil, salt, and pepper.
Seal and cook on Pasta for 24 minutes.
Depressurize quickly and serve.

192. Stuffed Artichokes
Preparation Time: 30 MIN
Servings: 4
Ingredients:
4 large artichokes
1 cup chopped mushrooms of your choice
1 cup dry breadcrumbs
¼ cup vegan Parmesan cheese
¼ cup chopped fresh flat-leaf parsley
3 garlic cloves, minced
2 tablespoons nutritional yeast
1 tablespoon olive oil (optional
Juice of 2 lemons
Salt and freshly ground black pepper
Directions:
Warm the oil in your instant pot with the lid off.
Add the garlic and cook a few seconds.
Add the mushrooms and cook for 3 minutes.
Put in a bowl and add the crumbs, nutritional yeast, parmesan, and parsley.
Pour half the lemon juice into a bowl of cold water and set aside.
Remove the stem and some of the top of each artichoke. Remove the tips of the leaves with scissors. Open the artichokes and use a knife to remove the middle leaves. Put them in lemon water before moving to the next one.
When they're all cored, add the stuffing and put them one by one in the steamer basket of your instant pot. Pour the water in the base.
Seal, set to steam, and cook for 20 minutes.

193. Collards and Pot Likker
Preparation Time: 2H 35 MIN
Servings: 8
Ingredients:
1½ pounds collard greens, trimmed of thick stems
1 small yellow onion, chopped
3 large garlic cloves, minced
1 cup vegetable broth
1 tablespoon cider vinegar
1 teaspoon liquid smoke
2 teaspoons olive oil (optional
¼ teaspoon red pepper flakes
Salt and freshly ground black pepper
Directions:
Cut the collards into thin strips.
Warm the oil in the base of your instant pot.
Add the onion and soften for 5 minutes.
Add the garlic and cook another minute.
Add the collards, red pepper flakes, salt and pepper.
Pour in the broth.
Set to Slow Cook for 2 hours and 25 minutes.
Release the pressure quickly and serve.

194. Creamed Corn
Preparation Time: 25 MIN
Servings: 8

Ingredients:
2 pounds fresh or thawed frozen corn kernels
1 (16-ouncecan creamed corn
1 cup plain unsweetened nondairy milk
½ cup vegan cream cheese, at room temperature
1 medium-size yellow onion, minced
1 tablespoon cornstarch or tapioca starch
2 teaspoons vegetable oil or vegan butter
Salt and freshly ground black pepper
Directions:
Warm the oil in your instant pot.
Add the onion and soften for 5 minutes. Turn off the heat.
Add the corn kernels and the creamed corn. Salt and pepper.
In a bowl, whisk together the cream cheese, cornstarch, and milk until smooth.
Pour the cream cheese mix in with the corn and combine.
Seal and cook on Stew for 18 minutes.
You may want to take some of the corn out, blend it, then add it back in for a thicker creamed corn.

195. Golden Ratatouille
Preparation Time: 30 MIN
Servings: 10
Ingredients:
1 large eggplant, peeled and cut into ½-inch dice
4 summer squashes, cut into ½-inch dice
1 yellow bell pepper, seeded and cut into ½-inch dice
6 ripe yellow tomatoes, peeled and diced
1 medium-size yellow onion, chopped
3 garlic cloves, minced
¼ cup chopped fresh basil or flat-leaf parsley
2 teaspoons olive oil
½ teaspoon dried marjoram
½ teaspoon dried basil
Salt and freshly ground black pepper
Directions:
Warm the oil in your instant pot.
Soften the onion for 5 minutes.
Add the garlic, dry basil, and marjoram for a minute.
Add the remaining ingredients except for the fresh basil.
Seal and cook for 25 minutes on Stew.
Depressurize quickly and stir in the fresh basil.

196. Country Green Beans and Tomato
Preparation Time: 35 MIN
Servings: 4
Ingredients:
1 pound green beans, trimmed and cut into 1-inch pieces
4 or 5 ripe plum tomatoes, chopped
4 garlic cloves, minced
2 teaspoons olive oil
2 tablespoons minced fresh basil
Salt and freshly ground black pepper
Directions:
Warm the oil in the instant pot.
Soften the garlic for a minute.
Add the remaining ingredients except for the basil.
Seal the instant pot and cook on Stew for 30 minutes.
Release the pressure fast and sprinkle with basil.

197. Taters And Sweets
Preparation Time: 35 MIN
Servings: 8
Ingredients:
2 to 4 russet or other baking potatoes
2 to 4 medium-size sweet potatoes
1 cup water
Directions:
Rinse your potatoes. Prick the skin with a fork.
Wrap them each individually in foil.
Put in the steamer basket of your instant pot.
Pour the water into your instant pot and lower the steamer basket.
Steam for 30 minutes.
Depressurize naturally and serve with vegetable spread.

198. Garlicky Mash
Preparation Time: 25 MIN
Servings: 6
Ingredients:
2 pounds Yukon Gold or russet potatoes, peeled and cut into 1-inch chunks
2 cups water or vegetable broth
½ cup vegan sour cream, purchased or homemade
¼ cup plain unsweetened nondairy milk, heated
3 garlic cloves, crushed
2 tablespoons vegan butter, plus more if needed
2 tablespoons minced fresh chives or 1 tablespoon dried chives
Salt and freshly ground black pepper
Directions:
Put the garlic and potatoes in your instant pot. Cover with water and a little salt and pepper.
Seal and cook for 20 minutes.
Depressurize quickly and drain.
Mash the potatoes with the remaining ingredients.

199. Granny Smith Sweet Potatoes
Preparation Time: 45 MIN
Servings: 4
Ingredients:
3 large sweet potatoes (about 2 pounds, peeled and thinly sliced
2 or 3 large Granny Smith apples, peeled, cored, and sliced
¼ to ⅓ cup packed light brown sugar
1 tablespoon vegan butter
1 tablespoon freshly squeezed lemon juice
¼ teaspoon ground cinnamon
¼ teaspoon salt
Directions:
In a bowl combine the sugar, cinnamon and salt.
Oil the inside of your instant pot.
Layer the sweet potatoes and apples alternately, sprinkling the sugar between each layer.
Top with butter and lemon.
Seal and cook on Stew for 35 minutes.

200. Scalloped Potatoes
Preparation Time: 45 MIN
Servings: 6
Ingredients:

2 pounds russet potatoes, peeled and cut into ⅛-inch-thick slices
1 cup vegetable broth, or as needed
1 cup vegan cream cheese
1 cup plain unsweetened nondairy milk
1 small onion, minced
3 garlic cloves, minced
2 teaspoons vegan butter or olive oil
2 tablespoons cornstarch or potato starch
1 teaspoon Dijon mustard
½ teaspoon dried thyme
Salt and freshly ground black pepper
Directions:
Melt the butter in your instant pot.
Add the onion and soften for 5 minutes.
Add the garlic and thyme and cook another minute.
Put in a blender and blend with the cream cheese, cornstarch, milk, mustard, salt, and pepper.
Add broth as you blend to make the sauce smooth.
Layer the potatoes with a drizzle of cream sauce between each layer.
Pour the remaining cream sauce over.
Seal and cook for 35 minutes on Stew.
Release the pressure quickly and serve.

201. Tomatoes, Potatoes, and Beans
Preparation Time: 40 MIN
Servings: 4
Ingredients:
1½ pounds Yukon Gold potatoes, peeled and thinly sliced
2 cups cooked butter beans
1½ pounds ripe tomatoes, diced
4 garlic cloves, minced
1 tablespoon tomato paste
1 tablespoon soy sauce
2 teaspoons olive oil
½ teaspoon dried basil
½ teaspoon dried marjoram
¼ teaspoon red pepper flakes
Salt and freshly ground black pepper
2 tablespoons chopped fresh basil or flat-leaf parsley, for garnish
Directions:
Warm the oil in your instant pot.
Add the garlic and soften a minute.
Add the tomato paste, basil, marjoram, red pepper flakes, and soy sauce.
Remove the mix and layer half the potatoes in the base.
Top with half the beans, tomatoes, and garlic mix.
Repeat the layers.
Seal and cook on Stew for 30 minutes.
Release the pressure naturally.
Top with basil and serve.

202. Maple Glazed Root Veg
Preparation Time: 65 MIN
Servings: 4
Ingredients:
4 large carrots, peeled and cut into 1-inch pieces
1 large parsnip, peeled and cut into 1-inch pieces
1 medium-size turnip, peeled and cut into 1-inch pieces
4 shallots, halved
3 tablespoons maple syrup
2 tablespoons water
1 tablespoon Dijon mustard
2 teaspoons olive oil
Salt and freshly ground black pepper
Directions:
Oil your instant pot and put the veg in it.
In a bowl, mix the remaining ingredients and pour over the vegetables.
Seal and cook on Stew for 60 minutes.
Release the pressure naturally.

203. Lemon Herb Beets
Preparation Time: 20 MIN
Servings: 4
Ingredients:
1-pound beets, peeled and chopped
1 teaspoon dried rosemary
1 teaspoon dried oregano
1/4 teaspoon thyme
Juice of one lemon
1/2 cup water
1/4 teaspoon salt
Directions:
Spray the instant pot with nonstick spray. Add the beets, water, and seasonings.
Seal the lid and cook on high 4 minutes, then quick release the pressure and remove the lid.
Drizzle with the lemon juice and serve.

204. Rutabagas with Apples and Pears
Preparation Time: 20 MIN
Servings: 8
Ingredients:
3 medium-size rutabagas, peeled and chopped
3 apples, peeled, and chopped
2 pears, peeled, and chopped
1 large onion, chopped
1/2 cup apple cider
Zest of 1/2 lemon
1/4 teaspoon thyme
1/4 teaspoon salt
1/4 teaspoon pepper
Directions:
Add all the ingredients to the instant pot, except the lemon zest.
Seal the lid and cook on high 3 minutes, then let pressure release naturally.
Remove the lid and serve topped with lemon zest.

205. Mashed Cauliflower and Parsnips
Preparation Time: 25 MIN
Servings: 4
Ingredients:
1 large head cauliflower, chopped
4 parsnips, peeled and chopped
1 shallot, minced
2 cloves garlic, minced
1/4 cup nondairy butter
1 cup unsweetened nondairy milk
1/4 teaspoon salt

1/4 teaspoon fresh ground pepper
1/4 cup water
1 tablespoon olive oil
Directions:
Heat the oil in the instant pot on the sauté setting and cook the shallot for 5 minutes. Add the garlic and cook an additional minute.
Add the water, parsnips, and cauliflower to the instant pot. Seal the lid and cook on high 3 minutes, then quick release the pressure.
Remove the lid and check the water levels. If there is too much water, remove some of it. Remember that you want the final product to be creamy, not runny. Add the nondairy butter and half of the milk. Puree with an immersion blender, and add more milk as needed until the mixture resembles the texture of mashed potatoes. Season with salt and pepper and serve.

206. Garlic Potatoes Au Gratin
Preparation Time: 20 MIN
Servings: 6
Ingredients:
1-pound potatoes, peeled and thinly sliced
1/2 cup cashews
1/2 cup nutritional yeast
3 cloves garlic
3/4 cups unsweetened nondairy milk
1/2 teaspoon salt
Pepper, to taste
1/2 cup vegan cheddar cheese
Directions:
Combine the cashews, yeast, milk, garlic, salt and pepper in a food processor and blend until smooth. Spray the instant pot with nonstick spray. Pour a third of the sauce into the instant pot, then layer with potatoes. Repeat the layers until you've used all the sauce and potatoes.
Seal the lid and cook on high 5 minutes. Allow the pressure to release naturally.
Top with cheese. Allow the cheese to melt, then serve.

207. Sesame Ginger Kale
Preparation Time: 10 MIN
Servings: 6
Ingredients:
3/4-pound kale, rinsed and chopped
2 cloves garlic, minced
1 teaspoon grated ginger
1 tablespoon soy sauce
1 teaspoon rice wine vinegar
1 tablespoon sesame oil
3 tablespoons chopped scallions
1
Directions:
Oil the instant pot with the sesame oil, then add the rest of the ingredients.
Seal the lid and cook on high for one minute, then let the pressure release naturally. Remove the lid and serve. Try this recipe with spinach or collard greens!

208. Mashed Sweet Potatoes with Sweet Pecan Topping
Preparation Time: 20 MIN
Servings: 6
Ingredients:
8 large sweet potatoes, peeled and chopped
2 tablespoons nondairy butter
1/2 cup plus 3 tablespoons nondairy milk
1/2 cup pecans, chopped
3 tablespoons olive oil
3/4 cup packed brown sugar
1/4 cup whole wheat flour
1/4 teaspoon nutmeg
1/2 teaspoon cinnamon
1/4 teaspoon ginger
1/8 teaspoon ground cloves
1 1/4 cups water
Directions:
Mix together the nondairy butter, brown sugar, olive oil, flour, and 3 tablespoons nondairy milk in a large bowl to make the topping.
Spray the instant pot with nonstick spray. Pour in the water and the sweet potatoes. Seal the lid and cook on high for 5 minutes before letting the pressure release naturally.
Mash the sweet potatoes together with the spices and half of the nondairy milk. Add more milk if needed, until the right texture is reached. Turn off the heat and spread the topping over the sweet potatoes, followed by the pecans.

209. Herb Roasted Mixed Vegetables
Preparation Time: 15 MIN
Servings: 6
Ingredients:
8 ounces cauliflower, chopped into florets
8 ounces brussels sprouts
4 carrots, peeled and chopped
4 ounces baby mushrooms
2 shallots, diced
1/4 cup water
2 tablespoons vegan chicken-flavored bouillon
2 tablespoons olive oil
2 teaspoons dried thyme
1 clove garlic, minced
1 teaspoon dried rosemary
1 teaspoon rubbed sage
1/2 teaspoon salt
1/2 teaspoon fresh ground pepper
Directions:
Spray instant pot with nonstick spray.
Combine all the ingredients in the instant pot. Seal the lid and cook on high 4 minutes, then let the pressure release naturally.

210. Corn with Creamy Truffle Sauce
Preparation Time: 20 MIN
Servings: 4
Ingredients:
1-pound frozen sweet corn kernels
1 tablespoon truffle oil
1 tablespoon dry white wine
1 shallot, minced
1/2 teaspoon salt
1/2 teaspoon fresh ground pepper
1/2 cup nondairy milk
1 tablespoon cornstarch

1 tablespoon warm water
Directions:
Spray the instant pot with nonstick spray.
Combine the cornstarch and warm water in a small bowl and set aside.
Add the rest of the ingredients to the instant pot. Seal the lid and cook on high 1 minute, then let pressure release naturally and remove the lid.
Switch to the sauté setting and add the cornstarch mixture. Cook an additional 10 minutes, or until the mixture has thickened.

211. Seared Maple Balsamic Brussels Sprouts
Preparation Time: 20 MIN
Servings: 4
Ingredients:
8 ounces brussels sprouts, halved
1 tablespoon balsamic vinegar
2 tablespoons red wine
1/2 teaspoon or maple syrup
1/4 cup water
1/4 teaspoon salt
1/4 teaspoon pepper
1 tablespoon olive oil
Directions:
Heat the oil in the instant pot using the sauté setting. Brown the brussels sprouts for about 5 minutes, until you start seeing some brown on the edges.
Add the rest of the ingredients, seal the lid, and cook on high 4 minutes. Let the pressure release naturally, and serve.

212. Smoky Cajun Green Beans
Preparation Time: 10 MIN
Servings: 4
Ingredients:
1-pound fresh green beans
1 teaspoon Cajun seasoning
1/4 cup water
1 teaspoon liquid smoke
1/4 teaspoon seasoned salt
1/4 teaspoon fresh ground pepper
Pinch of cayenne pepper
Directions:
Spray the instant pot with nonstick spray.
Combine the rest of the ingredients in the instant pot. Seal the lid and cook on high 3 minutes. Let the pressure release naturally and serve.

213. Dill Carrots in White Wine
Preparation Time: 10 MIN
Servings: 4
Ingredients:
1-pound carrots, peeled and quartered
2 tablespoons white wine
2 tablespoons vegan chicken-flavored bouillon
1/4 cup water
Zest of one lemon
1 teaspoon olive oil
2 teaspoons dill
1/4 teaspoon salt
1/4 teaspoon pepper

Directions:
Combine all the ingredients except for the lemon zest in the instant pot.
Seal the lid and cook on high 2 minutes. Let the pressure release naturally, remove the lid, and sprinkle with lemon zest before serving.

214. Sriracha Ginger Eggplant
Preparation Time: 12 MIN
Servings: 4
Ingredients:
1 1/2 pounds eggplant, chopped
1 teaspoon sriracha chili sauce
2 tablespoons fresh grated ginger
4 cloves garlic, minced
1 cup water
1 1/2 tablespoons vegan chicken-flavored bouillon
2 tablespoons hoisin sauce
2 tablespoons soy sauce
2 to 3 tablespoons agave nectar
Sesame oil, for serving
Directions:
Make the sauce by combining all the ingredients except for the eggplant and sesame oil in a bowl.
Oil the instant pot and pour in the sauce, followed by the eggplant pieces. Seal the lid and cook on high for 3 minutes.
Serve drizzled with a bit of sesame oil.

215. Mint Rum Black Beans
Preparation Time: 10 MIN
Servings: 4
Ingredients:
2 15-ounce cans pinto beans
1/4 cup dark rum
1/2 tablespoon vegan chicken-flavored bouillon
1 small onion, diced
1 tablespoon tomato paste
1/2 teaspoon cumin
Juice of 1 lime
Zest of 1 lime
1/4 teaspoon salt
1/4 teaspoon fresh ground peppercorns
1/2 cup water
Chopped fresh mint, for serving
Directions:
Combine all the ingredients except the mint and lime zest in the instant pot, seal the lid, and cook on high 6 minutes.
Serve topped with mint and lime zest.

216. Basic Baked Potatoes
Preparation Time: 8 MIN
Servings: 4
Ingredients:
4 large russet potatoes
Directions:
Poke holes in the potatoes with a fork, then place them in an oiled instant pot.
Seal the lid and cook for 3-4 minutes on high.
Serve as a side dish or top with beans or chili to make a complete meal.

SEAFOOD

217. Keto Lobster Tails in Butter Sauce
Preparation Time: 15 Minutes
Servings: 4
Ingredients:
1 lb fresh lobster tails; cleaned
5 tbsp butter; unsalted
1/4 cup fish stock
1 cup water
1 tbsp apple cider vinegar
1/2 cup mayonnaise
1/4 tsp dried rosemary
1/4 tsp garlic powder
1/2 tsp black pepper; freshly ground
1/4 tsp dried thyme
1 tsp salt
Directions:
Place lobster tails in the steam basket and transfer to the pot. Pour in one cup of water and seal the lid. Set the steam release handle to the *Sealing* position and press the *Steam* button. Cook for 5 minutes on high pressure
When done; preform a quick pressure release and open the lid. Remove the lobster tails from the pot and press the *Sauté* button
Pour in the stock and bring it to a boil. Stir in butter and mayonnaise and sprinkle with apple cider. Season with salt, pepper, thyme, rosemary, and garlic powder. Cook for 2 - 3 minutes.
Press the *Cancel'* button and remove the sauce from the pot. Drizzle over steamed lobster tails and serve immediately. Optionally, sprinkle with fresh dill.
Nutrition Values: Calories: 347; Total Fats: 25.3g; Net Carbs: 7.1g; Protein: 22.3g; Fiber: 0g

218. Delicious Mussels with Thyme
Preparation Time: 20 Minutes
Servings: 4
Ingredients:
1 lb mussels; cleaned
2 tbsp lemon juice; freshly squeezed
3 tbsp butter
1/4 cup Parmesan cheese; grated
2 cups fish stock
5 garlic cloves; crushed
1/2 tsp chili flakes
2 tbsp fresh parsley; finely chopped.
1 tsp dried thyme
Directions:
Rinse well the mussels under running water and remove any dirt. Drain and set aside
Plug in the instant pot and press the *Sauté* button. Grease the inner pot with butter and add garlic. Sauté for 2 - 3 minutes and then pour in the stock. Drizzle with lemon juice and season with thyme, chili flakes, and parsley
Place mussels in a steam basket and transfer to the pot. Seal the lid and set the steam release handle to the *Sealing* position
Press the *Manual* button and set the timer for 5 minutes on high pressure
When done; perform a quick release and open the lid. Remove any mussels that didn't open and transfer to serving bowls. Drizzle with the sauce from the pot and serve immediately
Nutrition Values: Calories: 207; Total Fats17.1g; Net Carbs: 5.6g; Protein: 17.1g; Fiber: 0.1g

219. Keto Tuna Steak with Mushrooms
Preparation Time: 50 Minutes
Servings: 4
Ingredients:
2 large tuna steaks; about 8 oz each
1/4 cup Parmesan cheese
4 tbsp butter
2 tbsp olive oil
2 cups mushrooms
2 cups fish stock
1 large onion; finely chopped.
1/2 cup heavy cream
1 tsp white pepper; freshly ground
1 tsp dried marjoram
1 tsp sea salt
Directions:
Plug in the instant pot and press the *Sauté* button. Grease the inner pot with butter and heat up.
Add onions and stir-fry for 3 - 4 minutes, or until translucent. Now; add tuna steaks and continue to cook for 2 - 3 minutes on each side
Pour in the stock and season with salt. Seal the lid and set the steam release handle to the *Sealing* position. Press the *Manual* button and set the timer for 5 minutes
When done; perform a quick pressure release and open the lid. Remove the steaks and place them to a bowl. Cover and set aside
Now; press the *Sauté* button and simmer the stock until the liquid has reduced in half. Add mushrooms and cook for 7 - 8 minutes, stirring occasionally
Season with salt, pepper, and marjoram and stir in the heavy cream and Parmesan cheese
Give it a good stir and add tuna steaks. Drizzle with olive oil. Press the *Cancel'* button to turn off the pot and serve immediately
Nutrition Values: Calories: 470; Total Fats: 32.6g; Net Carbs: 3.9g; Protein: 39.1g; Fiber: 1.2g

220. Tasty Cod Chowder with Bacon
Preparation Time: 25 Minutes
Servings: 5
Ingredients:
1 lb cod fillets
2 cups cauliflower; cut into florets
3 cups fish stock
3 tbsp butter
1/4 cup heavy cream
5 bacon slices; chopped.
1 cup button mushrooms; sliced
1/4 cup fish sauce
1/2 cup onions; finely chopped.
1 cup full-fat milk
1 tsp dried basil
1/2 tsp black pepper; freshly ground

1 tsp salt
Directions:
Plug in the instant pot and press the *Sauté* button. Grease the inner pot with butter and heat up. Add onions and mushrooms and stir well. Cook for 5 minutes, stirring occasionally
Now add the fish stock and cauliflower. Add cod fillets and season with salt, pepper, and basil. Add bacon and stir well again
Seal the lid and set the steam release handle to the *Sealing* position. Press the *Manual* button and set the timer for 8 minutes on high pressure
When done; perform a quick pressure release and carefully open the lid
Stir in the milk and heavy cream. Drizzle with the fish sauce and chill for a while. Serve with some freshly chopped parsley
Nutrition Values: Calories: 333; Total Fats: 20.7g; Net Carbs: 5.6g; Protein: 30.1g; Fiber: 1.4g

221. Onion Prawn Stew
Preparation Time: 45 Minutes
Servings: 6
Ingredients:
7oz chicken breast; chopped into bite-sized pieces
20 king prawn tails; peeled
1/2 cup olive oil
1 cup cherry tomatoes; chopped.
1 spring onion; chopped.
3 tbsp fresh parsley; chopped.
5 cups fish stock
1 cup onions; chopped.
1 small green bell pepper; finely chopped.
2 celery stalks; chopped.
3 garlic cloves; crushed
1 tsp stevia powder
1 tsp chili powder
1/2 tsp black pepper; freshly ground
2 tsp cayenne pepper; ground
1 tbsp dried celery
1 tsp white pepper; freshly ground
1 tsp sea salt
Directions:
Rinse well and clean prawns. Place in a deep bowl and season with salt and pepper, Set aside
Rinse the meat and pat-dry with some kitchen paper. Place on a large cutting board and cut into bite-sized pieces. Season with the remaining salt and pepper and set aside
Plug in the instant pot and grease the inner pot with some oil. Add onions, spring onions, celery stalk, and green pepper. Stir well and cook for 5 - 6 minutes, stirring constantly
Now add the meat and prawns. Give it a good stir and season with the remaining spices
Continue to cook for another 5 - 6 minutes. Pour in the fish stock and the remaining olive oil. Press the *Cancel'* button
Seal the lid and set the steam release handle to the *Sealing* position. Press the *Manual* button and set the timer for 20 minutes on high pressure
When done; perform a quick pressure release and open the lid. Stir in garlic and parsley. Let it sit for 5 minutes and serve

Nutrition Values: Calories: 418; Total Fats: 21.9g; Net Carbs: 6.4g; Protein: 46.8g; Fiber: 1.3g

222. Keto Fish Stew
Preparation Time: 25 Minutes
Servings: 4
Ingredients:
7 oz trout fillets; chopped into bite-sized pieces
3 garlic cloves; crushed
7 oz cod fillets; chopped into bite-sized pieces
2 cups shrimps; cleaned and deveined
2 cups fish stock
3 tbsp extra virgin olive oil
1 ½ cups tomatoes; chopped.
2 spring onions; finely chopped.
1 small green bell pepper; chopped.
1/2 tsp black pepper; freshly ground
2 bay leaves
1 tsp sea salt
Directions:
Plug in the instant pot and press the *Sauté* button. Grease the inner pot with olive oil and add onions, chopped pepper, garlic, and bay leaves. Stir well and cook for 5 minutes
Now add chopped fish fillets and shrimps. Give it a good stir and continue to cook for another 5 minutes. Pour in about 1/4 cup of the fish stock and add tomatoes. Bring it to a boil and simmer until softened
Season with salt and pepper. Optionally, add some dried herbs to taste. Stir well and seal the lid
Set the steam release handle to the *Sealing* position. Press the *Manual* button and set the timer for 10 minutes on high pressure
When done; press the *Cancel'* button and release the pressure naturally. Carefully, open the lid and serve immediately
Nutrition Values: Calories: 403; Total Fats: 22g; Net Carbs: 5.3g; Protein: 43.7g; Fiber: 1.5g

223. Keto Salmon Macaroni
Preparation Time: 20 Minutes
Servings: 4
Ingredients:
8oz salmon steak; thinly sliced
1 cup fresh celery; finely chopped.
3 tbsp almond flour
3 tbsp butter
2 cups cauliflower; chopped.
1 onion; finely chopped.
1 cup heavy cream
1 cup cottage cheese
3 cups chicken stock
1/2 tsp black pepper; freshly ground
2 tsp salt
Directions:
Rinse well the steaks and pat-dry with a kitchen towel. Place on a large cutting board and cut into bite-sized pieces
Plug in the instant pot and pour in the chicken stock. Add cauliflower and sprinkle with salt and pepper. Make a layer of thinly sliced salmon and seal the lid. Set the steam release handle to the *sealing* position and press the *Manual* button. Set the timer for 5 minutes on high pressure

When done; perform a quick release and open the pot. Remove the salmon and cauliflower and set aside
Press the *Sauté* button and grease the inner pot with butter. Add onions and cook for 2 - 3 minutes. Now add cottage cheese and heavy cream. Stir in celery and almond flour
Briefly cook, for 3 - 4 minutes, stirring constantly. Remove from the pot and serve with salmon macaroni.
Nutrition Values: Calories: 351; Total Fats: 25.7g; Net Carbs: 7.4g; Protein: 21.8g; Fiber: 2.4g

224. Shrimp Cauliflower Risotto
Preparation Time: 15 Minutes
Servings: 4
Ingredients:
1 lb fresh shrimps; peeled and deveined
3 garlic cloves; crushed
2 cups cauliflower florets
2 tbsp olive oil
4 tbsp butter
1 cup cherry tomatoes; chopped.
1/4 cup tomato puree; sugar-free
¾ cup fish stock
1/2 tsp black pepper
2 tbsp fresh parsley; finely chopped.
2 tsp smoked paprika
1 tsp salt
Directions:
Clean and rinse shrimps. Place in the instant pot and drizzle with olive oil. Press the *Sauté* button and briefly fry for 1 - 2 minutes.
Add cauliflower, garlic, and tomatoes. Stir well and season with smoked paprika, salt, and pepper. Continue to cook for a couple of minutes more
Now pour in the fish stock and add the tomato puree. Seal the lid and set the steam release handle to the *Sealing* position
Press the *Manual* button and set the timer for 6 minutes on high pressure
When done; perform a quick release by moving the pressure valve to the *Venting* position.
Carefully open the lid and stir in the butter. Sprinkle with fresh parsley and serve immediately
Nutrition Values: Calories: 334; Total Fats: 21g; Net Carbs: 6.2g; Protein: 28.7g; Fiber: 21g

225. Easy Creamy Mussel Soup
Preparation Time: 15 Minutes
Servings: 4
Ingredients:
2 cups mussels; defrosted
1/4 cup Parmesan cheese
1 lb cauliflower; chopped into florets
2 tbsp butter; unsalted
1 tbsp soy sauce
1 cup broccoli; chopped.
2 cups fish stock
1 cup heavy cream
1/2 tsp fresh pepper; ground
2 bay leaves
Directions:
Place mussels in a large sieve and rinse thoroughly under cold running water. Drain and place in a deep bowl. Season with pepper and set aside
Plug in the instant pot and press the *Sauté* button. Add cauliflower and broccoli. Stir well and cook for 5 minutes
Now add mussels and pour in the fish stock. Drizzle with soy sauce and add bay leaves
Seal the lid and set the steam release handle to the *Sealing* position. Press the *Manual* button and set the timer for 5 minutes on high pressure
When done; perform a quick release and open the lid. Remove the bay leaves and stir in the heavy cream and Parmesan. Chill for a while before serving
Nutrition Values: Calories: 283; Total Fats: 20g; Net Carbs: 8g; Protein: 15.9g; Fiber: 3.5g

226. Keto Chili Lime Salmon
Preparation Time: 15 Minutes
Servings: 1
Ingredients:
7 oz salmon fillets
1 tbsp swerve
1 jalapeno pepper; chopped.
1 tbsp olive oil
1 cup fish stock
1 tbsp freshly squeezed lime juice
2 garlic cloves; crushed
1/4 tsp cumin powder
1/2 tsp smoked paprika
1 tbsp fresh parsley; finely chopped.
1 tsp sea salt
1/2 tsp black pepper
Directions:
Rinse the fillets under cold running water and rub with salt and pepper. Place in the steam basket and pour in one cup of water
Seal the lid and set the steam release handle to the *Sealing* position. Press the *Steam* button and set the timer for 4 minutes on high pressure
When done; perform a quick release and open the lid
Meanwhile; in a small bowl, combine olive oil, swerve, garlic, lime juice, cumin powder, paprika, and parsley
Press the *Sauté* button and pour the mixture in the pot. Heat up and add chopped pepper. Stir in the salmon and cook for 2 minutes.
Press the *Cancel'* button to turn off the pot. To enjoy Serve it immediately
Nutrition Values: Calories: 399; Total Fats: 26.5g; Net Carbs: 2.5g; Protein: 39.2g; Fiber: 0.6g

227. Spicy Keto Shrimp Pasta
Preparation Time: 15 Minutes
Servings: 4
Ingredients:
7 oz shrimps; cleaned
3 cups chicken stock
1 tsp apple cider vinegar
2 cups cauliflower; chopped into florets
2 garlic cloves; crushed
2 tbsp olive oil
1 cup cream cheese
1/4 cup mayonnaise
1/2 tsp red pepper flakes

1/2 tsp onion powder
1 tsp smoked salt
Directions:
Place shrimps and cauliflower in the pot. Add garlic and pour in the stock. Sprinkle with olive oil and apple cider and stir well
Seal the lid and set the steam release handle to the *Sealing* position. Press the *Manual* button and cook for 9 minutes on high pressure
When done; perform a quick release and open the lid. Remove the shrimp mixture and drain the remaining liquid in the pot. Transfer to a deep bowl and set aside
Now press the *Sauté* button and heat up the inner pot. add cream cheese and mayonnaise. Season with smoked salt, onion powder, and red pepper flakes. Briefly cook, for about a minute and stir in the shrimp mixture. Mix well and press the *Cancel'* button.
Serve immediately and optionally sprinkle with some shredded mozzarella or grated parmesan.
Nutrition Values: Calories: 401; Total Fats: 33.5g; Net Carbs: 8.2g; Protein: 17.4g; Fiber: 1.3g

228. Lobster Tomato Stew
Preparation Time: 15 Minutes
Servings: 4
Ingredients:
4 lobster tails; defrosted
2 cups fish stock
2 cups cherry tomatoes; chopped.
2 cups heavy cream
3 tbsp olive oil
2 tbsp butter
1 cup celery; finely chopped.
2 shallots; diced
1 tsp black pepper; freshly ground
1/2 tsp smoked paprika
1 tbsp Old Bay seasoning
1 tsp dill
Directions:
In a large bowl, combine tomatoes, celery, shallots, olive oil, and dill. Mix until well incorporated and set aside
Plug in the instant pot and press the *Sauté* button. Grease the inner pot with butter and add lobster tails. Season with salt, pepper, and Old Bay seasoning. Cook for 3 - 4 minutes on each side
Pour in the tomato mixture, fish stock, and sprinkle with smoked paprika
Give it a good stir and seal the lid. Set the steam release handle and press the *Manual* button. Set the timer for 5 minutes on high pressure
When done; press the *Cancel'* button and release the pressure naturally. Carefully open the lid and stir in the heavy cream. Chill for a while and serve
Nutrition Values: Calories: 468; Total Fats: 40.3g; Net Carbs: 5.3g; Protein: 21.2g; Fiber: 1.5g

229. Teriyaki Shrimps
Preparation Time: 20 Minutes
Servings: 2
Ingredients:
2 cups shrimps, peeled and deveined
2 tbsp avocado oil
1 cup fish stock
1/4 cup soy sauce
1 tbsp rice vinegar
2 tsp stevia powder
1 tsp sea salt
1 tbsp fresh ginger, grated
1 tsp garlic powder
Directions:
Plug in the instant pot and add shrimps. Pour in the fish stock and stir well. Seal the lid and set the steam release handle to the *Sealing* position. Press the *Manual* button and set the timer for 4 minutes on high pressure
When done; perform a quick release and open the lid. Press the *Sauté* button and bring the stock to a boil. Stir in the soy sauce, avocado oil, and rice vinegar
Sprinkle with salt, stevia, garlic, and ginger. Continue to cook for 10 minutes. To enjoy Serve it immediately
Nutrition Values: Calories: 262; Total Fats: 5.6g; Net Carbs: 4.9g; Protein: 43.5g; Fiber: 0.9g

230. Tilapia Curry Recipe
Preparation Time: 15 Minutes
Servings: 4
Ingredients:
10 oz tilapia fillets; chopped.
3 garlic cloves; crushed
2 cups coconut milk; full-fat
1 small onion; finely chopped.
3 tbsp olive oil
1 tsp lemon juice
1/2 cup Thai basil; chopped.
1/2 cup cherry tomatoes; chopped.
1 small chili pepper; chopped.
2 tsp chili powder
1 tsp cumin powder
1/2 tsp turmeric powder
2 tsp fresh ginger; grated
1 tsp coriander powder
1 tsp sea salt
Directions:
Plug in the instant pot and grease the inner pot with oil. Press the *Sauté* button and add onions, garlic, ginger, coriander, chili, cumin powder, turmeric, and salt. Give it a good stir and cook for 3 - 4 minutes or until translucent
Now; pour in the coconut milk and give it a good stir. Add cherry tomatoes, tilapia fillets, and chopped chili pepper
Seal the lid and set the steam release handle to the *Sealing* position. Press the *Manual* button and set the timer for 4 minutes on high pressure
When you hear the end signal, perform a quick pressure release and open the pot. Sprinkle with Thai basil and serve immediately
Nutrition Values: Calories: 440; Total Fats: 39.9g; Net Carbs: 6.7g; Protein: 16.6g; Fiber: 3.4g

231. Spicy and Sweet Trout
Preparation Time: 15 Minutes
Servings: 2
Ingredients:
1 lb trout fillet; chopped.

2 chili peppers; finely chopped.
1/4 cup fish stock
3 tbsp butter
2 tbsp swerve
1 tbsp fish sauce
3 garlic cloves; crushed
1 tbsp ginger; freshly grated
1/2 tsp cumin powder
1 tsp salt
1 tsp black pepper; freshly ground
Directions:
Generously rub fillets with salt and pepper. Place on a large plate and cover with aluminum foil, Set aside
In a small bowl, whisk together fish stock, swerve, and fish sauce. Add grated ginger and cumin powder and stir well again
Plug in the instant pot and set the steam basket. Place the fish fillets in the basket and generously brush with the previously prepared mixture on all sides
Pour in one cup of water and seal the lid. Set the steam release handle to the *Sealing* position and press the *Manual* button. Set the timer for 5 minutes on high heat
When done; perform a quick release and carefully open the lid. Remove the fish and set aside
Melt the butter over medium heat and drizzle over fish. To enjoy Serve it immediately
Nutrition Values: Calories: 600; Total Fats: 36.8g; Net Carbs: 2g; Protein: 62g; Fiber: 0.2g

232. Salmon with Vegetables
Preparation Time: 45 Minutes
Servings: 4
Ingredients:
4 medium-sized salmon steaks
7 oz broccoli; chopped.
1 garlic clove; crushed
7 oz kale; chopped.
2 tbsp rice vinegar
1 cup chicken stock
2 tbsp soy sauce
2 tbsp sesame oil
2 tsp ginger; freshly grated
1/4 tsp chili powder
1/2 tsp black pepper; freshly ground
1 tsp sea salt
Directions:
Rub steaks with garlic, ginger, and chili powder. Sprinkle with some salt and pepper place in a small baking dish. Loosely cover with the aluminum foil and set aside
Plug in the instant pot and add vegetables. Pour in the chicken stock and season with salt and some pepper. Seal the lid and set the steam release handle
Press the *Manual* button and set the timer for 10 minute
When done; perform a quick release and open the lid. Remove the vegetables and drain. Place in a deep bowl and drizzle with some sesame oil, soy sauce, and rice vinegar, Set aside
Position a trivet in the inner pot and place the baking dish on top. Pour in 2 cups of water and seal the lid

Set the steam release handle again and press the *Manual* button. Set the timer for 8 minutes on high pressure
When done; perform a quick release and open the lid. Remove the steaks from the pot and set aside
Now press the *Sauté* button and add the vegetable mixture. Briefly cook – for 3 - 4 minutes, stirring constantly. Press the *Cancel'* button.
Remove the vegetables from the pot and place on a large serving platter. Top with salmon steaks and optionally season with some more salt or pepper to taste. To enjoy Serve it immediately
Nutrition Values: Calories: 313; Total Fats: 16.4g; Net Carbs: 7.4g; Protein: 32.7g; Fiber: 2.1g

233. Mussels with Asparagus
Preparation Time: 15 Minutes
Servings: 4
Ingredients:
1 lb mussels; cleaned
1 large green bell pepper; finely chopped.
7 oz asparagus; chopped into bite-sized pieces
1 cup sun-dried tomatoes
3 tbsp avocado oil
2 tsp lemon juice; freshly squeezed
4 cups fish stock
1/2 tsp garlic powder
1 ½ tsp smoked paprika
1/2 tsp pepper
1 tsp sea salt
Directions:
Plug in the instant pot and press the *Sauté* button. Grease the stainless steel insert with avocado oil and heat up. Optionally, use olive oil
Add asparagus and stir-fry for 2 - 3 minutes. Now add sun dried tomatoes and mussels. Sprinkle with salt, pepper, garlic powder, and smoked paprika
Continue to cook for 4 - 5 minutes
Finally add bell peppers and pour in the stock. Stir well and seal the lid. Set the steam release handle to the *Sealing* position and press the *Manual* button
Set the timer for 5 minutes on high pressure
When done; perform a quick release and open the lid. To enjoy Serve it immediately
Nutrition Values: Calories: 179; Total Fats: 6g; Net Carbs: 8.2g; Protein: 20.7g; Fiber: 2.5g

234. Quick Shrimp Soup
Preparation Time: 40 Minutes
Servings: 5
Ingredients:
2 lbs shrimps; tail-on
4 garlic cloves; minced
1 cup broccoli; cut into florets
3 tbsp olive oil
3 tbsp butter
4 cups fish stock
1 large tomato; roughly chopped.
1/2 cup fresh parsley; finely chopped.
1 tsp dried rosemary
2 tsp sea salt
Directions:
Plug in the instant pot. Heat up the olive oil on the *Sauté* mode and add broccoli. Stir well and cook

until golden brown. Sprinkle with garlic and cook for one more minute
Now add tomatoes and pour in some fish stock – about three tablespoons will be enough. Cook for 7 - 8 minutes, or until most of the liquid evaporates
Now add shrimps and briefly brown. Stir well and season with salt and rosemary
Add the remaining ingredients and give it a good stir. Seal the lid and set the steam release handle and press the *Manual* button
Set the timer for 15 minutes
When done; perform a quick pressure release and open the lid. Optionally, sprinkle with some more herbs or spices and serve immediately
Nutrition Values: Calories: 399; Total Fats: 20.1g; Net Carbs: 5.4g; Protein: 46.8g; Fiber: 1.2g

235. Delicious Pepper Salmon
Preparation Time: 20 Minutes
Servings: 4
Ingredients:
4 salmon fillets; about 1 lb
1 small chili pepper; finely chopped.
1 medium-sized red bell pepper; finely chopped.
3 tbsp butter
1 tbsp olive oil
1 cup fish stock
1/4 zucchini; cubed
2 tsp black pepper; freshly ground
1 tsp dried parsley
1 tsp sea salt
Directions:
Rinse the salmon fillet under cold running water and pat dry with a kitchen paper. Place on a large cutting board and slice in 4 equal pieces, Set aside
In a small bowl, whisk together olive oil, salt, pepper, and dried parsley. Generously brush fillets with this mixture and place in the steam basket
Pour in 2 cups of water in the inner pot and seal the lid. Set the steam release handle to the *Sealing* position and press the *Steam* button. Set the timer for 4 minutes on high pressure
When done; perform a quick release and open the lid. Using oven mitts remove the steam basket and set aside
Now press the *Sauté* button and melt the butter in the inner pot. Add red bell pepper, chili pepper, and zucchini. Stir well and cook for 3 - 4 minutes
Pour in the stock and stir well. Seal the lid and set the steam release handle. Press the *Manual* button and set the timer for 4 minutes on high pressure
When done; release the pressure naturally and open the lid. Add the previously prepared salmon and coat well with the sauce
Optionally, sprinkle with few drops of Tabasco sauce and serve immediately
Nutrition Values: Calories: 364; Total Fats: 23.7g; Net Carbs: 2.2g; Protein: 36.4g; Fiber: 0.6g

236. Keto Green Pesto Tuna Steak
Preparation Time: 40 Minutes
Servings: 4
Ingredients:
2 tuna steaks; about 1-inch thick
1 cup cauliflower; finely chopped.
3 tbsp mozzarella; shredded
1 cup basil leaves; finely chopped.
1/4 cup olive oil
2 garlic cloves
3 tbsp butter
1 tsp sea salt
Directions:
Plug in the instant pot and set the steam basket. Pour in one cup of water and add tuna steaks in the basket. Season with salt and seal the lid. Set the steam release handle to the *Sealing* position and press the *Manual* button. Cook for 7 minutes on high pressure
When done; perform a quick release and open the lid. Using oven mitts, gently remove the steam basket and set aside
Remove the water from the pot and add butter. Press the *Sauté* button and heat up
Briefly cook each tuna steak for 3 - 4 minutes on each side
Remove from the pot and set aside
Now; prepare the pesto. Combine the remaining ingredients in a food processor and process until completely smooth. Coat each tuna steak with pesto and place on a small baking sheet lined with some parchment paper.
Bake for 15 minutes at 400 degrees or until lightly brown and crispy. To enjoy Serve it immediately
Nutrition Values: Calories: 484; Total Fats: 32.9g; Net Carbs: 2g; Protein: 44.3g; Fiber: 0.8g

237. Simple Catfish Stew
Preparation Time: 10 Minutes
Servings: 2
Ingredients:
10 oz catfish fillets; cut into bite-sized pieces
2 cups collard greens; finely chopped [can be replaced with spinach or kale
3 tbsp olive oil
2 cups fish stock
2 cups cherry tomatoes; chopped.
1 tsp garlic powder
1/2 tsp sea salt
1 tsp dried dill
1 tsp Italian seasoning
1/4 tsp chili flakes
Directions:
Combine the ingredients in the instant pot and stir well. Seal the lid and set the steam release handle to the *Sealing* position
Press the *Manual* button and set the timer for 7 minutes on high pressure
When done; release the pressure for about 10 minutes and then move the pressure valve to the *Venting* position
Carefully open the lid and optionally sprinkle with some fresh parsley or grated Parmesan before serving.
Nutrition Values: Calories: 456; Total Fats: 34.3g; Net Carbs: 5.8g; Protein: 29.9g; Fiber: 3.7g

238. Steamed Salmon Recipe
Preparation Time: 15 Minutes

Servings: 4
Ingredients:
1 lb salmon fillets; sliced into 4 pieces
1/4 cup Parmesan cheese; freshly grated
2 lemons; juiced
2 cups fish stock
4 tbsp butter
1 tsp white pepper; freshly ground
1 tsp smoked salt
Directions:
Plug in the instant pot and pour in the stock. Drizzle with lemon juice and set the steam basket
Rinse the salmon fillets and sprinkle with salt and pepper. Place in the basket and seal the lid
Set the steam release handle to the *Sealing* position and press the *Manual* button
Set the timer for 5 minutes.
When done; perform a quick release and open the lid. Remove the salmon fillets and set asideRemove the stock from the pot.
Press the *Sauté* button and melt the butter. Add salmon steaks and cook for 2 - 3 minutes on each side
Sprinkle with grated parmesan and serve immediately
Nutrition Values: Calories: 257; Total Fats: 18.9g; Net Carbs: 0.1g; Protein: 22.7g; Fiber: 0g

239. Tilapia Fillets
Preparation Time: 40 Minutes
Servings: 2
Ingredients:
1 lb tilapia fillets; chopped.
1 spring onion; finely chopped.
1/4 cup celery leaves; finely chopped.
3 tbsp soy sauce
1 tbsp rice vinegar
1 cup fish stock
2 tbsp peanut oil
1 tsp garlic powder
1 tbsp fresh ginger; grated
1 tsp sea salt
Directions:
In a small bowl, whisk together peanut oil, soy sauce, rice vinegar, ginger, garlic powder, and sea salt. Rub the fish with this mixture and place in a large Ziploc bag. Seal the bag and refrigerate for at least 30 minutes
Plug in the instant pot and pour in the stock. Remove the fish from the refrigerator and place in the pot along with the marinade. Sprinkle with celery and seal the lid
Set the steam release handle to the *Sealing* position and press the *Manual* button. Set the timer for 6 minutes on high pressure
Nutrition Values: Calories: 348; Total Fats: 16.5g; Net Carbs: 2.2g; Protein: 46.6g; Fiber: 0.6g

240. Keto Seafood Stew
Preparation Time: 20 Minutes
Servings: 5
Ingredients:
2 lbs sea bass fillets; cut into chunks
1 large onion; finely chopped.
7oz shrimps; peeled and deveined
2 small tomatoes; roughly chopped.
3 tbsp soy sauce
5 cups fish stock
4 tbsp olive oil; extra-virgin
3 celery stalks; finely chopped.
2 bay leaves
1 tsp black pepper; freshly ground
1 tbsp Creole seasoning
2 tsp sea salt
Directions:
Clean and rinse fish fillets. Pat dry with some kitchen paper and set aside
In a small bowl, combine Creole seasoning with salt and pepper. Rub the fish with this mixture making sure to coat on all sides
Plug in the instant pot and press the *Sauté* button. Grease the inner pot with olive oil and heat up. Add the prepared fish and cook for 4 - 5 minutes, stirring occasionally
When the fish has nicely browned, gently remove from the pot and set aside
Grease the inner pot with some more oil and add onions and celery stalk. Season with some salt and stir well. Continue to cook for 2 - 3 minutes
Now press the *Cancel'* button and add the fish, shrimps, and tomatoes. Drizzle with soy sauce and pour in the stock.
Seal the lid and set the steam release handle to the *Sealing* position. Press the *Manual* button and set the timer for 5 minutes on high pressure
When done; release the pressure naturally and open the lid. Optionally, stir in some fresh parsley and serve
Nutrition Values: Calories: 433; Total Fats: 18.5g; Net Carbs: 4.6g; Protein: 58.5g; Fiber: 1.3g

241. Jamaican Jerk Fish
Preparation Time: 35 Minutes
Servings: 4
Ingredients:
2 lbs cod fillets; cut into 1-inch slices
1/4 cup fish stock
2 cups cherry tomatoes; chopped.
2 tbsp butter
2 tbsp swerve
3 tbsp soy sauce
1 tbsp Jamaican Jerk seasoning
2 tsp chili powder
Directions:
Rinse the fillets under cold running water and pat dry with a kitchen paper, Set aside
Plug in the instant pot and grease the inner pot with butter. Add fish fillets and cook for 4 - 5 minutes on each side. You will probably have to do this in several batches
Remove from the pot and transfer to a plate, Set aside
Now add cherry tomatoes and pour in the stock. Bring it to a boil and drizzle with soy sauce. Season with Jamaican Jerk seasoning and chili powder. Add swerve and cook until tomatoes soften
Add fish fillets and coat well with the sauce

Press the *Cancel'* button and remove from the pot. To enjoy Serve it immediately
Nutrition Values: Calories: 507; Total Fats: 25.3g; Net Carbs: 3.2g; Protein: 62.3g; Fiber: 1.2g

242. Adobo Shrimps Recipe
Preparation Time: 50 Minutes
Servings: 4
Ingredients:
1 lb shrimps; peeled and deveined
1/4 cup soy sauce
1/4 cup olive oil
1/4 cup rice vinegar
1 small onion; finely chopped.
1 red chili pepper; finely chopped.
2 cups fish stock
2 tbsp green onions; finely chopped.
5 garlic cloves; crushed
2 tbsp fish sauce
1 tbsp peppercorn
1 tsp stevia powder
2 tsp salt
Directions:
In a large bowl, whisk together olive oil, rice vinegar, soy sauce, green onions, garlic, fish sauce, chopped onion, chili pepper, salt, peppercorn, and stevia
Add shrimps and give it a good stir making sure to coat shrimps well in the marinade. Transfer to a large Ziploc bag and refrigerate for at least 30 minutes [up to 2 hours
Plug in the instant pot and pour in the stock. Remove the shrimps from the Ziploc and place in the pot along with 1/4 cup of the marinade
Stir well and seal the lid. Set the steam release handle to the *Sealing* position and press the *Manual* button.
Set the timer for 10 minutes. When done; perform a quick release and serve immediately
Nutrition Values: Calories: 298; Total Fats: 15.5g; Net Carbs: 5.7g; Protein: 30.4g; Fiber: 0.7g

243. Tasty Trout Casserole
Preparation Time: 40 Minutes
Servings: 4
Ingredients:
1 lb trout fillets; without skin
1 cup cherry tomatoes; halved
1/2 zucchini; sliced
1 cup cauliflower; chopped into florets
1 small onion; sliced
4 tbsp olive oil
1 tsp dried thyme
1/2 tsp garlic powder
2 tsp sea salt
1 tsp dried rosemary
Directions:
Line a small square pan with some parchment paper and sprinkle with two tablespoons of olive oil.
Arrange onions at the bottom of the pan and make a layer with sliced zucchini. Top with cherry tomatoes and onions. Sprinkle with some salt and drizzle with the remaining olive oil
Top with trout fillets and season with some more salt, rosemary, thyme, and garlic powder

Tightly wrap with aluminum foil and set aside
Plug in the instant pot and pour in 2 cups of water.
Set the trivet at the bottom of the inner pot and place the pan on top
Seal the lid and set the steam release handle to the *Sealing* position. Press the *Manual* button and set the timer for 20 minutes on high pressure
When done; perform a quick release and open the lid. Carefully remove the pan and chill for a while
Remove the aluminum foil and optionally, bake for 15 minutes at 450 degrees F. To enjoy Serve it immediately
Nutrition Values: Calories: 361; Total Fats: 23.8g; Net Carbs: 3.7g; Protein: 31.6g; Fiber: 1.8g

244. Surprising Shrimp Delight
Cooking Time:30 minutes
Servings:4
Ingredients:
18 oz. shrimp, peeled and deveined
1/2 tbsp. mustard seeds
3 oz. mustard oil
1 tsp. turmeric powder
2 onions; finely chopped
4 oz. curd, beaten
2 green chilies, cut into halves lengthwise
1-inch ginger; chopped.
Salt to the taste
Already cooked rice for serving
Directions:
Put mustard seeds in a bowl, add water to cover, leave aside for 10 minutes, drain and grind very well
Put shrimp in a bowl, add mustard oil, turmeric, mustard paste, salt, onions, chilies, curd and ginger, toss to coat and leave aside for 10 minutes.
Transfer everything to your instant pot, seal the instant pot lid and cook on Low for 10 minutes.
Quick release the pressure, divide among plates and serve with boiled rice

245. Tuna & Pasta Casserole.
Cooking Time:10 minutes
Servings:2
Ingredients:
1 can cream of mushroom soup
2 ½ cups. macaroni pasta
1/2 tsp. salt
1/2 tsp. pepper
1 cup. cheddar cheese, shredded.
1 cups. frozen peas
2 cans tuna
3 cups. water
Directions:
Mix the soup with the water in the Instant Pot.
Except for the cheese, add the rest of the ingredients. Stir to combine. Lock the lid and turn the steam valve to "Sealing". Press "Manual", set the pressure to "High", and set the timer for 4 minutes.
When the timer beeps, turn the steam valve to "Venting" to quickly release the pressure. Unlock and open the lid.
Sprinkle the cheese on top. Close the lid and let sit for 5 minutes or until the cheese is melted and the sauce is thick

246. Almond Cod.
Cooking Time: 45 minutes
Servings: 4
Ingredients:
8 oz. cod
3 tbsp. almond flakes
1 tsp. minced garlic
3 tbsp. soy sauce
1 tbsp. lime zest
1/4 cup. fish sauce
1/2 cup. almond milk
1 tbsp. butter
Directions:
Choose the roughly and transfer it to the mixing bowl
Add fish sauce and soy sauce. Stir the mixture.
Ager this, sprinkle the fish with the lime zest and minced garlic. Stir it.
Then add almond milk and leave the fish for 10 minutes to marinate.
Then toss the butter in the Instant Pot and melt it.
Then add the almond milk cod in the Instant Pot.
Close the lid and cook the dish at the "Sauté" mode for 10 minutes
When the time is over - open the Instant Pot lid and add almond flakes.
Stir the dish gently and cook it for 3 minutes.
Then remove the dish from the Instant Pot.
Serve it immediately. Enjoy!

247. Mussels and Spicy Sauce
Cooking Time: 15 minutes
Servings: 4
Ingredients:
2 lb. mussels, scrubbed and debearded
1/2 tsp. red pepper flakes
2 tsp. oregano; dried
2 tbsp. extra virgin olive oil
14 oz. tomatoes; chopped.
2 tsp. garlic; minced.
1/2 cup chicken stock
1 yellow onion; chopped.
Directions:
Set your instant pot on Sauté mode; add oil and heat it up.
Add onions, stir and cook for 3 minutes
Add pepper flakes and garlic, stir and cook for 1 minute
Add stock, oregano and tomatoes and stir well.
Add mussels; then stir well. seal the instant pot lid and cook on Low for 2 minutes
Quick release the pressure, discard unopened mussels, divide among bowls and serve

248. Tomato Mussels
Cooking Time: 15 minutes
Servings: 3
Ingredients:
28 oz. canned tomatoes, crushed.
2 lb. mussels, cleaned and scrubbed
1/4 cup extra virgin olive oil
1/4 cup balsamic vinegar
1/2 cup white onion; chopped.
2 jalapeno peppers; chopped.
2 tbsp. red pepper flakes
2 garlic cloves; minced.
1/4 cup dry white wine
1/2 cup basil; chopped.
Lemon wedges for serving
Salt to the taste
Directions:
Set your instant pot on Sauté mode; add tomatoes, onion, jalapenos, wine, oil, vinegar, garlic and pepper flakes, stir and bring to a boil.
Add mussels; then stir well. seal the instant pot lid and cook on Low for 4 minutes.
Quick release the pressure, carefully open the lid; discard unopened mussels, add salt and basil; then stir well. divide among bowls and serve with lemon wedges

249. Cheesy Tuna Dish.
Cooking Time: 15 minutes
Servings: 6
Ingredients:
28 oz. canned cream mushroom soup
3 cups. water
1 can (5 oz.tuna, drained
1 cup. frozen peas
1/4 cup. bread crumbs (optional
16 oz. egg noodles
4 oz. cheddar cheese
Directions:
Put the noodles in the Instant Pot. Pour in the water to cover the noodles.
Add the frozen peas, tuna, and the soup on top of the pasta layer. Cover and lock the lid
Press the "Manual" key, set the pressure to "High", and set the timer for 4 minutes. When the Instant Pot timer beeps, press the "Cancel" key and unplug the Instant Pot. Turn the steam valve to quick release the pressure.
Unlock and carefully open the lid. Stir in the cheese. If desired, you can pour the pasta mixture in a baking dish, sprinkle the top with bread crumbs, and broil for about 2 to 3 minutes. Serve.

250. Poached Salmon Dish
Cooking Time: 15 minutes
Servings: 4
Ingredients:
16 oz. salmon fillet, skin on
Zest from 1 lemon
1/2 cup dry white wine
1 tsp. white wine vinegar
2 cups chicken stock
1/2 tsp. fennel seeds
1 bay leaf
4 scallions; chopped.
3 black peppercorns
1/4 cup dill; chopped
Salt and black pepper to the taste
Directions:
Put salmon in the steamer basket of your instant pot and season with salt and pepper.
Add stock, scallions, lemon zest, peppercorns, fennel, vinegar, bay leaf, wine, stock and dill to your pot.
Cover and cook at High for 5 minutes.

Quick release the pressure, carefully open the lid and divide salmon among plates
Set the pot on Simmer mode and cook the liquid for a few minutes more
Drizzle over salmon and serve

251. Salmon and Veggies Dish
Cooking Time:20 minutes
Servings:2
Ingredients:
2 salmon fillets, skin on
1 bay leaf
2 cups broccoli florets
1 cinnamon stick
3 cloves
1 tbsp. canola oil
1 cup water
1 cup baby carrots
Salt and black pepper to the taste
Lime wedges for serving
Directions:
Pour the water in your instant pot
Add bay leaf, cinnamon stick and cloves.
Place salmon fillets in the steamer basket of your pot after you've brushed them with canola oil
Season with salt and pepper, add broccoli and carrots, seal the instant pot lid and cook at High for 6 minutes
Release the pressure naturally for 4 minutes, then release remaining pressure by turning the valve to 'Venting', and carefully open the lid.
Divide salmon and veggies among plates.
Drizzle the sauce from the pot after you've discarded cinnamon, cloves and bay leaf and serve with lime wedges on the side.

252. Salmon Dish
Cooking Time:25 minutes
Servings:4
Ingredients:
4 salmon fillets
4 thyme springs
3 tomatoes, sliced
1 lemon, sliced
1 white onion; chopped.
2 cups water
3 tbsp. extra virgin olive oil
4 parsley springs
Salt and black pepper to the taste
Directions:
Drizzle the oil on a parchment paper
Add a layer of tomatoes, salt and pepper.
Drizzle some oil again, add fish and season them with salt and pepper
Drizzle some more oil, add thyme and parsley springs, onions, lemon slices, salt and pepper
Fold and wrap packet, place in the steamer basket of your instant pot
Add 2 cups water to the pot, seal the instant pot lid and cook on Low for 15 minutes.
Quick release the pressure, carefully open the lid; open packet, divide fish mix among plates and serve.

253. Crispy Salmon Fillet
Cooking Time:15 minutes
Servings:2
Ingredients:
2 salmon fillets, frozen
2 tbsp. extra virgin olive oil
1 cup water
Salt and black pepper to the taste
Directions:
Pour the water in your instant pot.
Place salmon in the steamer basket, seal the instant pot lid and cook on Low for 3 minutes.
Quick release the pressure, transfer salmon to paper towels and pat dry them.
Heat up a pan with the oil over medium high heat, add salmon fillets skin side down, season with salt and pepper to the taste and cook for 2 minutes.
Divide among plates and serve with your favorite salad on the side

254. Steamed Fish Recipe
Cooking Time:20 minutes
Servings:4
Ingredients:
4 white fish fillets
1 lb. cherry tomatoes, cut into halves
A pinch of thyme; dried
1 garlic clove; minced.
A drizzle of olive oil
1 cup olives, pitted and chopped.
1 cup water
Salt and black pepper to the taste
Directions:
Pour the water in your instant pot.
Put fish fillets in the steamer basket of the pot.
Add tomatoes and olives on top
Also add garlic, thyme, oil, salt and pepper
Cover the pot and cook on Low for 10 minutes.
Quick release the pressure, carefully open the lid; divide fish, olives and tomatoes mix among plates and serve.

255. Spicy Salmon Dish
Cooking Time:15 minutes
Servings:4
Ingredients:
4 salmon fillets
2 tbsp. assorted chili pepper
1 lemon, sliced
1 cup water
Juice of 1 lemon
Salt and black pepper to the taste
Directions:
Place salmon fillets in the steamer basket of your pot, add salt, pepper, lemon juice, lemon slices and chili pepper.
Add 1 cup water to the pot, seal the instant pot lid and cook at High for 5 minutes.
Quick release the pressure, divide salmon and lemon slices among plates and serve

256. Tuna and Noodle
Cooking Time:30 minutes
Servings:4
Ingredients:
8 oz. egg noodles
1/2 cup red onion; chopped.
1 ¼ cups water

8 oz. artichoke hearts, drained and chopped.
1 tbsp. parsley; chopped.
1 tbsp. extra-virgin olive oil
14 oz. canned tomatoes; chopped and mixed with oregano, basil and garlic
14 oz. canned tuna, drained
Salt and black pepper to the taste
Crumbled feta cheese
Directions:
Set your instant pot on Sauté mode; add oil and heat it up
Add onion, stir and cook for 2 minutes
Add tomatoes, noodles, salt, pepper and water, set the pot on Simmer and cook for 10 minutes.
Add tuna and artichokes; then stir well. seal the instant pot lid and cook at High for 5 minutes.
Quick release the pressure, divide tuna and noodles among plates, sprinkle cheese and parsley on top and serve

257. Delicious Shrimp Paella
Cooking Time:15 minutes
Servings:4
Ingredients:
20 shrimps, deveined
1 ½ cups water
4 garlic cloves; minced.
1 cup jasmine rice
1/4 cup butter
1/4 cup parsley; chopped.
A pinch of saffron
A pinch of red pepper, crushed.
Juice of 1 lemon
Melted butter for serving
Salt and black pepper to the taste
Parsley; chopped for serving
Hard cheese, grated for serving
Directions:
Put shrimp in your instant pot.
Add rice, butter, salt, pepper, parsley, red pepper, saffron, lemon juice, water and garlic.
Stir, seal the instant pot lid and cook at High for 5 minutes.
Quick release the pressure, carefully open the lid; takes shrimps and peel them
Return to pot, stir well and divide into bowls
Add melted butter, cheese and parsley on top and serve.

258. Crispy Skin Salmon Fillets.
Cooking Time:20 minutes
Servings:2
Ingredients:
2 salmon fillets, frozen (1-inch thickness
2 tbsp. olive oil
1 cup. tap water, running cold
Salt and pepper, to taste
Directions:
Pour 1 cup. water in the Instant Pot.
Set the steamer rack and put the salmon fillets in the rack. Lock the lid and close the steamer valve.
Press "Manual", set the pressure on "Low", and set the timer for 1 minute

When the timer beeps, turn off the pot and quick release the pressure
Carefully open the lid. Remove the salmon fillets and pat them dry using paper towels.
Over medium-high heat, preheat a skillet.
Grease the salmon fillet skins with 1 tablespoon olive oil and generously season with black pepper and salt.
When the skillet is very hot, with the skin side down, put the salmon fillet in the skillet.
Cook for 1 to 2 minutes until the skins are crispy.
Transfer the salmon fillets into serving plates and serve with your favorite side dishes.
This dish is great with rice and salad.
Tips: You can use a nonstick skillet to make sure the skin does not stick to the skillet. If you do not like the skin on your salmon, you can remove it after pressure cooking. Increase the cooking time to 2 minutes

259. Salmon Burger
Cooking Time:20 minutes
Servings:4
Ingredients:
1 lb. salmon meat; minced.
1 tsp. extra virgin olive oil
1/2 cup panko
2 tbsp. lemon zest
Tomatoes slices for serving
Mustard for serving
Salt and black pepper to the taste
Arugula leaves for serving
Directions:
Put salmon in your food processor and blend it.
Transfer to a bowl, add panko, salt, pepper and lemon zest and stir well.
Shape 4 patties and place them on a working surface.
Set your instant pot on Sauté mode; add oil and heat it up
Add patties, cook for 3 minutes on each side and divide them on buns.
Serve with tomatoes, arugula and mustard.

260. Miso Mackerel
Cooking Time:60 minutes
Servings:4
Ingredients:
2 lb. mackerel, cut into big pieces
1 cup water
1 garlic clove, crushed.
2 celery stalks, sliced
1/3 cup mirin
1/4 cup miso
1/3 cup sake
1 sweet onion, thinly sliced
1 tbsp. rice vinegar
1 tsp. Japanese hot mustard
1 tsp. sugar
1 shallot, sliced
1-inch ginger piece; chopped
Salt to the taste
Directions:
Set your instant pot on Sauté mode; add mirin, sake, ginger, garlic and shallot, stir and boil for 2 minutes.
Add miso and water and stir.

Add mackerel, seal the instant pot lid and cook at High for 45 minutes.
Meanwhile, put onion and celery in a bowl and cover with ice water.
In another bowl, mix vinegar with salt, sugar and mustard and stir well
Release the pressure from the pot naturally for 10 minutes and divide mackerel among plates.
Drain onion and celery well and mix with mustard dressing.
Divide along mackerel and serve

261. Shrimp with Herbs and Risotto
Cooking Time:30 minutes
Servings:4
Ingredients:
1 lb. shrimp, peeled and deveined
4 tbsp. butter
2 garlic cloves; minced.
1 ½ cups Arborio rice
2 tbsp. dry white wine
4 ½ cups chicken stock
3/4 cup parmesan, grated
1/4 cup tarragon and parsley; chopped
1 yellow onion; chopped.
Salt and black pepper to the taste
Directions:
Set your instant pot on Sauté mode; add 2 tablespoon butter and melt.
Add garlic and onion, stir and cook for 4 minutes
Add rice, stir and cook for 1 minute
Add wine, stir and cook 30 seconds more.
Add 3 cups stock, salt, and pepper; then stir well. seal the instant pot lid and cook at High for 9 minutes.
Quick release the pressure, carefully open the lid; add shrimp, the rest of the stock, set the pot on Sauté mode again and cook for 5 minutes stirring from time to time.
Add cheese, the rest of the butter, tarragon and parsley; then stir well. divide among plates and serve.

262. Fish with Orange Sauce
Cooking Time:17 minutes
Servings:4
Ingredients:
4 white fish fillets
1 cup fish stock
Juice and zest from 1 orange
A drizzle of extra virgin olive oil
A small piece of ginger; chopped.
4 spring onions; chopped.
Salt and black pepper to the taste
Directions:
Pat dry fish fillets, season with salt, pepper and rub them with the olive oil
Put stock, ginger, orange juice, orange zest and onions in your instant pot.
Put fish fillets in the steamer basket, seal the instant pot lid and cook at High for 7 minutes.
Quick release the pressure, divide fish among plates and drizzle the orange sauce on top.

263. Simple Clams
Cooking Time:25 minutes
Servings:4
Ingredients:
15 small clams
30 mussels, scrubbed and debearded
2 tbsp. parsley; chopped.
1 tsp. extra virgin olive oil
1 yellow onion; chopped.
10 oz. beer
2 chorizo links, sliced
1 lb. baby red potatoes
Lemon wedges for serving
Directions:
Set your instant pot on Sauté mode; add oil and heat it up
Add chorizo and onions, stir and cook for 4 minutes.
Add clams, mussels, potatoes and beer; then stir well. seal the instant pot lid and cook at High for 10 minutes.
Quick release the pressure, carefully open the lid; add parsley; then stir well. divide among bowls and serve with lemon wedges on the side.

264. Crab Legs and Garlic Butter Sauce.
Cooking Time:15 minutes
Servings:2
Ingredients:
2 lb. frozen or fresh crab legs
1 tsp. olive oil
1 minced garlic clove
1 cup. water
1 halved lemon
4 tbsp. salted butter
Directions:
Pour water in your Instant Pot and lower in the steamer basket. Add the crab legs.
Choose the "steam" option adjust time to 3 minutes for fresh, and 4 for frozen. In the meantime, heat the oil in a skillet.
Cook garlic for just 1 minute, stirring so it doesn't burn
Add the butter and stir to melt. Squeeze the halved lemon in the butter.
By now, the crab will be done, so hit "cancel" and quick-release the pressure
Serve crabs with the garlic butter on the side

265. Shrimp and Potatoes Dish
Cooking Time:25 minutes
Servings:4
Ingredients:
2 lb. shrimp, peeled and deveined
8 potatoes, cut into quarters
4 tbsp. extra virgin olive oil
4 onions; chopped.
1 lb. tomatoes; peeled and chopped.
1 tbsp. watercress
1 tsp. coriander, ground.
1 tsp. curry powder
Juice of 1 lemon
Salt to the taste
Directions:
Put potatoes in the steamer basket of the pot, add some water to the pot, seal the instant pot lid and cook at High for 10 minutes.

Quick release the pressure, transfer potatoes to a bowl and clean up your pot.
Set the pot on Sauté mode; add oil and heat it up
Add onions, stir and cook for 5 minutes.
Add salt, coriander and curry, stir and cook for 5 minutes
Add tomatoes, shrimp, lemon juice and return potatoes as well.
Stir, seal the instant pot lid and cook at High for 3 minuets
Release the pressure again, divide among bowls and serve with watercress on top

266. Shrimp and Fish
Cooking Time:20 minutes
Servings:4
Ingredients:
1/2 lb. shrimp, cooked, peeled and deveined
4 lemon wedges
2 tbsp. butter
2 lb. flounder
1/2 cup water
Salt and black pepper to the taste
Directions:
Season fish with salt and pepper and place in the steamer basket of the pot
Add water to the pot, seal the instant pot lid and cook at High for 10 minutes.
Release the pressure carefully open the lid; transfer fish to plates and leave aside
Discard water, clean pot and set on Sauté mode. Add butter and melt it.
Add shrimp, salt and pepper, stir and divide among plates on top of fish and serve with lemon wedges on the side

267. Shrimp and Sausage Boil
Cooking Time: 35 minutes
Servings: 4
Ingredients:
1/2 lb. shrimp; peeled and deveined
4 baby red potatoes, halved
4 ears sweet corn, cut into thirds
4 shakes hot sauce
8 ounces smoked sausage, cut into 4 pieces each
1 tbsp. minced garlic
1 tbsp. Louisiana-style shrimp and crab boil seasoning
6 tbsp. (¾ sticksalted butter
Juice of ½ lemon
1/4 tsp. Old Bay seasoning
⅛ tsp. Cajun seasoning
⅛ tsp. lemon-pepper seasoning
Lemon slices
Directions:
In your Instant Pot, combine the sausage, corn and potatoes. Add water to cover. Add the shrimp and crab boil seasoning.
Now secure the lid on the pot and close the valve.
Now Press "Manual" and set the pot at "High" pressure for 4 minutes
Meanwhile; in a small saucepan, melt the butter over medium-high heat. Add the garlic and cook, stirring continuously, until fragrant, 1 to 2 minutes

Add the lemon juice, Old Bay, Cajun seasoning, lemon-pepper seasoning and hot sauce. Stir until warmed through; keep warm
After completing the cooking time, quick release the pressure. Open the lid carefully and check to ensure the potatoes are cooked. If they are not done, you can boil them for a few minutes using the "Sauté" setting. Gently stir in the shrimp. As soon as the shrimp turn pink, drizzle everything with the spiced garlic-butter sauce. Add the lemon slices to the pot. Stir gently until everything is well coated.

268. Tuna and Crushed Crackers Casserole.
Cooking Time:25 minutes
Servings:8
Ingredients:
8 oz. fresh tuna
3 tbsp. butter
3 tbsp. all-purpose flour
1 cup. frozen peas
1 cup. cheddar, shredded.
1 cup. celery
3 ½ cups. chicken stock
2 tsp. salt
2 cups. pasta (I used elbow mac
1/4 cup. heavy cream
1 cup. onion
1 cup. buttery crackers, crushed.
Fresh ground black pepper
Directions:
Press the "Sauté" key of the Instant Pot to preheat it. When hot, put the celery and onion
Sauté until the onion is translucent. Pour in the chicken stock and pasta, and season with salt and pepper.
Stir to combine for a bit. Put the fresh tuna on top of the pasta mix. Press "Cancel" to stop the sauté function. Close and lock the lid.
Press "Manual" and set the timer for 5 minutes. Meanwhile, heat the sauté pan over medium-high. Put the butter in the pan and melt. Stir in the flour and cook for 2 minutes. Remove the pan from the heat and set aside.
When the timer of the Instant Pot beeps, turn the steam valve to "Venting" to quick release the pressure. Transfer the tuna onto a plate and set aside. Pour the butter mix into the Instant Pot. Press the "Sauté" key. Stir until the mixture is thick. Turn off the Instant Pot. Stir in the heavy cream, the peas, and the tuna
Cover the mix with the crackers and then with the grated cheese
Cover and let stand for 5 minutes. Serve

269. Shrimp Coconut Soup
Cooking Time: 21 minutes
Servings: 4
Ingredients:
1/2 lb. medium shrimp; peeled (tails left onand deveined
1/4 cup fresh lime juice
1 cup canned straw mushrooms; undrained
6 thin slices fresh ginger

1 (13.5-ouncecan full-fat coconut milk
Grated zest of 1 lime
3 cups chicken broth
2 tbsp. fish sauce
1 tbsp. minced fresh lemongrass
1 tsp. honey
1/2 tsp. salt or as your liking
Chopped fresh cilantro, for garnish
Lime wedges, for serving
Directions:
In your Instant Pot, combine the broth, shrimp, mushrooms and their liquid, half the coconut milk, the ginger, chiles (if using, 1 tbsp. of the fish sauce, the lemongrass, honey and salt
Now secure the lid on the pot and close the valve.
Now Press "Manual" and set the pot at "Low" pressure for 1 minute
After completing the cooking time, quick release the pressure. Stir in the remaining 1 tbsp. fish sauce, remaining coconut milk, the lime zest and lime juice
Divide the soup among four serving bowls. Garnish with cilantro and serve with lime wedges alongside for squeezing.

270. Shrimp Teriyaki Recipe
Cooking Time:15 minutes
Servings:4
Ingredients:
1 lb. shrimp, peeled and deveined
1/2 lb. pea pods
3/4 cup pineapple juice
1 cup chicken stock
3 tbsp. vinegar
3 tbsp. sugar
2 tbsp. soy sauce
Directions:
Put shrimp and pea pods in your instant pot.
In a bowl, mix soy sauce with vinegar, pineapple juice, stock and sugar and stir well.
Pour this into the pot; then stir well. seal the instant pot lid and cook at High for 3 minutes.
Quick release the pressure, carefully open the lid; divide among plates and serve

271. Instant Shrimp Boil
Cooking Time:15 minutes
Servings:4
Ingredients:
1 ½ lb. shrimp, head removed
1 lb. potatoes, cut into medium chunks
8 garlic cloves, crushed.
1 tbsp. old bay seasoning
12 oz. Andouille sausage, already cooked and chopped.
4 ears of corn, each cut into 3 pieces
1 tsp. red pepper flakes, crushed.
2 sweet onions, cut into wedges
16 oz. beer
Salt and black pepper to the taste
French baguettes for serving
Directions:
In your instant pot, mix beer with old bay seasoning, red pepper flakes, salt, black pepper, onions, garlic, potatoes, corn, sausage pieces and shrimp.
Cover the pot and cook at High for 5 minutes
Quick release the pressure, carefully open the lid; divide shrimp boil into bowls and serve with French baguettes on the side.

272. Cheesy Tilapia.
Cooking Time:35 minutes
Servings:4
Ingredients:
5 oz. Cheddar cheese
12 oz. tilapia
1 tbsp. butter
1 tsp. ground ginger
1 onion
1/3 tsp. ground black pepper
1/2 cup. cream
Directions:
Cut the tilapia into the medium fillets.
Then combine the ground ginger and ground black pepper together. Mix up the mixture.
After this, rub the tilapia fillets with the spice mixture. Leave the fish for 5 minutes
After this, grate Cheddar cheese.
Peel the onion and slice it. Toss the butter in the Instant Pot and melt it at the "Manual" mode.
Then add the tilapia fillets and cook them for 2 minutes from each side.
After this, cover the tilapia fillets with the sliced onion
Sprinkle the dish with the grated cheese and pour cream
Close the lid and cook the dish at the STEW mode for 10 minutes.
When the time is over - open the Instant Pot lid. Let the fish chill little
Serve the tilapia fillets immediately. Enjoy!

273. Mediterranean Fish
Cooking Time:20 minutes
Servings:4
Ingredients:
17 oz. tomatoes, cut into halves
4 cod fillets
1 cup olives, pitted and chopped.
2 tbsp. capers, drained and chopped.
1 tbsp. extra-virgin olive oil
1 tbsp. parsley; chopped.
1 garlic clove, crushed.
Salt and black pepper to the taste
Directions:
Put tomatoes on the bottom of a heat proof bowl.
Add parsley, salt and pepper and toss to coat
Place fish fillets on top, add olive oil, salt, pepper, garlic, olives and capers
Place the bowl in the steamer basket of the pot, seal the instant pot lid and cook at High for 5 minutes.
Release the pressure naturally, divide among plates and serve.

274. Delicious Salmon and Raspberry Sauce
Cooking Time: 2 hours and 5 minutes
Servings: 6
Ingredients:

6 salmon steaks
2 tbsp. parsley; chopped.
1 cup clam juice
2 tbsp. lemon juice
2 tbsp. extra virgin olive oil
4 leeks, sliced
2 garlic cloves; minced
1 tsp. sherry
1/3 cup dill; finely chopped
Salt and white pepper to the taste
Raspberries for serving
For the raspberry vinegar:
1-pint cider vinegar
2 pints red raspberries
Directions:
Mix red raspberries with vinegar and stir well
Add salmon steaks and leave aside in the fridge for 2 hours
Set your instant pot on Sauté mode; add oil and heat it up.
Add parsley, leeks and garlic, stir and cook for 2 minutes
Add clam and lemon juice, sherry, salt, pepper and dill and stir
Add salmon steaks, seal the instant pot lid and cook at High for 3 minutes
Quick release the pressure, carefully open the lid; divide salmon among plates and serve with leeks and fresh raspberries

275. Sesame Honey Salmon
Cooking Time: 20 minutes
Servings: 4
Ingredients:
1 lb. salmon fillet
2 cups water
1 tbsp. dark soy sauce
1 tbsp. toasted sesame oil
2 tbsp. sesame seeds
1 tbsp. honey
2 tsp. minced fresh ginger
1 tsp. minced garlic
1/2 tsp. red pepper flakes
Salt and black pepper to taste
Directions:
Place the salmon in a 6-inch round heatproof pan. In a small bowl, combine the honey, soy sauce, sesame oil, ginger, garlic and red pepper flakes and season with salt and black pepper. Whisk to combine.
Pour the mixture over the salmon. Allow the salmon to sit at room temperature for 15 to 30 minutes.
Pour the water into the Instant Pot. Place a steamer rack in the pot. Place the pan with the salmon on the rack
Now secure the lid on the pot and close the valve.
Now Press "Manual" and set the pot at "Low" pressure for 3 minutes
After completing the cooking time, allow the pot to sit undisturbed for 5 minutes, then release any remaining pressure. Sprinkle with the sesame seeds. Serve the salmon immediately.

276. Crab Quiche
Cooking Time: 60 minutes
Servings: 4
Ingredients:
1 cup half-and-half
4 large eggs
2 cups water
8 ounces imitation crabmeat, real crabmeat
1 cup shredded Swiss cheese
1 cup chopped scallions
Vegetable oil
1 tsp. smoked paprika
1 tsp. herbes de Provence
1 tsp. black pepper
1 tsp. salt or as your liking
Directions:
Grease a 6-inch or 7-inch nonstick springform pan with vegetable oil. Set the pan on a sheet of aluminum foil that is larger than the pan and crimp the foil around the bottom of the pan.
In a large bowl, whisk together the eggs and half-and-half. Add the cheese, scallions, pepper, paprika, herbes de Provence and salt. Stir with a fork to combine. Add the imitation crabmeat and stir to combine
Pour the egg mixture into the prepared pan. Cover the pan loosely with foil. Pour the water into the Instant Pot. Set a steamer rack in the pot. Place the pan on the steamer rack
Now secure the lid on the pot and close the valve.
Now Press "Manual" and set the pot at "High" pressure for 25 minutes
After completing the cooking time, allow the pot to sit undisturbed for 10 minutes, then release any remaining pressure. Using silicone oven mitts, very carefully remove the pan from the pot. Using a knife, loosen the sides of the quiche from the pan, then remove the springform ring. Serve warm.

277. Shrimp with Tomatoes, Spinach
Cooking Time: 31 minutes
Servings: 4
Ingredients:
1 lb. shrimp (21 to 25 count; peeled and deveined
4 cups chopped baby spinach
1 ½ cups chopped yellow onions
1/4 cup shredded Parmesan cheese
1 (14.5-ouncecan diced tomatoes; undrained
1/4 cup chopped fresh basil
1 tbsp. minced garlic
2 tbsp. salted butter
1 tsp. dried oregano
1/2 tsp. red pepper flakes
1 tsp. salt or as your liking
1 tsp. black pepper
Directions:
Now Press "Sauté" on the Instant Pot. When the pot is hot, add the butter. When the butter has melted, add the garlic and red pepper flakes.
Cook, stirring, for 1 minute. Add the spinach, shrimp, onions, tomatoes and their juices, oregano, salt and pepper. Stir to combine. Now Press "Cancel"
Secure the lid on the pot. Close the pressure release valve. Now Press "Manual" and set the pot at "Low" pressure for 1 minute
After completing the cooking time, quick release the pressure. Allow the mixture to cool for 5 minutes. Stir in the basil. Divide the mixture among four shallow bowls. Top with Parmesan and serve immediately.

278. Seafood Stew
Cooking Time: 43 minutes
Servings: 4
Ingredients:
1 cup chopped carrots
1 cup chicken broth
1 cup diced yellow onions
1 cup water
1 (14.5-ouncecan fire-roasted diced tomatoes
2 bay leaves
4 cups mixed seafood, such as white fish chunks; peeled shrimp, bay scallops, shelled mussels and calamari rings
1 tbsp. tomato paste
2 tbsp. minced garlic
1 tbsp. fresh lemon juice
2 tsp. fennel seeds, toasted and ground
1 tsp. dried oregano
1 tsp. red pepper flakes, plus more for garnish
Salt or as your liking
Crusty bread, toasted
Directions:
In your Instant Pot, combine the tomatoes and their juices, onions, carrots, water, wine, garlic, fennel seeds, tomato paste, oregano, red pepper flakes and bay leaves. Season with salt. Stir to combine.
Now secure the lid on the pot and close the valve.
Now Press "Manual" and set the pot at "High" pressure for 15 minutes
After completing the cooking time, allow the pot to sit undisturbed for 10 minutes, then release any remaining pressure. Remove the lid from the Instant Pot. Now Press "Sauté" and bring the soup to a boil.
Add the mixed seafood and cook until the fish and shellfish are cooked through, 3 to 4 minutes. Stir in the lemon juice. Now Press "Cancel"
Discard the bay leaves. Serve the stew garnished with red pepper flakes, with crusty bread alongside to mop up the delicious, savory broth.

279. Fresh Catfish with Herbs.
Cooking Time:20 minutes
Servings:6
Ingredients:
14 oz. catfish
1 tsp. fresh parsley
1 tsp. dill
2 tbsp. soy sauce
1 tbsp. olive oil
1/4 cup. fresh thyme
3 garlic cloves
1/4 cup. water
1 tbsp. salt
Directions:
Wash the fresh parsley and fresh thyme. Chop the greens.
Combine the chopped greens with the dill and salt. Stir the mixture.
After this, peel the garlic cloves and slice them. Pour the olive oil in the Instant Pot.
Add the sliced garlic and "Sauté" it for 1 minute
Then combine the catfish with the green mixture.
Add soy sauce and water.
Stir the mixture and transfer it to the Instant Pot.
"Sauté" the dish for 4 minutes on each side.
When the dish is cooked - you will get the light golden brown color of the fish.
Serve the dish hot! Enjoy!

280. Steamed Scallion Ginger Fish
Cooking Time: 32 minutes
Servings: 4
Ingredients:
For Fish:
1 lb. firm white-fleshed fish, such as tilapia, cut into large pieces
2 cups water
2 tbsp. rice wine
1 tbsp. Chinese black bean paste
3 tbsp. soy sauce
1 tsp. minced fresh ginger
1 tsp. minced garlic
For Sauce:
1/4 cup chopped fresh cilantro
1/4 cup julienned scallions
2 tbsp. julienned fresh ginger
1 tbsp. peanut oil
Directions:
For fish: Place the fish pieces on a rimmed plate. In a small bowl, combine the soy sauce, rice wine, black bean paste; minced ginger and garlic. Whisk to combine. Pour over the fish, turning to coat
Allow the fish to stand at room temperature for 20 to 30 minutes. Pour the water into the Instant Pot. Place a steamer basket in the pot. Transfer the fish to the steamer basket, reserving the marinade
Now secure the lid on the pot and close the valve.
Now Press "Manual" and set the pot at "Low" pressure for 2 minutes. After completing the cooking time, quick release the pressure. Transfer the fish to a serving platter.
Meanwhile; for the sauce: In a small saucepan, heat the peanut oil over medium-high heat. When the oil shimmers, add the julienned ginger and cook, stirring, for 10 seconds
Add the scallions and cilantro. Cook, stirring, until the ginger and scallions are just softened, about 2 minutes.
Add the reserved marinade and bring to a boil. Boil vigorously for 1 to 2 minutes. Pour the vegetable mixture over the fish and serve immediately.

281. Delicious Cod and Peas
Cooking Time:20 minutes
Servings:4
Ingredients:
10 oz. peas
9 oz. wine
1/2 tsp. oregano; dried
16 oz. cod fillets
1 tbsp. parsley; chopped.
2 garlic cloves; chopped.
1/2 tsp. paprika
Salt and pepper to the taste
Directions:
In your food processor mix garlic with parsley, oregano and paprika and blend well.
Add wine, blend again and leave aside for now.
Place fish fillets in the steamer basket of your instant pot, add salt and pepper, seal the instant pot lid and cook at High for 2 minutes.
Release the pressure and divide fish among plates
Add peas to the steamer basket, seal the instant pot lid again and cook at High for 2 minutes.
Release the pressure again and arrange peas next to fish fillets.
Serve with herbs dressing on top

282. Instant Pot Steamed Mussels
Cooking Time: 15 minutes
Servings: 4
Ingredients:
2 lb. mussels, cleaned and scrubbed
1 radicchio, cut into thin strips
1/2 cup dry white wine
1 lb. baby spinach
1/2 cup water
1 garlic clove, crushed.
1 white onion; chopped.
A drizzle of extra virgin olive oil

Directions:
Arrange baby spinach and radicchio on appetizer plates
Set instant pot on Sauté mode; add oil and heat it up
Add garlic and onion, stir and cook for 4 minutes.
Add wine, stir and cook for 1 minute.
Place mussels in the steamer basket of the pot, seal the instant pot lid and cook on Low for 1 minute.
Release the pressure and divide mussels on top of spinach and radicchio
Add cooking liquid all over and serve

POULTRY

283. Creamy Basil Chicken Breasts
Cooking Time: 30 minutes
Servings: 4
Ingredients
4 Chicken Breasts, skinless and boneless
½ cup Heavy Cream
⅓ cup Chicken Broth
⅓ tsp minced Garlic
Salt and Black Pepper to taste
⅓ tsp Italian Seasoning
¼ cup Roasted Red Peppers
1 tbsp Basil Pesto
1 tbsp Arrowroot Starch
Directions
Place the chicken at the bottom of the Instant Pot. Pour in broth, and add Italian seasoning, garlic, salt, and pepper. Seal the lid, select Poultry and cook on High pressure for 15 minutes.
Once ready, do a natural pressure release for 5 minutes, then a quick pressure release to let the remaining steam out, and open the pot. Use a spoon to remove the chicken onto a plate; select Sauté mode. Scoop out any fat or unwanted chunks from the sauce.
In a bowl, add cream, arrowroot starch, red peppers, and pesto. Mix with a spoon. Pour the creamy mixture in the pot and whisk for 4 minutes until well-mixed and thickened.
Put the chicken back to the pot and let simmer for 3 minutes. Press Cancel and dish the sauce onto a serving platter. Serve with sauce over a bed of mixed spiralized zoodles.
Nutrition Values: Calories 238, Protein 25g, Net Carbs 1g, Fat 12g

284. Lemon Chicken
Cooking Time: 30 minutes
Servings: 4
Ingredients
4 Chicken Thighs
1 ½ tbsp Olive oil
½ tsp Garlic Powder
Salt and Black Pepper to taste
½ tsp Red Pepper Flakes
½ tsp smoked Paprika
1 small Onion, chopped
2 cloves Garlic, sliced
¼ cup Chicken Broth
1 tsp Italian Seasoning
1 Lemon, zested and juiced
1 ½ tbsp Heavy Cream
Lemon slices and chopped Parsley to garnish
Directions
Heat oil on Sauté, and brown the chicken thighs on each side for 3 minutes. Remove the browned chicken to a plate. Melt the butter, add the garlic, onions, and lemon juice. Stir with a spoon to deglaze the bottom of the pot and cook for 1 minute. Add the Italian seasoning, chicken broth, lemon zest, and the chicken. Seal the lid, select Poultry and cook on High pressure for 15 minutes. Once ready, do a quick pressure release.
Open the lid. Remove the chicken onto a plate and add in the heavy cream. Select Sauté and stir the cream into the sauce until it thickens. Press Cancel and add the chicken. Coat the chicken with sauce. Serve with steamed kale and spinach mix. Garnish with the lemons slices and parsley.
Nutrition Values: Calories 358, Protein 28g, Net Carbs 0g, Fat 36g

285. Coq Au Vin
Cooking Time: 50 minutes
Servings: 4
Ingredients
3 Chicken Legs, cut into drumsticks and thighs
2 Bacon Slices, chopped in ¾-inch pieces
1 ½ cups Dry White Wine
Salt and Black Pepper to taste
½ bunch Thyme, divided
8 oz Shiitake Mushrooms, cut into 4 pieces
3 Shallots, peeled
3 tbsp Unsalted Butter, divided
3 skinny Carrots, cut into 4 crosswise pieces each
2 cloves Garlic, crushed
1 tbsp Almond flour
3 tbsp chopped Parsley for garnishing
Directions
Season the chicken on both sides with salt and pepper.
In a plastic zipper bag, pour the wine. Add half of the thyme and chicken.
Zip the bag and shake to coat the chicken well with the wine. Place in the fridge. After 8 hours, turn on the Instant Pot on Sauté, and add the bacon to it. Fry until brown for 8 minutes; then remove to a plate. Pour in the mushrooms, season with salt and cook for 5 minutes. Remove to the side of the bacon. Remove the chicken from the fridge. Discard the thyme but reserve the marinade. Pat the chicken dry with paper towels. In the the pot, melt half of the butter, and place in the chicken. Cook until dark golden brown color on each side for 12 minutes. Add the bacon, mushrooms, shallots, garlic, and carrots. Cook for 4 minutes and top with the wine and remaining thyme. Seal the lid, select Poultry and cook on High pressure for 15 minutes.
Add almond flour and the remaining butter in a bowl and smash together with a fork; set aside. Once ready, do a natural pressure release for 10 minutes and open the pot. Plate the chicken and vegetables with a slotted spoon and set the Instant Pot on Sauté mode. Discard the thyme.
Add the almond flour mixture to the sauce in the pot, stir until is well incorporated. Cook for 4 minutes. Spoon the sauce over the chicken. Garnish with parsley and serve with steamed asparagus.
Nutrition Values: Calories 268, Protein 32g, Net Carbs 2g, Fat 12g

286. Coconut Chicken Curry
Cooking Time: 32 minutes
Servings: 4
Ingredients
4 Chicken Breasts

4 tbsp Red Curry Paste
2 cups Coconut Milk
4 tbsp Swerve Sugar
Salt and Black Pepper to taste
2 Red Bell pepper, seeded and cut in 2-inch sliced
2 Yellow Bell pepper, seeded and cut in 2-inch slices
2 cup Green Beans, cut in Half
2 tbsp Lime Juice
Directions
Add the chicken, red curry paste, salt, pepper, coconut milk, and swerve. Seal the lid, select Poultry and cook on High pressure for 15 minutes. Once ready, do a quick pressure release. Remove to a cutting board and select Sauté on the pot. Add bell peppers, green beans, and lime juice. Stir the sauce with a spoon and let simmer for 4 minutes.
Slice the chicken with a knife and add back to the pot. Stir and simmer for 1 minute. Dish the chicken with sauce and vegetable into a serving bowl and serve with coconut flatbread.
Nutrition Values: Calories 368, Protein 32g, Net Carbs 0g, Fat 24g

287. Chicken Taco Bowls
Cooking Time: 25 minutes
Servings: 4
Ingredients
4 Chicken Breasts
1 cup Chicken Broth
2 ¼ packets Taco Seasoning
2 cups Cauli Rice
2 Green Bell peppers, seeded and diced
2 Red Bell peppers, seeded and diced
2 cups Salsa
Salt and Black Pepper to taste
To serve:
Grated Cheese, of your choice
Chopped Cilantro
Sour Cream
Avocado Slices
Directions
Pour the chicken broth in the pot, add the chicken, and pour the taco seasoning over. Add the salsa and stir lightly with a spoon.
Seal the lid, select Poultry and cook on High for 15 minutes. Once ready, do a quick pressure release. Add the cauli rice and bell peppers, and use a spoon to push them into the sauce.
Seal the lid, select Steam and cook on High pressure for 4 minutes. Once ready, do a quick pressure release. Gently stir the mixture, adjust the taste with salt and pepper and spoon the chicken dish into serving bowls. Top with sour cream, avocado slices, cilantro and cheese.
Nutrition Values: Calories 240, Protein 34g, Net Carbs 0g, Fat 22g

288. Sweet Spicy Shredded Chicken
Cooking Time: 35 minutes
Servings: 4
Ingredients
4 Chicken Breasts, skinless
¼ cup Sriracha Sauce
2 tbsp unsalted Butter
1 tsp grated Ginger
2 cloves Garlic, minced
½ tsp Cayenne Pepper
½ tsp Red Chili Flakes
½ cup Monk Fruit Syrup
⅓ cup Chicken Broth
Salt and Black Pepper to taste
Chopped Scallion to garnish
Directions
In a bowl, pour the broth. Add the monk fruit syrup, ginger, Sriracha sauce, red pepper flakes, cayenne pepper, and garlic. Use a spoon to mix them well and set aside.
Put the chicken on a plate and season with salt and pepper. Set aside too. Melt the butter on Sauté, and add the chicken in 2 batches; cook to brown on both sides for 3 minutes.
Add all the chicken back to the pot and pour the pepper sauce over. Seal the lid, select Poultry and cook on High pressure for 20 minutes. Once ready, do a natural pressure release for 5 minutes, then a quick pressure release to let the remaining steam out. Remove the chicken on a cutting board and shred with two forks. Transfer to a serving bowl, pour the sauce over and garnish with the scallions. Serve with a side of zoodles.
Nutrition Values: Calories 160, Protein 37g, Net Carbs 0g, Fat 16g

289. Chicken in Tomato Sauce
Cooking Time: 30 minutes
Servings: 4
Ingredients
4 Chicken Thighs, skinless but with Bone
4 tbsp Olive oil
1 cup Crushed Tomatoes
1 large Red Bell pepper, seeded and diced
1 large Green Bell pepper, seeded and diced
1 Red Onion, diced
Salt and Black Pepper to taste
1 tbsp chopped Basil
1 Bay Leaf
½ tsp dried Oregano
Directions
Place the chicken on a clean flat surface and season with salt and pepper. Heat oil on Sauté, and brown the chicken on both sides for 6 minutes. Then, add the onions and bell peppers.
Cook to soften them for 5 minutes. Add the tomatoes, bay leaf, salt, pepper, and oregano. Stir using a spoon. Seal the lid, select Poultry and cook on High pressure for 20 minutes.
Once ready, do a natural pressure release for 5 minutes, then a quick pressure release to let the remaining steam out. Discard the bay leaf. Dish the chicken with the sauce into a serving bowl and garnish with basil. Serve over a bed of steamed squash spaghetti.
Nutrition Values: Calories 133, Protein 14g, Net Carbs 6.5g, Fat 3g

290. Spinach Feta Stuffed Chicken
Cooking Time: 30 minutes
Servings: 4

Ingredients
4 Chicken Breasts, skinless
Salt and Black Pepper to taste
1 cup Baby Spinach, frozen
½ cup crumbled Feta Cheese
½ tsp dried Oregano
½ tsp Garlic Powder
2 tbsp Coconut Oil
tsp dried Parsley
1 cup Water
Directions
Cover the chicken in plastic wrap and put them on a cutting board. Use a rolling pin to pound them flat to a quarter inch thickness. Then, remove the plastic wrap. In a bowl, add spinach, salt, and feta cheese. Use a spoon to mix well and scoop the mixture onto the chicken breasts.
Wrap the chicken to secure the spinach filling in it. Use toothpicks to secure the wrap firmly from opening. Season the chicken pieces with the oregano, parsley, garlic powder, and pepper. Turn on the Instant Pot, open the lid, and select Sauté mode. Add the coconut oil and chicken, and sear to golden brown on each side. Work in 2 batches. After, remove the chicken onto a plate and set aside.
Pour the water into the pot and use a spoon to scrape the bottom of the pot to let loose any chicken pieces or seasoning that is stuck to the bottom of the pot. Then, fit the steamer rack into the pot with care as the pot will still be hot. Use a pair of tongs to transfer the chicken onto the steamer rack. Close the lid, secure the pressure valve, and select Poultry mode on High pressure for 15 minutes.
Once ready, do a quick pressure release. Plate the chicken and serve with side of sautéed broccoli, asparagus, and some slices of tomatoes.
Nutrition Values: Calories 225, Protein 33g, Net Carbs 2g, Fat 17g

291. Meatballs Primavera
Cooking Time: 30 minutes
Servings: 4
Ingredients
1 lb Ground Chicken
1 Egg, cracked into a bowl
6 tsp Coconut Flour
Salt and Black Pepper to taste
2 tbsp chopped Basil + Extra to garnish
1 tbsp Avocado Oil + ½ tbsp Avocado Oil
1 ½ tsp Italian Seasoning
1 Red Bell pepper, seeded and sliced
2 cups chopped Green Beans
½ lb chopped Asparagus
1 cup chopped Tomatoes
1 cup Chicken Broth
Directions
In a mixing bowl, add the chicken, egg, coconut flour, salt, pepper, 2 tbsp of basil, 1 tbsp of avocado oil, and Italian seasoning. Use your hands to mix well and make 16 large balls.
Set the meatballs aside. Select Sauté mode on the pot. Heat ½ a tsp of avocado oil and add bell pepper, green beans, and asparagus. Cook them for 3 minutes while stirring frequently.

After 3 minutes, use a spoon to remove the veggies to a plate; set aside. Heat the remaining oil and fry the meatballs in batches. Cook for 2 minutes on each side to brown lightly.
Put all the meatballs back into the pot as well as the vegetables. Pour the chicken broth over. Seal the lid, select Poultry and cook on High pressure for 15 minutes. Once ready, do a quick pressure release. Dish the meatballs with sauce into bowls and garnish with basil.
Nutrition Values: Calories 135, Protein 16g, Net Carbs 0g, Fat 16.4g

292. Buffalo Chicken Soup
Cooking Time: 37 minutes
Servings: 4
Ingredients
4 Chicken Breasts, Boneless and skinless
½ cup Hot Sauce
2 large White Onion, finely chopped
2 cups finely chopped Celery
1 tbsp Olive oil
1 tsp dried Thyme
3 cups Chicken Broth
1 tsp Garlic Powder
½ cup crumbled Blue Cheese + extra for serving
4 oz Cream Cheese, cubed in small pieces
Salt and Pepper to taste
Directions
Put the chicken on a clean flat surface and season with pepper and salt; set aside. Heat oil on Sauté, and add onion and celery. Cook, constantly stirring, until soft for 5 minutes.
Stir in garlic and thyme. Cook for about a minute, and add the chicken, hot sauce, and broth. Season with salt and pepper. Seal the lid, select Poultry and cook on High for 20 minutes.
Meanwhile, put the blue cheese and cream cheese in a bowl, and use a fork to smash them together. Set the resulting mixture aside. Once ready, do a quick pressure release.
Shred the chicken inside the pot and select Sauté mode. Mix in the cheese; press Cancel. Dish the soup into bowls. Sprinkle the remaining cheese and serve with low-carb baguette.
Nutrition Values: Calories 114, Protein 4.1g, Net Carbs 0g, Fat 4.3g

293. Balsamic Chicken
Cooking Time: 50 minutes
Servings: 4
Ingredients
2 lb Chicken Thighs, Bone in and skin on
2 tbsp Olive oil
Salt and Pepper to taste
1 ½ cups diced Tomatoes
¾ cup Yellow Onion
2 tsp minced Garlic
½ cup Balsamic Vinegar
3 tsp chopped fresh Thyme
1 cup Chicken Broth
2 tbsp chopped Parsley
Directions

Put the chicken thighs on a cutting board and use paper towels to pat dry. Season with salt and pepper. Heat oil on Sauté, and put the chicken with skin side down.
Cook until golden brown on each side for 9 minutes. Remove on a clean plate. Add the onions and tomatoes, and sauté for 3 minutes stirring occasionally. Top the onions with the garlic too and cook for 30 seconds, then, stir in the broth, salt, thyme, and balsamic vinegar.
Add the chicken back to the pot. Seal the lid, select Poultry and cook on High pressure for 20 minutes. Meanwhile, preheat an oven to 350 F.
Once ready, do a quick pressure release. Select Sauté mode. Remove the chicken onto a baking tray using tongs and leave the sauce in the pot to thicken for about 10 minutes.
Tuck the baking tray in the oven and let the chicken broil on each side to golden brown for about 5 minutes. Remove and set aside to cool slightly. Adjust the salt and pepper and when cooked to your desired thickness, press Cancel.
Place the chicken in a serving bowl and spoon the sauce all over it. Garnish with parsley and serve with thyme roasted tomatoes, carrots, and radishes.
Nutrition Values: Calories 277, Protein 34g, Net Carbs 2g, Fat 10g

294. Tuscan Chicken
Cooking Time: 30 minutes
Servings: 4
Ingredients
4 Chicken Thighs, cut into 1-inch pieces
1 tbsp Olive oil
1 ½ cups Chicken Broth
Salt to taste
1 cup chopped Sun-Dried Tomatoes with Herbs
2 tbsp Italian Seasoning
2 cups Baby Spinach
¼ tsp Red Pepper Flakes
10 oz softened Cream Cheese, cut into small cubes
1 cup shredded Pecorino
Directions
Pour in chicken broth and add the Italian seasoning, chicken, tomatoes, salt, and red pepper flakes. Stir them with a spoon. Seal the lid, select Poultry and cook on High for 15 minutes.
Once ready, do a quick pressure release. Add and stir in the spinach, parmesan cheese, and cream cheese until the cheese melts and is fully incorporated. Let in the warm for 5 minutes. Dish the Tuscan chicken over a bed of zoodles or a side of steamed asparagus and serve.
Nutrition Values: Calories 385, Protein 45g, Net Carbs 2g, Fat 24g

295. Barbecue Chicken
Cooking Time: 30 minutes
Servings: 4
Ingredients
2 lb Chicken Drumsticks, Bone in and skin in
½ cup Chicken Broth
¼ tbsp Monk Fruit Powder
½ tsp Dry Mustard
½ tsp sweet Paprika
½ tbsp. Cumin Powder
½ tsp Onion Powder
¼ tsp Cayenne Powder
Salt and Pepper to taste
1 stick Butter, sliced in 5 to 7 pieces
Low Carb BBQ Sauce, to taste
Cooking Spray
Directions
Pour the chicken broth in and fit the steamer rack at the bottom of the pot. In the zipper bag, pour in the monk fruit powder, dry mustard, cumin powder, onion powder, cayenne powder, salt, and pepper. Add the chicken, then zip, close the bag and shake to coat the chicken well.
Remove the chicken from the bag and lay on the steamer rack and place the butter slices on the drumsticks. Seal the lid, select Poultry and cook on High pressure for 20 minutes.
Meanwhile, preheat an oven to 350 F. Once ready, do a quick pressure release. Remove chicken onto a clean flat surface and brush with Barbecue sauce. Grease a baking tray with cooking spray and arrange the chicken pieces on it. Tuck the tray into the oven and broil the chicken for 4 minutes while paying close attention to prevent burning. Serve warm.
Nutrition Values: Calories 234, Protein 28.4g, Net Carbs 2.6g, Fat 11.3g

296. Quick Chicken Fajitas
Cooking Time: 30 minutes
Servings: 4
Ingredients
2 lb Chicken Breasts, skinless and cut in 1-inch slices
¼ cup Chicken Broth
1 Yellow Onion, sliced
1 Green Bell peppers, seeded and sliced
1 Yellow Bell pepper, seeded and sliced
1 Red Bell pepper, seeded and sliced
2 tbsp Cumin Powder
2 tbsp Chili Powder
Salt to taste
Half a Lime
Cooking Spray
Fresh cilantro, to garnish
Assembling:
Low Carb Tacos
Guacamole
Sour Cream
Salsa
Cheese
Directions
Grease the pot with cooking spray and line the bottom with the bell peppers and onion. Lay the chicken on the bed of peppers and sprinkle with salt, chili powder, and cumin powder.
Squeeze some lime juice and pour in the broth. Seal the lid, select Poultry and cook on High pressure for 20 minutes. Once ready, do a quick pressure release. Dish the chicken with the vegetables and juice onto a large serving platter. Add the sour cream, cheese, guacamole, salsa, and tacos in one layer on the side of the chicken.

Nutrition Values: Calories 352, Protein 19.7g, Net Carbs 0g, Fat 12.1g

297. Stuffed Full Chicken
Cooking Time: 51 minutes
Servings: 6
Ingredients
4 lb Whole Chicken
1 tbsp Herbes de Provence Seasoning
1 tbsp Olive oil
Salt and Black Pepper to season
2 cloves Garlic, peeled
1 tsp Garlic Powder
1 Yellow Onion, peeled and quartered
1 Lemon, quartered
1 ¼ cup Chicken Broth
Directions
Put the chicken on a clean flat surface and pat dry using paper towels. Sprinkle the top and cavity of the chicken with salt, black pepper, Herbes de Provence, and garlic powder. Stuff the onion, lemon quarters, and garlic cloves into the cavity of the chicken.
Open the Instant Pot and fit the steamer rack in it. Pour the chicken broth in and put the chicken on the rack. Seal the lid, select Poultry and cook on High pressure for 30 minutes.
Meanwhile, get a baking pan ready. Once ready, do a natural pressure release for 12 minutes, then a quick pressure release to let the remaining steam out, and press Cancel.
Open the pot and use two tongs to remove the chicken onto a prepared baking pan. Preheat an oven to 350 F and place the baking pan with the chicken in when it is ready.
Broil the chicken for 5 minutes to ensure that it attains a golden brown color on each side.
Dish the chicken on a bed of steamed mixed veggies for dinner. Right here, the choice is yours to whip up some good keto veggies together as your appetite instructs you.
Nutrition Values: Calories 370, Protein 43g, Net Carbs 2g, Fat 14g

298. Chicken Wings
Cooking Time: 35 minutes
Servings: 5
Ingredients
3 Chicken breasts, cubed
1 tsp Garlic powder
1 cup Almond flour
2 tbsp Coriander, chopped
½ tsp Salt
½ tsp Chili Pepper
½ tsp Cinnamon powder
1 cup Olive oil
¼ cup Water
Directions
In a bowl, mix flour, salt, chili powder, cumin powder, coriander and toss well. Add water and make a thick paste. Heat oil on Sauté mode.
Dip each chicken piece into the flour mixture and then put into the oil. Fry until golden and place on a paper towel to drain. Transfer to a dish and serve with mint sauce.

Nutrition Values: Calories 456, Protein 31g, Net Carbs 0.9g, Fat 34g

299. Whole Chicken
Cooking Time: 70 minutes
Servings: 6
Ingredients
1 white Chicken
1 tsp Garlic paste
1 tsp Ginger paste
1 tsp salt
1 tsp Cayenne Pepper
¼ tsp Chili powder
½ tsp black Pepper
½ tsp Cinnamon powder
½ tsp Cumin powder
3 tbsp Lemon juice
2 tbsp Apple Cider Vinegar
2 tbsp Soya sauce
3 tbsp Olive oil
Directions
In a bowl, combine vinegar, cayenne, lemon juice, ginger garlic paste, salt, pepper, chili, olive oil, cumin powder and cinnamon powder; mix well.
Pour over the chicken and rub with hands. Place the chicken in your greased Instant Pot and seal the lid. Set on Poultry for 45 minutes on High pressure. Do a quick release.
Nutrition Values: Calories 245, Protein 33g, Net Carbs 1.2g, Fat 13g

300. Broccoli Chicken
Cooking Time: 45 minutes
Servings: 3
Ingredients
¼ lb Chicken, Boneless, cut into small pieces
1 cup Broccoli florets
2 Garlic cloves, minced
1 tsp salt
½ tsp black Pepper
3 tbsp Butter
1 cup Chicken broth
2 cup Cream
Directions
Melt butter on Sauté and fry garlic for 1 minute. Add the chicken and stir-fry until golden.
Season with salt and pepper. Add broccoli and cream and pour in chicken broth. Seal the lid, and cook for 10 minutes on High pressure. Once ready, quick release the pressure.
Nutrition Values: Calories 432, Protein 13g, Net Carbs 5.5g, Fat 42g

301. Simple Chicken Wings
Cooking Time: 20 minutes
Servings: 4
Ingredients
2 lb Chicken wings
1 cup BBQ sauce
Directions
Put the chicken wings in the Instant pot and cover them with the BBQ sauce. Seal the lid and cook on High pressure for 20 minutes. When ready, do a quick release.

Nutrition Values: Calories 305, Protein 51g, Net Carbs 3.3g, Fat 9g

302. Asian-Style Chicken Thighs
Cooking Time: 20 minutes
Servings: 4
Ingredients
1 tsp Olive oil
1 lb Chicken thighs
1 Onion, chopped
2 tsp Ginger, minced
2 tsp Garlic, minced
2 ½ cups Chicken broth
½ cup sugar-free Ketchup
2 tsp Wine Vinegar
Directions
Heat oil on Sauté. Cook ginger and garlic for 1 minute. Add the chicken thighs and cook for 10 minutes. Add onion and chicken broth, seal the lid and press Manual.
Cook for 10 minutes on High pressure. Meanwhile, mix ketchup, mirin and wine vinegar in a bowl. When the pot beeps, quick-release the pressure. Serve hot with the sauce.
Nutrition Values: Calories 276, Protein 19g, Net Carbs 2.6g, Fat 21g

303. Chicken with Sesame oil
Cooking Time: 20 minutes
Servings: 3
Ingredients
1 tsp flaxseed meal
2 egg whites
1 lb Chicken, sliced
½ cup Water
1 tsp soy sauce
1 tsp sesame oil
1 tsp Wine Vinegar
1 tsp Ginger, grated
2 tsp Garlic cloves, minced
Salt and Pepper, to taste
Directions
Mix flaxseed meal and egg whites, in a bowl. Add the mixture into the instant pot. Stir in the chicken, soy sauce, sesame oil, vinegar, ginger, garlic, water, salt and pepper.
Seal the lid, press Manual and cook for 20 minutes on High. When ready, release the pressure quickly.
Nutrition Values: Calories 214, Protein 33g, Net Carbs 2.5g, Fat 7.4g

304. Hot Garlic Chicken Breasts
Cooking Time: 35 minutes
Servings: 4
Ingredients
2 Chicken breasts
2 tbsp Apple Cider Vinegar
1 cup Tomato Ketchup
1 tsp Garlic powder
¼ tsp salt
½ tsp Chili powder
3 tbsp Olive oil
Directions
Combine vinegar, ketchup, chili powder, salt, and garlic powder, in a bowl. Drizzle over the chicken and toss well. Set the Instant Pot on Sauté mode and heat the oil.
Transfer the chicken breasts to the pot. Cook for 25 minutes, turning multiple times until well cooked.

Nutrition Values: Calories 254, Protein 23g, Net Carbs 1.2g, Fat 19g

305. Chicken Tenders with Garlic
Cooking Time: 15 minutes
Servings: 2
Ingredients
1 lb Chicken tenders
2 Garlic cloves, minced
2 tsp Paprika
2 tsp Oregano powder
2 tsp Olive oil
1 Onion, chopped
2 cups green Beans, frozen
1 cup Almond flour
1 cup Chicken stock
1 Egg, raw
Salt and Pepper, to taste
Directions
Mix chicken tenders, garlic, paprika, oregano, onion, green beans, flour and chicken stock, in a bowl. Add egg, and stir well. Season with salt and pepper. Seal the lid, press the Manual and cook for 10 minutes on High pressure. When ready, release the pressure quickly and serve hot.
Nutrition Values: Calories 436, Protein 53g, Net Carbs 9.1g, Fat 18g

306. Tropic Shredded Chicken
Cooking Time: 30 minutes
Servings: 4
Ingredients
3 Chicken breasts, shredded, boiled
½ tsp Garlic paste
½ tsp salt
½ tsp soy sauce
2 tbsp Barbecue sauce
½ tsp Chili powder
2 tbsp Olive oil
Directions
Heat oil on Sauté mode and fry garlic for a minute. Add chicken breasts and brown until lightly golden. Add soy sauce, barbecue sauce, salt, and chili powder and fry well. Serve with mashed cauliflower and green salad.
Nutrition Values: Calories 487, Protein 53g, Net Carbs 4.5g, Fat 28g

307. Hot Butter Chicken
Cooking Time: 40 minutes
Servings: 4
Ingredients
¼ lb Chicken, Boneless, pieces
1 cup Tomato puree
1-inch Ginger slice
1-2 red Chilies, diced
½ tsp Garlic paste
1 tsp salt
¼ tsp black Pepper
4 tbsp Butter
Directions
In a blender, add tomato puree, chilies, ginger, garlic, salt, and pepper and blend well. Melt butter on Sauté mode and fry the chicken for 5-10 minute. Transfer the tomato mixture and combine. Simmer for 10-15 minutes until the chicken tenders.
Nutrition Values: Calories 154, Protein 10g, Net Carbs 4.3g, Fat 9.4g

MEAT

308. Cheesy Pork Chops
Cooking Time: 55 Minutes
Servings: 5
Ingredients:
5 pork chops; boneless
1/2 cup cottage cheese
2 garlic cloves; crushed
1 onion; finely chopped.
4 tablespoon olive oil
1/2 cup diced canned tomatoes; sugar-free
3-ounce prosciutto
2 tablespoon balsamic vinegar
1 teaspoon dried basil
1/2 teaspoon black pepper; freshly ground.
1 teaspoon salt
Directions:
Rinse well the meat and pat dry with a kitchen towel. Place on a cutting board and remove the bones. Rub well with some olive oil, salt, pepper, and basil. Let it sit for 15 minutes
Plug in the instant pot and position a trivet at the bottom of the inner pot. Pour in one cup of water and set aside
Transfer the meat into a small baking pan. Drizzle with some more olive oil and add cheese and prosciutto. Loosely cover with aluminum foil and place in the pot.
Press the *Manual* button and set the steam release handle. Set the timer for 20 minutes on high pressure
When done, perform a quick pressure release and open the lid. Remove the pan and set aside
Now press the *Saute* button and grease the inner pot with some oil. Add onions and cook until translucent. Pour in tomatoes and cook for 10-12 minutes, stirring occasionally. Optionally, season with some more salt or dried basil
Remove from the pot and drizzle over meat. Serve and enjoy.
Nutrition Info: Calories: 416; Total Fats: 19g; Net Carbs: 3.6g; Protein: 54.6g; Fiber: 0.7g

309. Portobello Pork Butt Recipe
Cooking Time: 45 Minutes
Servings: 2
Ingredients:
1-pound pork butt
1/2 cup dried shiitake
4 tablespoon soy sauce
2 garlic cloves; crushed
1 cup Portobello mushrooms; sliced
3 tablespoon oil
2 tablespoon apple cider vinegar
1 teaspoon turmeric powder
2 teaspoon stevia powder
1 teaspoon salt
Directions:
Place the meat on a cutting board and cut 2-inch long strips, Set aside.
Place shiitake in a bowl and pour in enough water to cover. Soak for 10-15 minutes. Drain and set aside

Plug in the instant pot and heat the oil. Add the meat and season with salt, turmeric, and stevia. Stir well and cook for 10 minutes.
Stir in Portobello mushrooms, soaked shiitake, and garlic. Continue to cook for 7-8 minutes, stirring constantly
Finally, pour in the soy sauce and give it a good stir. Continue to cook for another 5 minutes. If necessary, add about 2-3 tablespoons of water. Press the *Cancel'* button and serve immediately.
Nutrition Info: Calories: 545; Total Fats: 28.4g; Net Carbs: 6.1g; Protein: 62.4g; Fiber: 0.8g

310. Ground Pork Burgers
Cooking Time: 15 Minutes
Servings: 6
Ingredients:
1-pound ground pork
2 onions
3 tablespoon almond flour
1/2 cup fresh parsley; finely chopped
1 red chili pepper
1/4 teaspoon black pepper; freshly ground.
1/4 teaspoon garlic powder
1/2 teaspoon salt
Directions:
Place the onions and chili pepper in a food processor and process for 30 seconds. Transfer to a bowl and add the meat. Sprinkle with parsley, almond flour, and spices
Mix well and shape burgers, about 2-inch in diameter. Place burgers in the steam basket and pour in one cup of water in the inner pot.
Seal the lid and set the steam release handle to the *Sealing* position. Press the *Manual* button and set the timer for 7 minutes on high pressure
When done, perform a quick pressure release and open the lid. Remove burgers from the pot and serve immediately.
Nutrition Info: Calories: 198; Total Fats: 4.9g; Net Carbs: 4.4g; Protein: 30.9g; Fiber: 1.7g

311. Sweet Coconut Pork
Cooking Time: 1 hour
Servings: 6
Ingredients:
4 pork chops; with bones
1 chili pepper; finely chopped
1 large onion; finely chopped.
3 tablespoon almond flour
2 tablespoon butter
1/4 cup coconut milk
2 tablespoon coconut cream
1 cup cauliflower; chopped into florets
1 cup heavy cream
1/2 teaspoon white pepper; freshly ground.
1 teaspoon rum extract
2 teaspoon stevia powder
1 teaspoon salt
Directions:
In a medium-sized bowl, combine heavy cream, coconut milk, coconut cream, salt, pepper, stevia, and rum. Add the meat and coat well with the mixture.

Transfer to a large Ziploc bag. Seal the bag and refrigerate overnight.
Plug in the instant pot and set the trivet at the bottom of the inner pot. Remove the pork from the refrigerator and place in a deep oven-safe bowl along with the marinade
Place the bowl in the pot and pour in about one cup of water in the inner pot. Seal the lid and set the steam release handle to the *Sealing* posisiton. Press the *Manual* button and set the timer for 20 minutes on high pressure
When done, perform a quick pressure release and open the lid. Remove the bowl with the pork and press the *Saute* button
Grease the inner pot with butter and heat up. Add onions, peppers, and cauliflower. Stir well and cook for 6-7 minutes.
Now add the pork along with its sauce and stir in almond flour. Continue to cook for another 3-4 minutes, coating the meat well with the sauce. Press the *Cancel'* button and serve immediately
Nutrition Info: Calories: 462; Total Fats: 24.6g; Net Carbs: 7.9g; Protein: 49.4g; Fiber: 1.6g

312. Pork Shoulder Recipe
Cooking Time: 40 Minutes
Servings: 4
Ingredients:
2 -pounds pork shoulder roast
2 shallots; sliced
4 garlic cloves; crushed
3 tablespoon olive oil
3 tablespoon Dijon mustard
1 tablespoon fresh rosemary; finely chopped
1/2 teaspoon white pepper; freshly ground
1 teaspoon salt
Directions:
Rinse well the meat and sprinkle with salt and pepper, Set aside.
Take a round oven-safe bowl and coat with olive oil. Make a layer with shallots and sprinkle with garlic and fresh rosemary
Place the meat on top and generously brush with Dijon mustard. Loosely cover with aluminum foil and set aside
Plug in the instant pot and set the trivet in the inner pot. Pour in one cup of water and place the bowl on the trivet.
Seal the lid and set the steam release handle to the *Sealing* position and press the *Manual* button. Set the timer for 25 minutes on high pressure
When done; release the pressure naturally and open the lid. Remove the bowl from the pot and chill for a while. Serve and enjoy.
Nutrition Info: Calories: 430; Total Fats: 19g; Net Carbs: 2g; Protein: 60.2g; Fiber: 0.5g

313. Meatloaf Recipe
Cooking Time: 70 Minutes
Servings: 6
Ingredients:
2 -pounds ground pork
2 small onions; finely chopped.
2 spring onions; finely chopped
1 cup almond flour
1/2 cup celery stalk; finely chopped.
3 garlic cloves; crushed
2 tablespoon butter
3 tablespoon olive oil
1 cup cherry tomatoes; chopped
2 teaspoon dried celery
1/2 teaspoon white pepper; ground.
1 teaspoon salt
Directions:
In a large bowl, combine the ground pork with onions, spring onions, celery stalk, and garlic. Sprinkle with salt, celery, and pepper
Now add about one cup of almond flour and mix well agan. Optionally, add a handful of finely chopped almonds for a crunchy taste.
Transfer the mixture to a large piece of plastic foil and wrap tightly Refrigerate for 30 minutes. Meanwhile, place cherry tomatoes in a food processor and process until smooth. Add olive oil and mix well. Set aside.
Remove the meat from the refrigerator and place back in the mixing bowl. Add tomatoes and butter. Mix well again and shape the meatloaf using a large piece of plastic foil. Place in a baking dish and loosely cover with aluminum foil
Plug in the instant pot and set the trivet at the bottom of the inner pot. Pour in one cup of water and place the baking dish on top
Seal the lid and set the steam release handle to the *Sealing* position. Press the *Manual* button and set the timer for 20 minutes on high pressure.
When done, perform a quick pressure release and open the lid. Remove the pan from the pot and chill for a while. Serve and enjoy!
Nutrition Info: Calories: 358; Total Fats: 18.5g; Net Carbs: 3.8g; Protein: 41.4g; Fiber: 1.7g

314. Mushroom Pork Recipe
Cooking Time: 40 Minutes
Servings: 4
Ingredients:
1-pound pork fillet; sliced into half-inch thick slices
1 cup tomato sauce; sugar-free
2 garlic cloves; crushed
1 small chili pepper; chopped
1 cup mushrooms; sliced
1 small onion; finely chopped
3 tablespoon oil
3 tablespoon balsamic vinegar
1/2 teaspoon red pepper flakes
1 teaspoon smoked paprika
1/4 teaspoon black pepper; freshly ground.
2 teaspoon dried celery
1/2 teaspoon salt
Directions:
Remove the fillets from the fridge about 20 minutes before cooking. Sprinkle with salt and pepper and set aside.
Plug in the instant pot and heat up the oil. Add fillets and briefly brown on both sides, for 2-3 minutes. Remove from the pot and set aside
Now add onions and mushrooms. Sprinkle with salt, pepper, and celery. Cook for 5-6 minutes and then

add balsamic vinegar, chili, tomato, and garlic. Sprinkle with red pepper flakes and smoked paprika. Continue to cook for 1-2 minutes and add the meat. Coat the meat with the sauce and continue to cook for another 10-12 minutes.
When done, press the *Cancel'* button and remove form the pot. Optionally, sprinkle with some grated Parmesan cheese and serve immediately.
Nutrition Info: Calories: 385; Total Fats: 24.8g; Net Carbs: 4.6g; Protein: 33.2g; Fiber: 1.6g

315. Pork Loin with Leeks Recipe
Cooking Time: 45 Minutes
Servings: 4
Ingredients:
1-pound pork loin; boneless
2 large leeks; chopped.
2 cups beef broth
1 celery stalk; chopped
1 onion; finely chopped.
1/4 cup apple cider vinegar
4 tablespoon olive oil
1/4 teaspoon dried thyme
1/4 teaspoon chili powder
2 teaspoon dried celery
2 tablespoon stevia crystal (or powder
1 ½ teaspoon sea salt
Directions:
Rub the meat with salt and place in the pot. Pour in enough water to cover and seal the lid
Set the steam release handle and press the *Manual* button. Set the timer for 25 minutes on high pressure
When done; perform a quick pressure release and open the lid. Transfer the meat to a bowl and remove the water, Set aside
Press the *Saute* button and heat up the oil. Add onions, leeks, and celery. Give it a good stir and cook for 3-4 minutes.
Meanwhile, place the meat on a cutting board and chop into bite-sized pieces. Add to the pot and stir well. Drizzle with apple cider vinegar and season with spices
Brown for 4-5 minutes, stirring occasionally Press the *Cancel'* button and serve immediately.
Nutrition Info: Calories: 456; Total Fats: 30.6g; Net Carbs: 8.1g; Protein: 34.4g; Fiber: 1.5g

316. Classic Pork Ribs
Cooking Time: 30 Minutes
Servings: 5
Ingredients:
2 -pounds pork ribs
1 cup portobello mushrooms; chopped.
2 tablespoon hot chili sauce; sugar-free
2 garlic cloves; whole
1 teaspoon apple cider vinegar
1 cup cauliflower; chopped into florets
1 cup tomatoes; diced
3 tablespoon butter
5 cups beef broth
2 celery stalks; chopped
2 red bell peppers; chopped.
1/2 cup onions; finely chopped
1 teaspoon dried celery
2 teaspoon onion powder
1/2 teaspoon black pepper; freshly ground.
2 teaspoon salt
Directions:
Place the ribs in the pot and pour in enough water to cover. Add celery stalks and seal the lid. Set the steam release handle to the *Sealing* position and press the *Meat* button
Set the timer for 15 minutes on high pressure
When done, perform a quick pressure release and open the lid.
Now stir in the remaining ingredients and sprinkle with salt, pepper, celery, and onion powder. Stir all well and seal the lid again.
Set the steam release handle to the *Sealing* position and continue to cook for another 7 minutes.
When done, perform a quick pressure release and open the lid. Serve hot and enjoy!
Nutrition Info: Calories: 633; Total Fats: 40.7g; Net Carbs: 7.1g; Protein: 54.9g; Fiber: 2.1g

317. Steamed Pork Neck Recipe
Cooking Time: 40 Minutes
Servings: 3
Ingredients:
1-pound pork neck; cut into 3 pieces
2 cups cauliflower florets
4 tablespoon olive oil
3 tablespoon apple cider vinegar
3 garlic cloves; crushed
1 tablespoon dried celery
1 tablespoon cayenne pepper
1 teaspoon white pepper; freshly ground.
2 teaspoon sea salt
Directions:
Rinse the meat under cold running water and place on a cutting board. Using a sharp cutting knife, cut into 3 equal pieces. Rub each piece with salt, white pepper, cayenne pepper, and celery, Set aside
Grease a small round baking pan with oil and add cauliflower. Top with pork and sprinkle with apple cider vinegar.
Plug in the instant pot and position a trivet at the bottom of the inner pot. Place the baking pan on the trivet and pour in 2 cups of water in the inner pot. Seal the lid and set the steam release handle to the *Sealing* position. Press the *Manual* button and set the timer for 25 minutes on high pressure
When done; perform a quick pressure release and open the lid.
Remove the baking pan from the pot and chill for a while. Serve with some Greek yogurt or cottage cheese
Nutrition Info: Calories: 401; Total Fats: 24.1g; Net Carbs: 3g; Protein: 41.1g; Fiber: 1.7g

318. Slow Cooked Pork
Cooking Time: 8 hours
Servings: 6
Ingredients:
2 -pounds pork butt; chopped into smaller pieces
2 large leeks; chopped into 2-inch long pieces
5 cups beef broth
1 green bell pepper; sliced

1 cup cherry tomatoes; sliced
4 tablespoon olive oil
2 teaspoon cayenne pepper
3 bay leaves
1/2 teaspoon black pepper; freshly ground.
1 teaspoon salt
Directions:
Combine the ingredients in the pot and seal the lid
Set the steam release handle to the *Sealing* position and press the *Slow Cook* button
Set the timer for 8 hours on low pressure
When done, release the pressure naturally for 10-15 minutes and then move the pressure valve to release the remaining pressure
Carefully open the lid and serve immediately. Optionally, sprinkle with some Parmesan before serving
Nutrition Info: Calories: 434; Total Fats: 20.8g; Net Carbs: 6.4g; Protein: 52g; Fiber: 1.2g

319. Pork Neck with Soy Sauce and Sesame Seeds
Cooking Time: 45 Minutes
Servings: 4
Ingredients:
1-pound pork neck; chopped into bite-sized pieces
1 large onion; finely chopped
1/2 cup dark soy sauce
1/2 cup canned tomatoes; sugar-free
3 tablespoon sesame seeds
3 tablespoon oil
4 garlic cloves; whole
1/2 teaspoon ginger powder
2 teaspoon stevia powder
1 teaspoon salt
Directions:
Plug in the instant pot and press the *Saute* button. Grease the inner pot with oil and heat up. Add onions and cook until translucent.
Now add garlic and chopped meat. Pour in about 1/4 cup of water and cook for 20 minutes, stirring occasionally.
Finally, add tomatoes, soy sauce, and sesame seeds. Season with salt, ginger powder, and stevia powder. Give it a good stir and continue to cook for 10 minutes
Press the *Cancel'* button and serve immediately
Optionally, sprinkle with some freshly chopped parsley or spring onions
Nutrition Info: Calories: 328; Total Fats: 17.6g; Net Carbs: 8.3g; Protein: 31.8g; Fiber: 1.9g

320. Sweet Pork Ribs
Cooking Time: 45 Minutes
Servings: 5
Ingredients:
2 -pounds pork ribs; chopped
1 celery stalk; chopped.
2 red bell peppers; sliced
1 green bell pepper; sliced
1/4 cup soy sauce
1 tablespoon apple cider
1 tablespoon almond flour
3 tablespoon oil

1/2 teaspoon dried basil
1 rosemary sprig; fresh
1 bay leaf
1 teaspoon salt
Directions:
Place the ribs in the pot and pour in enough water to cover. Sprinkle with salt, add basil, bay leaf, and rosemary. Seal the lid.
Set the steam release handle to the *Sealing* position and press the *Manual* button. Cook for 25 minutes on high pressure
When done; release the pressure naturally and open the lid. Remove the ribs from the pot and chill for a while.
Grease the inner pot with oil and press the *Saute* button. Add bell peppers and celery stalks. Sauté for 5-6 minutes, stirring constantly
Rub the ribs with soy sauce and add to the pot. Pour in the remaining soy sauce and about 1/4 cup of water.
Stir in the almond flour and simmer for 4-5 minutes. Press the *Cancel'* button and serve immediately.
Nutrition Info: Calories: 367; Total Fats: 15g; Net Carbs: 5.8g; Protein: 49.1g; Fiber: 1.2g

321. Pork Steak in Mushroom Sauce Recipe
Cooking Time: 30 Minutes
Servings: 4
Ingredients:
4 pork steaks (about 8oz each
4 cups beef broth
1 celery stalk; chopped.
1/2 cup celery leaves; whole
1/4 cup apple cider vinegar
1 small onion; roughly chopped
1 cup button mushrooms; sliced
3 tablespoon butter
2 cups heavy cream
1/4 cup cottage cheese
1/4 cup crumbled feta cheese
3 tablespoon Parmesan; grated
1 tablespoon peppercorn
1 thyme sprig; fresh
2 bay leaves
2 teaspoon salt
Directions:
Rinse the meat under cold running water and place at the bottom of the instant pot. Pour in the broth and apple cider. Add salt, peppercorn, by leaves, thyme sprig, onion, celery stalk, and celery leaves. Seal the lid and set the steam release handle
Press the *Meat* button and cook for 15 minutes. When done, perform a quick pressure release and open the lid. Remove the meat along with the broth from the pot and set aside
Now press the *Saute* button and grease the inner pot with butter. Add pre-cooked onions from the broth and give it a good stir. Season with salt and add mushrooms.
Cook for 5-6 minutes and then add the cheese and heavy cream. Give it a good stir and remove from the pot. Drizzle over the meat and serve.

Nutrition Info: Calories: 721; Total Fats: 44g; Net Carbs: 5.6g; Protein: 71.8g; Fiber: 0.6g

322. Garlic Pork Recipe
Cooking Time: 45 Minutes
Servings: 6
Ingredients:
2 -pounds pork chops
1 cup cherry tomatoes
1/4 cup soy sauce
2 large onions; finely chopped
4 garlic cloves
3 tablespoon butter
1/2 cup celery stalks; chopped
3 tablespoon apple cider vinegar
1/2 teaspoon ginger powder
2 tablespoon stevia crystal
1/2 teaspoon chili flakes
1 teaspoon salt
Directions:
Rinse well the meat and pat dry each piece with some kitchen paper. Place on a large cutting board and remove the bones. Chop into bite-sized pieces and place in a deep bowl. Sprinkle with salt, ginger, and chili flakes. Drizzle with soy sauce and set aside.
Plug in the instant pot and press the *Saute* button. Grease the inner pot with butter and heat up. Add onions, garlic, and celery stalks. Cook for 3-4 minutes, stirring constantly. Now add cherry tomatoes and sprinkle with stevia. Continue to cook for 5 minutes or until soft.
Finally, add the meat and drizzle with apple cider vinegar. Stir fry for another 4-5 minutes and then pour in one cup of water.
Press the *Cancel'* button and seal the lid. Set the steam release handle to the *Sealing* position and press the *Manual* button
Set the timer for 10 minutes on high pressure. When done, release the pressure naturally and open the lid. Optionally, sprinkle with freshly chopped parsley and serve immediately.
Nutrition Info: Calories: 569; Total Fats: 43.5g; Net Carbs: 5.3g; Protein: 35.6g; Fiber: 1.7g

323. Thai Style Pork with White Pepper Gravy
Cooking Time: 15 Minutes
Servings: 2
Ingredients:
10-ounce pork fillet; cut into strips
1 small onion; sliced
2 tablespoon fish sauce
1 cup dried black mushrooms; chopped
3 garlic cloves
2 tablespoon oyster sauce
3 tablespoon peanut oil
2 spring onion; chopped.
1 teaspoon white pepper; freshly ground.
1/2 teaspoon sea salt
Directions:
Soak the mushrooms about 10-15 minutes before cooking
Plug in the instant pot and heat the oil. Add sliced pork, onions, and garlic. Cook 1-2 minutes and then add spring onions. Continue to cook for another 2-3 minutes, stirring constantly
Now add mushrooms and give it a good stir. Drizzle with fish sauce and oyster sauce. Continue to cook for 2-3 minutes, stirring constantly.
Sprinkle with white pepper and pour in about 1/4 cup of water. Gently simmer for 10 minutes, Press the *Cancel'* button and serve immediately.
Nutrition Info: Calories: 423; Total Fats: 25.4g; Net Carbs: 6.5g; Protein: 40.1g; Fiber: 1.6g

324. Pork with Cauliflower
Cooking Time: 40 Minutes
Servings: 6
Ingredients:
2 -pounds pork shoulder; cut into bite-sized pieces
2 cups cauliflower; cut into florets
5 bacon slices; chopped.
1 small onion; finely chopped.
2 celery stalks; chopped
4 tablespoon olive oil
4 cups beef broth
1 teaspoon onion powder
2 teaspoon peppercorn
1/4 cup stevia crystal
1/2 teaspoon garlic powder
1 ½ teaspoon salt
Directions:
Grease the bottom of the instant pot with oil and make the first layer with meat. Season with some salt and then add onions and celery stalks. Optionally, sprinkle with some more salt and add cauliflower. Top with bacon and gently pour in the broth.
Seal the lid and set the steam release handle to the *Sealing* position. Press the *Manual* button and set the timer for 15 minutes on high pressure.
When done, release the pressure naturally and open the lid. Remove the meat and vegetables from the pot but keep the broth
Now press the *Saute* button and add stevia crystal, some more salt, peppercorn, onion powder, and garlic powder.
Gently simmer until the liquid has reduced in half Remove the peppercorn from the pot and add the meat. Coat well with the sauce and serve with cauliflower. Drizzle with some more sweet sauce before serving
Nutrition Info: Calories: 647; Total Fats: 49.2g; Net Carbs: 2.7g; Protein: 45.1g; Fiber: 1.2g

325. Pork Chops with Onions
Cooking Time: 55 Minutes
Servings: 4
Ingredients:
4 pork chops; about 1-inch thick
2 large onions; chopped
4 garlic cloves; whole
3 tablespoon balsamic vinegar
3 tablespoon butter
2 tablespoon olive oil
1 teaspoon dried thyme
1 teaspoon salt
Directions:
Rub the meat with spices and set aside.

Grease a fitting baking pan with oil and place chops along with onions and whole garlic cloves. Drizzle with some more oil and tightly wrap with aluminum foil.
Plug in the instant pot and pour in two cups of water. Set the trivet at the bottom of the inner pot and place the pan on top.
Seal the lid and set the steam release handle. Press the *Manual* button and cook for 35 minutes on high pressure
When done; perform a quick pressure release. Carefully open the lid and remove the baking pan with pork.
Remove the trivet and the remaining water from the pot and press the *Saute* button
Grease the inner pot with butter and heat up. Add balsamic vinegar and briefly cook – for 1 minute.
Now add onions from the baking pan and give it a good stir. Cook for another minute and finally add the meat.
Brown for 2-3 minute on each side. When done, remove from the pot and serve immediately.
Nutrition Info: Calories: 429; Total Fats: 35.6g; Net Carbs: 6.4g; Protein: 19.1g; Fiber: 1.7g

326. Pork Curry
Cooking Time: 25 Minutes
Servings: 4
Ingredients:
1-pound pork neck; cut into thin strips
2 small onions; sliced
1 spring onion; chopped.
1 tablespoon rice vinegar
2 teaspoon sesame oil
1/4 cup olive oil
1 garlic clove; crushed
2 teaspoon curry powder
1 teaspoon fresh ginger; grated
1/2 teaspoon salt
Directions:
Plug in the instant pot and heat up the oil. Add the meat and cook for 4-5 mintues. Remove from the pot and set aside.
Now add onions, garlic, and spring onions. Sauté for 3-4 minuts, stirring constantly
Stir in ginger and garlic powder. Add the emat and season with salt. Cook for 2 more minutes
Press the *Cancel'* button. Remove the meat with the curry sauce from the pot and sprinkle with sesame oil before serving.
Nutrition Info: Calories: 540; Total Fats: 34.8g; Net Carbs: 4.1g; Protein: 48.7g; Fiber: 4.1g

327. Asian Pork Strips
Cooking Time: 55 Minutes
Servings: 4
Ingredients:
1-pound pork neck; cut into 2-inch long strips
1/2 cup canned bamboo; chopped.
2 red bell peppers; sliced into strips
2 tablespoon dark soy sauce
1 spring onion; finely chopped.
2 tablespoon light soy sauce
1 tablespoon rice vinegar
1-egg
3 tablespoon vegetable oil
1/2 teaspoon stevia powder
1/2 teaspoon salt
Directions:
Rinse the meat and place on a large cutting board. Using a sharp knife, cut into strips and place in a deep bowl. Add one egg, salt, and soy sauce. Cover with a lid and set it sit for 10-15 minutes
Plug in the instant pot and press the *Saute* button. Add half of the meat and cook for 6-7 minutes, stirring constantly. Repeat with the remaining meat and remove from the pot, Set aside.
Now; grease the inner pot with oil and heat up. Add bamboo and sliced bell peppers. Cook for 7-8 minutes, stirring constantly
Sprinkle with stevia and rice vinegar and add the meat. Give it a good stir and add onions
Continue to cook for another 2-3 minutes. Press the *Cancel'* button and serve immediately
Nutrition Info: Calories: 302; Total Fats: 15.5g; Net Carbs: 5.3g; Protein: 33g; Fiber: 1.3g

328. Marinated Pork Recipe
Cooking Time: 20 Minutes
Servings: 3
Ingredients:
1-pound pork butt; sliced
1 celery stalk; finely chopped.
1/2 cup sun-dried tomatoes
2 small onions; finely chopped
4 garlic cloves; whole
2 tablespoon lemon juice
2 tablespoon fresh parsley; finely chopped
1 cup olive oil
1/4 cup apple cider vinegar
1 teaspoon white pepper; freshly ground.
2 bay leaves
2 teaspoon fresh rosemary; finely chopped.
1 teaspoon chili pepper
2 teaspoon salt
Directions:
In a medium-sized bowl, combine olive oil, cider, chopped onions, garlic, celery, tomatoes, lemon juice, and parsley. Season with rosemary, chili pepper, salt, white pepper, and bay leaves.
Mix well and submerge the meat into this mixture. Tightly wrap with aluminum foil and marinate overnight.
Plug in the instant pot and position the trivet at the bottom of the inner pot. Place the meat directly on the trivet and drizzle with some of the marinade.
Seal the lid and set the steam release handle to the *Sealing* position
Press the *Manual* button and cook for 15 minutes on high pressure
When done, perform a quick pressure release and open the lid. Remove the meat from the pot and drizzle with some more marinade before serving
Nutrition Info: Calories: 381; Total Fats: 22.3g; Net Carbs: 3.1g; Protein: 40.3g; Fiber: 0.9g

329. Mushroom and Pepper Pork
Cooking Time: 40 Minutes

Servings: 4
Ingredients:
1-pound pork loin; cut into bite-sized pieces
1 cup button mushrooms; sliced
1 garlic clove; crushed
1/2 cup sun-dried tomatoes
2 red bell peppers; sliced
3 tablespoon olive oil
2 cups beef broth
1/2 teaspoon dried oregano
1/4 teaspoon black pepper; freshly ground.
1/2 teaspoon salt
Directions:
Rinse the meat and place on a cutting board. Chop into bite-sized pieces and set aside
Plug in the instant pot and press the *Saute* button. Grease the inner pot with oil and heat up. Add peppers and garlic. Cook for 4-5 minutes and then add the pork.
Brown on all sides for a couple of minutes, stirring constantly
Now season with salt, pepper, and oregano. Add mushrooms, tomatoes, and pour in the broth. Stir well and seal the lid.
Set the steam release handle to the *Sealing* position and press the *Manual* button. Set the timer for 15 minutes on high pressure
When done; release the pressure naturally for 15-20 minutes before serving
Nutrition Info: Calories: 299; Total Fats: 15.4g; Net Carbs: 5.4g; Protein: 33.5g; Fiber: 1.3g

330. Pork Shoulder with Sweet Potatoes
Cooking Time: 30 Minutes
Servings: 5
Ingredients:
2 -pounds pork shoulder; cut into bite-sized pieces
1 cup purple cabbage; shredded
4 garlic cloves; whole
1 celery stalk; chopped.
1 cup cauliflower; chopped into florets
2 chili peppers; sliced
1 large sweet potato; chopped into bite-sized chunks
4 tablespoon butter
2 bay leaves; whole
1 teaspoon white pepper; freshly ground.
1 teaspoon dried thyme
2 teaspoon salt
Directions:
Place the meat in the pot and pour in enough water to cover. Seal the lid and set the steam release handle. Press the *Meat* button
When done; perform a quick pressure release and open the lid
Now add the remaining ingredients and optionally pour in one more cup of water. Stir well and season with salt, pepper, thyme, and bay leaves
Seal the lid again and set the steam release handle to the *Sealing* position. Press the *Manual* button and set the timer for 7 minutes on high pressure.
When you hear the cooker's end signal, release the pressure naturally for 10-15 minutes and then carefully open the lid. Serve and enjoy.

Nutrition Info: Calories: 657; Total Fats: 48.1g; Net Carbs: 8.2g; Protein: 43.8g; Fiber: 2.2g

331. Keto Pork Fillets
Cooking Time: 30 Minutes
Servings: 4
Ingredients:
1-pound pork fillet; central cut
1 green bell pepper; finely chopped.
1 small chili pepper
2 tablespoon balsamic vinegar
1 pickle; sliced
2 boiled eggs
1/4 cup fresh parsley; finely chopped
3 tablespoon butter
2 small onions; finely chopped.
3 bacon slices; chopped.
2-ounce prosciutto
1 teaspoon smoked pepper
Directions:
Plug in the instant pot and press the *Saute* button. Heat the butter and add onions, bacon, prosciutto, bell pepper, and chili pepper
Cook for 3-4 minutes, stirring constantly and then add pickle and season with smoked pepper. Drizzle with balsamic vinegar and continue to cook for one minute.
Now add the fillets and pour in 1/2 cup of water. Simmer for 10-15 minutes, turning a couple of times. When done; press the *Cancel'* button. Transfer the fillets to serving plates and top with sliced eggs. Serve with the sauce from the pot
Nutrition Info: Calories: 396; Total Fats: 21.7g; Net Carbs: 5.4g; Protein: 41.7g; Fiber: 1.5g

332. Pork in Tomato Sauce
Cooking Time: 20 Minutes
Servings: 4
Ingredients:
1-pound pork loin; chopped.
2 cups cherry tomatoes; finely chopped
1 cup broccoli; finely chopped
1 large onion; finely chopped.
1/4 cup olive oil
1/2 teaspoon black pepper; freshly ground.
1/4 teaspoon chili powder
1 rosemary sprig; fresh
1 teaspoon salt
Directions:
Rinse well the meat and sprinkle with salt and pepper. Place in the pot and drizzle with oil. Pour in the broth and add onions, broccoli, and tomatoes. Season with come chili powder and add rosemary. Stir well and seal the lid. Set the steam release handle to the *Sealing* position and press the *Stew* button. When done; release the pressure naturally and open the lid.
Remove the rosemary sprig and optionally sprinkle with some more chili pepper.
Nutrition Info: Calories: 421; Total Fats: 28.1g; Net Carbs: 6g; Protein: 32.8g; Fiber: 2.5g

333. Pork Leg Roast Recipe
Cooking Time: 55 Minutes
Servings: 6

Ingredients:
3 -pounds pork leg
2 spring onions; finely chopped
2 tablespoon mustard
3 tablespoon soy sauce
4 tablespoon olive oil
1 teaspoon coriander seeds
1/2 teaspoon dried sage
1/2 teaspoon dried rosemary
2 bay leaves
1 teaspoon white peppercorn
Directions:
Grease the inner pot with two tablespoons of olive oil and press the *Saute* button. Heat up and add spring onions and coriander seeds. Cook for 2-3 minutes and then add the meat.
Pour in 5-6 cups of water and add bay leaves. Seal the lid. Set the steam release handle to the *Sealing* position and press the *Meat* button
Cook for 25 minutes on high pressure.
When done, release the pressure naturally and open the lid. Remove the meat from the pot and chill for a while
Preheat the oven to 450 degrees F. Grease a baking sheet with the remaining oil and set aside
Rub the meat with sage and rosemary and place on a baking sheet. Pour in about one cup of water.
Place in the oven and reduce the heat to 400. Roast for 20 minutes.
Nutrition Info: Calories: 428; Total Fats: 18.4g; Net Carbs: 1.6g; Protein: 60.9g; Fiber: 0.7g

334. Pork Chops and Cabbage
Cooking Time: 20 Minutes
Servings: 5
Ingredients:
4 thick-cut Pork Chops (about ¾-inch or 2 cm.
1 small head of cabbage (about a pound or 500g.
1 tablespoon vegetable oil
1 teaspoon fennel seeds
1 teaspoon salt
1 teaspoon pepper
3/4 cup meat stock
2 teaspoons; flour
Directions:
Unwrap the pork chops and sprinkle with fennel, salt and pepper
Prepare the cabbage by slicing the cabbage in half almost through the core, and then in thick 3/4 inch slices and set aside.
In the pre-heated pressure cooker, on medium-high heat without the lid, add oil, and brown all of the chops on one side only,-only two at a time may fit depending on the size of the pressure cooker base, or the chops
When all of the chops have been browned and set aside, add the cabbage slices into the empty pressure cooker
On top of the cabbage arrange the pork chops brown-side up, overlapping as needed. Pour any juice from the chops and meat stock around the edges.
Close and lock the lid of the pressure cooker. Cook for 8 minutes at high pressure
When time is up, open the pressure cooker with the Normal release-release pressure through the valve Using tongs, move the cabbage and pork chops to a serving platter and tent lightly with foil while preparing the gravy
Bring the left-over juices in the pressure cooker to a boil and whisk-in the flour
Pour thickened sauce on top of cabbage and pork chop platter and serve.
Nutrition Info: Calories: 490; Protein: 42g; Fat: 31g; Carbs: 8g

335. Pork Ribs Recipe
Cooking Time: 45 Minutes
Servings: 6
Ingredients:
2 -pounds pork ribs; chopped
1 large onion; finely chopped.
1 cup sun-dried tomatoes
4 cups beef broth
4 tablespoon butter
2 cups cherry tomatoes; whole
1 teaspoon dried thyme
1/2 teaspoon dried oregano
3 tablespoon stevia or swerve
1/2 teaspoon garlic powder
1 teaspoon sea salt
Directions:
Plug in the instant pot and add ribs. Pour in the broth and seal the lid. Set the steam release handle and press the *Manual* button
Set the timer for 20 minutes on high pressure.
When done, release the pressure naturally and open the lid. Remove the meat along with the broth from the pot and press the *Saute* button
Grease the inner pot with butter and add onions. Sprinkle with some salt and cook until translucent. Now add tomatoes and pour in 2 cups of broth. Sprinkle with the remaining spices and cook until tomatoes have softened. Stir occasionally
When done; press the *Cancel'* button and add the meat. Coat well with the sauce and cover. Let it sit for about 10 minute before serving
Nutrition Info: Calories: 532; Total Fats: 35.6g; Net Carbs: 4.9g; Protein: 44.4g; Fiber: 1.6g

336. Dijon Pork with Turmeric
Cooking Time: 30 Minutes
Servings: 4
Ingredients:
1-pound pork neck; chopped into bite-sized pieces
1 large onion; sliced
1 cup heavy cream
2 tablespoon Dijon mustard
4 tablespoon olive oil
3 cups beef broth
2 teaspoon dried celery
1/2 teaspoon red pepper; freshly ground.
1 teaspoon salt
Directions:
Plug in the instant pot and press the *Saute* button. Grease the inner pot with some oil and add onions. Sauté for 3-4 minutes and then add the meat.

Continue to cook for another 5-6 minutes, stirring occasionally
Season with salt, pepper, and celery and remove from the pot. Transfer to a deep bowl.
In a separate bowl, combine together heavy cream, Dijon mustard, and the remaining olive oil. Stir well and pour over the meat
Place back to the pot and pour in the broth. Stir well and seal the lid.
Set the steam release handle to the *Sealing* position and press the *Manual* button. Set the timer for 15 minutes on high pressure
When done, release the pressure naturally and open the lid. Serve and enjoy.
Nutrition Info: Calories: 435; Total Fats: 30.5g; Net Carbs: 4.3g; Protein: 34.7g; Fiber: 1.1g

337. Quick Pork Chops
Cooking Time: 25 Minutes
Servings: 4
Ingredients:
2 pork chops; 1-inch thick
3 garlic cloves; crushed
4 bacon slices; chopped
2 tablespoon oil
1 cup onions; finely chopped
1/2 teaspoon dried thyme
1 teaspoon black pepper; ground.
1/4 teaspoon garlic powder
1 teaspoon salt
Directions:
Plug in the instant pot and press the *Saute* button. Grease the inner pot with oil and heat up.
Rub the meat with salt, pepper, garlic and thyme, Set aside
Add onions and garlic to the pot. Sauté for 2-3 minutes and then add the bacon. Continue to cook for another 2 minutes, stirring constantly
Now add the seasoned meat and briefly brown for 2 minutes on each side.
Press the *Cancel'* button and pour in one cup of water. Seal the lid and set the steam release handle to the *Sealing* position.
Press the *Manual* button and set the timer for 13 minutes
When done, release the pressure naturally and open the lid
Optionally, brown the meat in a large non-stick skillet over medium-high heat before serving.
Nutrition Info: Calories: 340; Total Fats: 18.8g; Net Carbs: 3g; Protein: 37.2g; Fiber: 0.7g

338. Butterery Pork Chops
Cooking Time: 35 Minutes
Servings: 4
Ingredients:
4 pork chops; with bones
4 tablespoon butter
3 tablespoon almond flour
1 small onion; chopped.
1 cup vegetable stock
1 tablespoon tomato paste
2 tablespoon Dijon mustard
3 garlic cloves; crushed
2 teaspoon smoked paprika
1/2 teaspoon black pepper; freshly ground.
1 teaspoon salt
Directions:
Plug in the instant pot and press the *Saute* button. Grease the inner pot with butter and add onions. Sauté until translucent.
Now add garlic and continue to cook for another 1-2 mintues
Finally, add chops, two at the time, and cook for 2-3 minutes on each side. Remove from the pot and place on a large platter. Brush each piece with Dijon mustard and sprinkle generously with salt, pepper, and paprika.
Place the meat back in the pot and pour in the stock. Stir in tomato paste and seal the lid
Set the steam release handle to the *Sealing* position and press the *Manual* button
Cook for 22 minutes on high pressure.
When done; release the pressure naturally and open the lid. Stir in the almond flour and let it sit, covered, for 10 minutes before serving
Nutrition Info: Calories: 383; Total Fats: 18.9g; Net Carbs: 3g; Protein: 47.2g; Fiber: 1.2g

339. Keto Pork with Eggs
Cooking Time: 20 Minutes
Servings: 4
Ingredients:
7-ounce ground pork
4 large eggs
1 garlic clove; crushed
1 onion; finely chopped.
2 bacon slices; chopped
3 tablespoon butter
1/2 teaspoon pepper; freshly ground.
1/2 teaspoon salt
Directions:
Grease the bottom of the pot with butter and press the *Saute* button. Add onions and briefly cook – for 2-3 minutes.
Now add pork, bacon, and garlic. Season with salt and pepper
Continue to cook for 5 minutes.
Finally, crack the eggs and cook for 2-3 minutes.
Press the *Cancel'* button and serve immediately.
Nutrition Info: Calories: 282; Total Fats: 19.4g; Net Carbs: 2.8g; Protein: 23.2g; Fiber: 0.6g

340. Italian Style Pork Roast
Cooking Time: 45 Minutes
Servings: 4
Ingredients:
1-pound boneless pork loin; chopped into 4 pieces
1 cup olive oil
1 lemon; sliced
1/4 cup apple cider vinegar
2 tablespoon Dijon mustard
3 tablespoon butter
1 teaspoon white pepper; freshly ground
2 teaspoon smoked paprika
1/2 teaspoon dried thyme
1 tablespoon dried rosemary
2 teaspoon garlic powder

2 teaspoon salt
Directions:
In a medium-sized bowl, combine together olive oil, apple cider, Dijon, lemon slices, dried rosemary, garlic powder, smoked paprika, thyme, salt, and pepper. Mix well and add pork
Coat each piece with the mixture and place in a large Ziploc bag, refrigerate overnight.
Plug in the instant pot and pour in one cup of water. Set the trivet at the bottom of the stainless steel insert.
Remove the meat from the refrigerator about 30 minutes before cooking. Place in an oven-safe bowl and drizzle with some of the marinade – about 3 tablespoons
Loosely cover with aluminum foil and seal the lid. Set the steam release handle to the *Sealing* position and press the *Meat* button. Cook for 20 minutes. When done, release the pressure naturally and open the lid
Preheat the oven to 400 degrees. Line some parchment paper over a baking sheet and add the meat.
Generously brush with the marinade and roast for 15 minutes.
When done, remove from the oven and brush with butter. Serve and enjoy.
Nutrition Info: Calories: 351; Total Fats: 25.4g; Net Carbs: 0.2g; Protein: 29.9g; Fiber: 0.1g

341. Spring Onion Pork Recipe
Cooking Time: 30 Minutes
Servings: 2
Ingredients:
14oz pork neck; chopped into bite-sized pieces
1 cup beef stock
3 spring onions; finely chopped
3 tablespoon olive oil
2 tablespoon butter
1 teaspoon peppercorn
1/2 teaspoon black pepper; freshly ground.
2 teaspoon cayenne pepper
1 ½ teaspoon salt
Directions:
Plug in the instant pot and press the *Saute* button. Grease the inner pot with oil and heat up. Add onions and sprinkle with some salt
Cook for 2-3 minutes and then add the meat. Season with pepper, cayenne pepper, and sprinkle with peppercorn.
Cook for 5-6 minutes, stirring constantly. Add butter and pour in the stock.
Seal the lid and set the steam release handle. Press the *Manual* button and set the timer for 12 minutes. When done, release the pressure naturally and open the lid. Serve and enjoy.
Nutrition Info: Calories: 581; Total Fats: 39.8g; Net Carbs: 1.1g; Protein: 53.8g; Fiber: 0.6g

342. Tomato Pork Chops
Cooking Time: 40 Minutes
Servings: 2
Ingredients:
2 pork chops; with bones
1 small onion; finely chopped.
4 tablespoon olive oil
1 green bell pepper; sliced
1 cup cherry tomatoes
1 cup beef broth
1/2 teaspoon white pepper; freshly ground.
1/4 teaspoon garlic powder
1/2 teaspoon salt
Directions:
Place the meat in the pot and season with salt. Pour in the broth and seal the lid. Set the steam release handle to the *Sealing* position and press the *Manual* button
Set the timer for 15 minutes on high pressure. When done, release the pressure naturally and open the lid. Remove the meat from the pot and transfer to a deep bowl, Set aside.
Now; press the *Saute* button and grease the inner pot with olive oil. Heat up and add onions and peppers. Sprinkle with some more salt. Cook for 5-6 minutes and then add cherry tomatoes. Pour in about 1/4 cup of the broth and simmer for 10-12 minutes, stirring occasionally
Season with pepper and garlic powder. Optionally, add some red pepper flakes. Transfer the mixture to a food processor and process until smooth. Drizzle over pork chope and serve immediately.
Nutrition Info: Calories: 633; Total Fats: 37g; Net Carbs: 9.1g; Protein: 63.6g; Fiber: 2.6g

343. Pork Belly Recipe
Cooking Time: 110 Minutes
Servings: 3
Ingredients:
1 pound. pastured pork belly
1/2 cup of broth
1/4 cup sherry
2 tablespoon duck fat (or coconut oil.
1 teaspoon sea salt
1 teaspoon smoked paprika
1 teaspoon thyme
4 cloves of garlic (sliced or chopped.
Directions:
Rub the fatty side of the pork belly with the salt-spice mixture.
Pour the broth and the sherry into the Instant Pot.
Now place the pork belly in the instant pot, spice side up
Close and lock the lid. Set the pressure to *High* and the time to 80 minutes
A few minutes before the time is up, preheat your oven to 400 F. Place a couple tablespoons of duck fat in a cast iron pan. Transfer the pan to the oven to get nice and hot.
When the time is up, use two spatulas to lift the cooked pork belly out of the Instant Pot. It will be very tender and may fall apart if you use tongs.
Remove any large bits of garlic or spice and place the pork belly fat side down in the preheated cast iron pan
If your pork belly has curled, top it with another cast iron pan to weigh it down. Then pop into the preheated oven for 20 minutes, or to your desired crispness

Allow to cool slightly, then gently transfer to a cutting board.
Using a sharp chef's knife, cut into cubes. Sprinkle with a little more sea salt
Nutrition Info: Calories: 340; Protein: 6g; Fat: 33g; Carbs: 2

344. Apple Cider Pork Ribs Recipe
Cooking Time: 55 Minutes
Servings: 5
Ingredients:
2 -pounds pork ribs; cut into smaller pieces
2 celery stalks; chopped.
1/4 cup celery leaves; chopped
1/4 cup light soy sauce
1 onion; finely chopped
2 green bell peppers; sliced
2 eggs; whole
3 tablespoon apple cider vinegar
1/4 cup canned tomatoes; sugar-free
1 cup beef broth
1 teaspoon chili powder
1/4 cup swerve
2 teaspoon salt
Directions:
Place ribs in the pot and pour in enough water to cover. Seal the lid and set the steam release handle to the *Sealing* position. Press the *Meat* button and set the timer for 20 minutes on high pressure.
When done, perform a quick release and open the lid.
Transfer the ribs to a deep bowl and chill for a while
Remove the water press the *Saute* button
Now; whisk together eggs, apple cider, soy sauce, swerve, salt, and chili powder. Rub the meat with this mixture and let it sit for a while.
Add celery stalks, onions, and peppers to the pot and cook for 8-10 minutes, stirring constantly. Season with some more salt and add tomatoes. Pour in the broth and continue to cook until most of the liquid has evaporated
Now add the prepared pork and coat well with vegetables. Press the *Cancel'* button and sprinkle with fresh celery leaves. Let it sit for a while before serving
Nutrition Info: Calories: 321; Total Fats: 8.6g; Net Carbs: 6.1g; Protein: 51.7g; Fiber: 1.3g

345. Spicy Pork with Celery
Cooking Time: 40 Minutes
Servings: 4
Ingredients:
2 -pounds pork ribs; cut into smaller pieces
1/4 cup fresh parsley; finely chopped.
1 cup celery stalks; finely chopped.
1 large leek; finely chopped
1 large onion; sliced
4 cups beef broth
3 tablespoon olive oil
1 cup cauliflower florets
1 bay leaf
1 teaspoon chili powder
1/2 teaspoon red pepper flakes
1 teaspoon salt
Directions:

Plug in the instant pot and press the *Saute* button. Heat up the oil and then add ribs in several batches. Brown for 2-3 minutes on each side and remove from the pot. Repeat with the remaining meat.
Now add onions and celery stalk. Sprinkle with some salt and sauté for 4-5 minutes, stirring constantly
Finally, add the pork and the remaining ingredients. Pour in the broth and seal the lid. Set the steam release handle to the *Sealing* position and press the *Manual* button
Cook for 20 minutes on high pressure
When done, release the pressure naturally and serve immediately.
Nutrition Info: Calories: 493; Total Fats: 20g; Net Carbs: 7.5g; Protein: 65.7g; Fiber: 2.4g

346. Pork Chops with Peppers
Cooking Time: 35 Minutes
Servings: 5
Ingredients:
1-pound pork chops; cut into bite-sized pieces
2 tablespoon butter; unsalted
2 chili peppers; chopped.
2 red bell peppers; sliced
2 bacon slices; chopped
2 small onions; finely chopped
1 cup beef broth
2 teaspoon Italian seasoning
1/4 teaspoon salt
Directions:
Rinse the meat under cold running water and sprinkle with one teaspoon of Italian seasoning. Place in the instant pot and pour in the broth
Seal the lid and set the steam release handle. Press the *Manual* button and set the timer for 10 minutes on high pressure.
When done, release the pressure by moving the handle to the *Venting* position and carefully open the lid.
Remove the meat from the pot along with the broh and press the *Saute* button.
Grease the inner pot with butter and add onion. Sauté for 2 minutes and then add peppers. Sprinkle with salt and the remaining Italian seasoning and cook for 2-3 minutes
Now add bacon and stir well. Optionally, add some more salt or Italian seasoning and cook for 5 minutes. If necessary, add some beef broth – about 2 tablespoons at the time
Finally, add the meat and give it a good stir. Cook for 5 minutes. Press the *Cancel'* button and serve immediately.
Nutrition Info: Calories: 407; Total Fats: 30.8g; Net Carbs: 5.4g; Protein: 25g; Fiber: 1.3g

347. Balsamic Pork with Broccoli
Cooking Time: 50 Minutes
Servings: 4
Ingredients:
2 -pounds pork shoulder; boneless
10-ounce shiitake mushrooms; sliced
2 tablespoon oyster sauce
3 tablespoon balsamic vinegar
2 cups broccoli; cut into florets

3 tablespoon soy sauce
3 tablespoon butter
2 cups beef broth
2 teaspoon peppercorn
2 bay leaves
1 ½ teaspoon sea salt
Directions:
Rinse well the meat and place in the pot. Sprinkle with salt and peppercorn. Pour in the broth and one cup of water. Add bay leaves and seal the lid. Set the steam release handle and press the *Manual* button. Cook for 25 minutes on high pressure.
When done; perform a quick pressure release and open the lid. Remove half of the remaining liquid and add broccoli, shiitake, soy sauce, oyster sauce, balsamic vinegar, and butter
Seal the lid again and continue to cook for another 8 minutes on the *Manual* mode
When done, release the pressure naturally and serve immediately.
Nutrition Info: Calories: 483; Total Fats: 17.6g; Net Carbs: 11.7g; Protein: 65g; Fiber: 2.8g

348. Zucchini Pork
Cooking Time: 1 hour
Servings: 4
Ingredients:
1-pound pork neck; chopped into bite-sized pieces
1 cup button mushrooms; sliced
1 large tomato; roughly chopped
1 cup cauliflower florets
2 tablespoon apple cider vinegar
2 red bell peppers; chopped.
2 tablespoon butter
2 tablespoon soy sauce
1 zucchini; spiralized into noodles
1 small onion; finely chopped.
2 garlic cloves; crushed
1-egg white
1 tablespoon cayenne pepper
1/2 teaspoon ginger powder
2 bay leaves
2 tablespoon stevia powder
1 teaspoon salt
Directions:
In a small bowl, combine egg whites, soy sauce, apple cider, salt, stevia, half of the cayenne pepper, and ginger powder
Generously brush the meat with this mixture and let it sit for 15-20 minutes.
Plug in the instant pot and add butter. Heat up and add the meat. Cook for 4-5 minutes, stirring constantly
Remove the meat from the pot and add onions, garlic, mushrooms, peppers, tomato, and cauliflower. Continue to cook for 10-12 minutes.
Finally, add the meat, bay leaf, and pour in 1 cup of water. Seal the lid and set the steam release handle to the *Sealing* posisiton
Press the *Manual* button and set the timer for 13 minutes on high pressure
When done; perform a quick pressure release and open the lid. Stir in zucchini noodles and press the *Saute* button.

Cook for 7-8 minutes, stirring occasionally. Serve with grated Parmesan cheese or freshly chopped parsley
Nutrition Info: Calories: 277; Total Fats: 10.2g; Net Carbs: 9.5g; Protein: 34.1g; Fiber: 3.2g

349. Mint Lamb Chops
Preparation time: 10 minutes
Cooking time: 25 minutes
Servings: 4
Ingredients:
½ cup cilantro, chopped
4 lamb chops
2 green chilies, chopped
3 garlic cloves, minced
Juice of 2 limes
2 tablespoons olive oil
A pinch of salt and black pepper
½ cup mint, chopped
1 cup veggie stock
Directions:
Set your instant pot on Sauté mode, add the oil, heat it up, add the garlic, chilies and the lamb chops and brown for 5 minutes
Add the rest of the ingredients, put the lid on and cook on High for 25 minutes.
Release the pressure naturally for 10 minutes, divide the mix between plates and serve.
Nutrition Values: calories 143, fat 10.9, fiber 0.9, carbs 3, protein 15.6

350. Lamb Chops, Fennel and Tomatoes
Preparation time: 10 minutes
Cooking time: 25 minutes
Servings: 4
Ingredients:
4 lamb chops
1 tablespoon olive oil
4 garlic cloves, minced
A pinch of salt and black pepper
Zest of 1 lime, grated
2 bay leaves
1 tablespoon rosemary, chopped
1 fennel bulb, cut into 8 wedges
½ cup cherry tomatoes, halved
1 teaspoon sweet paprika
1 cup veggie stock
Directions:
Set your instant pot on Sauté mode, add the oil, heat it up, add the meat and the garlic and brown for 5 minutes.
Add the rest of the ingredients, put the lid on and cook on High for 20 minutes.
Release the pressure naturally for 10 minutes, divide everything between plates and serve.
Nutrition Values: calories 194, fat 7.9, fiber 2.3, carbs 5.3, protein 7.5

351. Italian Leg of Lamb
Preparation time: 10 minutes
Cooking time: 40 minutes
Servings: 4
Ingredients:

2 pounds leg of lamb, boneless
2 tablespoons olive oil
4 garlic cloves, minced
2 tablespoons rosemary, chopped
¼ teaspoon red pepper flakes
½ cup walnuts, chopped
5 ounces baby spinach
A pinch of salt and black pepper
½ cup mustard
Directions:
Set your instant pot on Sauté mode, add the oil, heat it up, add the garlic, pepper flakes, the lamb and the mustard, toss and cook for 5 minutes.
Add all the other ingredients except the spinach, put the lid on and cook on High for 30 minutes.
Release the pressure naturally for 10 minutes, set the pot on Sauté mode again, add the spinach, cook for 5 minutes more, divide the mix between plates and serve.
Nutrition Values: calories 367, fat 25.3, fiber 3.5, carbs 5.8, protein 25.4

352. Hot Curry Lamb and Green Beans
Preparation time: 10 minutes
Cooking time: 35 minutes
Servings: 4
Ingredients:
4 lamb chops
1 pound green beans, trimmed and halved
Juice of 1 lime
A pinch of salt and black pepper
½ cup beef stock
1 teaspoon rosemary, dried
1 tablespoon olive oil
1 tablespoon curry powder
Directions:
In your instant pot, combine all the ingredients, put the lid on and cook on High for 35 minutes.
Release the pressure naturally for 10 minutes, divide the mix between plates and serve.
Nutrition Values: calories 139, fat 7.7, fiber 3.4, carbs 4.6, protein 8.9

353. Lamb and Sun-dried Tomatoes Mix
Preparation time: 10 minutes
Cooking time: 40 minutes
Servings: 6
Ingredients:
6 lamb loins
2 garlic cloves, minced
2 teaspoons thyme, chopped
A pinch of salt and black pepper
2 tablespoons olive oil
2 tablespoons balsamic vinegar
½ cup parsley, chopped
½ cup sun-dried tomatoes, chopped
1 cup beef stock
Directions:
Set the instant pot on Sauté mode, add the oil, heat it up, add the lamb and garlic and brown for 5 minutes.
Add the rest of the ingredients, put the lid on and cook on High for 35 minutes.
Release the pressure naturally for 10 minutes, divide the mix between plates and serve.
Nutrition Values: calories 353, fat 23.7, fiber 0.5, carbs 1.5, protein 34.2

354. Cumin Lamb and Capers
Preparation time: 10 minutes
Cooking time: 35 minutes
Servings: 4
Ingredients:
4 lamb chops
2 tablespoons avocado oil
A pinch of salt and black pepper
2 tablespoons sweet paprika
2 tablespoons capers, drained
1 cup beef stock
2 teaspoons cumin, ground
1 tablespoon parsley, chopped
1 tablespoon cilantro, chopped
Directions:
Set the instant pot on Sauté mode, add the oil, heat it up, add the lamb chops, paprika and cumin and brown for 5 minutes.
Add the rest of the ingredients, put the lid on and cook on High for 30 minutes.
Release the pressure naturally for 10 minutes, divide the mix between plates and serve.
Nutrition Values: calories 110, fat 5.6, fiber 1.9, carbs 4.5, protein 7.9

355. Herbed Crusted Lamb Cutlets
Preparation time: 10 minutes
Cooking time: 30 minutes
Servings: 4
Ingredients:
8 lamb cutlets
4 tablespoons mustard
3 tablespoons olive oil
¼ cup parmesan, grated
1 tablespoon parsley, chopped
1 tablespoon thyme, chopped
1 tablespoon rosemary
1 cup tomato passata
Directions:
In a bowl, mix the lamb with the rest of the ingredients except the tomato passata.
Add the sauce to the instant pot, add the lamb, put the lid on and cook on High for 30 minutes.
Release the pressure naturally for 10 minutes, divide the mix between plates and serve.
Nutrition Values: calories 162, fat 14, fiber 3.3, carbs 6.5, protein 14.4

356. Pine Nuts Lamb Meatballs
Preparation time: 10 minutes
Cooking time: 30 minutes
Servings: 6
Ingredients:
2 pounds lamb, ground
½ cup almond milk
2 shallots, minced
2 garlic cloves, minced
1 tablespoon thyme, chopped
A pinch of salt and black pepper
½ cup pine nuts, toasted

1 egg
1 tablespoon olive oil
12 ounces canned tomatoes, crushed
Directions:
In a bowl, combine the lamb with the rest of the ingredients except the oil and the tomatoes, stir well and shape medium meatballs out of this mix
Set the instant pot on Sauté mode, add the oil, heat it up, add the meatballs and cook for 2 minutes on each side.
Add the tomatoes, put the lid on and cook on High for 25 minutes.
Release the pressure naturally for 10 minutes, divide the mix between plates and serve.
Nutrition Values: calories 363, fat 26.4, fiber 1.6, carbs 5.5, protein 24.8

357. Lamb Shoulder Roast
Preparation time: 10 minutes
Cooking time: 35 minutes
Servings: 6
Ingredients:
2 tablespoons ghee, melted
2 tablespoons olive oil
2 shallots, chopped
2 garlic cloves, minced
½ cup mint, chopped
2 pounds lamb shoulder, fat trimmed
1 cup veggie stock
Directions:
Set the instant pot on Sauté mode, add the oil and the ghee, heat it up, add the lamb shoulder, garlic and shallots and sear for 2 minutes on each side.
Add all the other ingredients, put the lid on and cook on High for 30 minutes.
Release the pressure naturally for 10 minutes, slice the roast, between plates and serve.
Nutrition Values: calories 378, fat 19.2, fiber 0.4, carbs 0.7, protein 27.5

358. Moroccan Lamb
Preparation time: 10 minutes
Cooking time: 30 minutes
Servings: 4
Ingredients:
8 lamb chops
1 cup Greek yogurt
3 tablespoons olive oil
1 tablespoon lemon zest, grated
A pinch of salt and black pepper
1 tablespoon cumin, ground
1 tablespoon coriander, ground
1 tablespoon turmeric powder
½ cup mint, chopped
4 garlic cloves, minced
2 tablespoons lemon juice
1 and ½ cups veggie stock
Directions:
Set the instant pot on Sauté mode, add the oil, heat it up, add the meat, cumin, coriander and turmeric and brown for 5 minutes.
Add the rest of the ingredients, put the lid on and cook on High for 25 minutes.
Release the pressure naturally for 10 minutes, divide everything between plates and serve.
Nutrition Values: calories 179, fat 14.9, fiber 1.5, carbs 5.5, protein 7.5

359. Spinach Pork Meatloaf
Preparation time: 10 minutes
Cooking time: 30 minutes
Servings: 6
Ingredients:
½ cup almond milk
½ cup almond flour
1 spring onion, chopped
A pinch of salt and black pepper
2 eggs, whisked
1 cup baby spinach
2 pounds pork meat, ground
½ cup tomato passata
1 tablespoon parsley, chopped
1 and ½ cups water
Directions:
In a bowl, mix pork with the rest of the ingredients except the tomato passata and the water, stir well, transfer to a loaf pan that fits the instant pot and brush it with the tomato passata.
Add the water to your instant pot, add the steamer basket, put the loaf pan inside, put the lid on and cook on High for 30 minutes.
Release the pressure naturally for 10 minutes, cool the meatloaf down, slice and serve.
Nutrition Values: calories 394, fat 26.8, fiber 1, carbs 2.7, protein 35.6

360. Ginger Lamb and Basil
Preparation time: 10 minutes
Cooking time: 30 minutes
Servings: 4
Ingredients:
1 and ½ pounds leg of lamb, boneless and cubed
1 tablespoon olive oil
2 tablespoons basil, chopped
1 tablespoon ginger, grated
A pinch of salt and black pepper
1 and ½ cups veggie stock
1 cup tomato passata
Directions:
Set the instant pot on Sauté mode, add the oil, heat it up, add the meat and brown for 5 minutes.
Add the rest of the ingredients, put the lid on and cook on High for 25 minutes.
Release the pressure naturally for 10 minutes, divide the mix between plates and serve.
Nutrition Values: calories 320, fat 13.6, fiber 0.9, carbs 4.4, protein 35.6

361. Coconut Lamb Chops
Preparation time: 10 minutes
Cooking time: 30 minutes
Servings: 6
Ingredients:
6 lamb chops
2 tablespoons olive oil
1 teaspoon rosemary, chopped
1 cup veggie stock
1 tablespoon garlic, minced

A pinch of salt and black pepper
1 cup coconut cream
1 tablespoon dill, chopped
Directions:
Set the instant pot on Sauté mode, add the oil, heat it up, add the lamb, garlic and rosemary and brown for 5 minutes.
Add the rest of the ingredients, put the lid on and cook on High for 25 minutes.
Release the pressure naturally for 10 minutes, divide everything between plates and serve.
Nutrition Values: calories 269, fat 25.1, fiber 1.6, carbs 5.9, protein 7.9

362. Spicy Beef, Sprouts and Avocado Mix
Preparation time: 10 minutes
Cooking time: 30 minutes
Servings: 4
Ingredients:
1 pound beef stew meat, cubed
1 avocado, peeled, pitted and cubed
2 cups Brussels sprouts, trimmed and quartered
½ teaspoon oregano, dried
A pinch of salt and black pepper
1 tablespoon avocado oil
1 cup beef stock
1 teaspoon sweet paprika
Directions:
Set the instant pot on Sauté mode, add the oil, heat it up, add the meat, oregano, paprika, salt and pepper and brown for 5 minutes
Add the rest of the ingredients except the avocado, put the lid on and cook on High for 25 minutes.
Release the pressure naturally for 10 minutes, divide the mix between plates and serve with the avocado on top.
Nutrition Values: calories 343, fat 17.5, fiber 3.3, carbs 6.7, protein 34.8

363. Beef and Creamy Sauce
Preparation time: 10 minutes
Cooking time: 35 minutes
Servings: 6
Ingredients:
2 pounds beef stew meat, cubed
2 shallots, minced
1 cup coconut cream
½ teaspoon rosemary, chopped
1 tablespoon olive oil
1 cup beef stock
1 tablespoon dill, chopped
A pinch of salt and black pepper
Directions:
Set your instant pot on Sauté mode, add the oil, heat it up, add the meat, shallots and the rosemary and brown for 5 minutes.
Add rest of the ingredients except the cream, put the lid on and cook on High for 25 minutes.
Release the pressure naturally for 10 minutes, set the pot on Sauté mode again, add the cream, toss and cook for 10 minutes more.
Divide the mix between plates and serve.

Nutrition Values: calories 397, fat 21.4, fiber 1, carbs 2.6, protein 32.4

364. Pork and Chives Asparagus
Preparation time: 10 minutes
Cooking time: 30 minutes
Servings: 6
Ingredients:
2 pounds pork stew meat, cubed
4 garlic cloves, minced
1 cup beef stock
1 bunch asparagus, trimmed
A pinch of salt and black pepper
1 teaspoon sweet paprika
1 teaspoon chives, chopped
1 tablespoon olive oil
Directions:
Set your instant pot on sauté mode, add the oil, heat it up, add the garlic and the beef stew meat and brown for 5 minutes
Add the rest of the ingredients except the asparagus, put the lid on and cook on High for 20 minutes.
Release the pressure naturally for 10 minutes, set the pot on Sauté mode again, add the asparagus, cook for 5 minutes more, divide everything between plates and serve.
Nutrition Values: calories 347, fat 17.1, fiber 0.2, carbs 0.9, protein 24.7

365. Oregano and Thyme Beef
Preparation time: 5 minutes
Cooking time: 30 minutes
Servings: 4
Ingredients:
1 pound beef stew meat, cubed
2 garlic cloves, minced
1 tablespoon olive oil
1 teaspoon thyme, dried
A pinch of salt and black pepper
1 tablespoon oregano, chopped
1 and ½ cups beef stock
Directions:
Set your instant pot on Sauté mode, add the oil, heat it up, add the garlic, thyme and the meat and brown for 5 minutes.
Add the rest of the ingredients, put the lid on and cook on High for 25 minutes.
Release the pressure naturally for 10 minutes, divide the mix between plates and serve.
Nutrition Values: calories 247, fat 10.7, fiber 0.6, carbs 1.4, protein 34.2

366. Almond Lamb Meatloaf
Preparation time: 10 minutes
Cooking time: 30 minutes
Servings: 4
Ingredients:
1 and ½ pound lamb, ground
2 shallots, minced
2 eggs, whisked
3 garlic cloves, minced
1 tablespoon almonds, chopped
1 tablespoon rosemary
A pinch of salt and black pepper
1 cup kale, chopped

¼ cup coconut milk
Cooking spray
2 cups water
Directions:
In a bowl, combine the meat with rest of the ingredients except the cooking spray and the water, and stir well.
Grease a loaf pan that fits the instant pot with the cooking spray, shape the meatloaf and put it in the pan.
Add the water to the instant pot, add the steamer basket, put the meatloaf inside, put the lid on and cook on High for 30 minutes.
Release the pressure naturally for 10 minutes, cool the meatloaf, slice and serve.
Nutrition Values: calories 301, fat 15.1, fiber 1.2, carbs 4.4, protein 35.4

367. Pork and Bok Choy
Preparation time: 10 minutes
Cooking time: 35 minutes
Servings: 6
Ingredients:
1 and ½ pounds pork stew meat, cubed
4 garlic cloves, minced
2 tablespoons chili powder
1 teaspoon red pepper flakes
1 pound bok choy, torn
1 tablespoon olive oil
A pinch of salt and black pepper
1 cup beef stock
Directions:
Set the instant pot on sauté mode, add the oil, heat it up, add the garlic, the meat, chili powder and pepper flakes and brown for 5 minutes.
Add the rest of the ingredients, put the lid on and cook on High for 30 minutes.
Release the pressure naturally for 10 minutes, divide the mix between plates and serve.
Nutrition Values: calories 365, fat 17.5, fiber 1.8, carbs 3.9, protein 34.6

368. Smoked Paprika Lamb
Preparation time: 10 minutes
Cooking time: 30 minutes
Servings: 4
Ingredients:
1 and ½ pounds leg of lamb, boneless and cubed
1 tablespoon smoked paprika
1 and ½ cups tomatoes, cubed
3 garlic cloves, minced
1 cup veggie stock
1 tablespoon ghee, melted
A pinch of salt and black pepper
1 tablespoon cilantro, chopped
Directions:
Set your instant pot on Sauté mode, add the ghee, heat it up, add the meat, smoked paprika and the garlic and brown for 6 minutes.
Add the rest of the ingredients except the cilantro, put the lid on and cook on High for 25 minutes.
Release the pressure naturally for 10 minutes, divide the mix between plates and serve with the cilantro sprinkled on top.

Nutrition Values: calories 306, fat 13.4, fiber 0.5, carbs 1.2, protein 43.2

369. Cajun Beef and Leeks Sauce
Preparation time: 10 minutes
Cooking time: 35 minutes
Servings: 6
Ingredients:
2 pounds beef sirloin, cut into steaks
1 tablespoon olive oil
2 tablespoons Cajun seasoning
1 and ½ cups beef stock
A pinch of salt and black pepper
1 teaspoon garlic, minced
1 leek, sliced
Directions:
Set your instant pot on sauté mode, add the oil, heat it up, add the garlic, the meat and Cajun seasoning and brown for 5 minutes.
Add the remaining ingredients, put the lid on and cook on High for 30 minutes.
Release the pressure naturally for 10 minutes, divide the mix between plates and serve.
Nutrition Values: calories 311, fat 11.8, fiber 0.3, carbs 2.3, protein 25.7

370. Beef and Savoy Cabbage Mix
Preparation time: 10 minutes
Cooking time: 25 minutes
Servings: 4
Ingredients:
1 pound beef stew meat, cubed
1 Savoy cabbage, shredded
2 garlic cloves, minced
1 tablespoon olive oil
A pinch of salt and black pepper
1 and ½ cups tomato passata
1 tablespoon parsley, chopped
Directions:
Set the instant pot on Sauté mode, add the oil, heat it up, add the meat and the garlic and brown for 5 minutes.
Add the rest of the ingredients, put the lid on and cook on High for 20 minutes.
Release the pressure naturally for 10 minutes, divide the mix between plates and serve.
Nutrition Values: calories 243, fat 10.6, fiber 0.1, carbs 0.6, protein 34.5

371. Pork and Mint Zucchinis
Preparation time: 10 minutes
Cooking time: 25 minutes
Servings: 6
Ingredients:
2 pounds pork stew meat, cubed
A pinch of salt and black pepper
1 cup beef stock
1 cup zucchinis, sliced
1 tablespoon balsamic vinegar
1 tablespoon olive oil
1 tablespoon garlic, minced
1 tablespoon mint, chopped
Directions:

Set the instant pot on Sauté mode, add the oil, heat it up, add the pork and the garlic and brown for 5 minutes.
Add the rest of the ingredients, put the lid on and cook on High for 20 minutes.
Release the pressure naturally for 10 minutes, divide everything between plates and serve.
Nutrition Values: calories 349, fat 17.1, fiber 0.3, carbs 1.2, protein 34.2

372. Beef and Walnuts Rice
Preparation time: 10 minutes
Cooking time: 35 minutes
Servings: 6
Ingredients:
1 and ½ pounds beef stew meat, cubed
2 garlic cloves, minced
1 cup beef stock
1 tablespoon walnuts, toasted and chopped
1 cup tomato passata
A pinch of salt and black pepper
1 tablespoon basil, chopped
1 tablespoon olive oil
Directions:
Set your instant pot on sauté mode, add the oil, heat it up, add the meat and the garlic and brown for 5 minutes.
Add the rest of the ingredients, put the lid on and cook on High for 30 minutes.
Release the pressure naturally for 10 minutes, divide everything between plates and serve.
Nutrition Values: calories 329, fat 12.7, fiber 0.9, carbs 4.2, protein 27.6

373. Bangers and Mash with Onion Gravy
Cooking Time: 30 minutes
Servings: 2
Ingredients:
2 lb Turnips, peeled and halved
5 Pork Sausages
1 cup Water + 2 tbsp Water
⅓ cup Green Onion, sliced
Salt and Pepper to taste
4 tbsp Milk
¼ cup + 4 tbsp Unsalted Butter
1 tbsp Arrowroot Starch
3 tbsp Balsamic Vinegar
1 Onion, sliced thinly
1 cup + 2 tbsp Beef Broth
Directions:
Place the turnips in the pot and pour the water over. Seal the lid, secure the pressure valve, and select Steam on High pressure for 5 minutes. Once ready, do a quick pressure release.
Remove the turnips to a bowl. Add a quarter cup butter to the turnip and use a masher to mash the turnips until the butter is well mixed into the turnip. Slowly add the milk and mix using a spoon. Add green onions, season with pepper and salt and fold in with the spoon. Set aside.
Pour out the liquid in the Instant Pot and use paper towels to wipe inside the pot dry. Select Sauté and melt 2 tbsp of butter. Add sausages and brown them on each side for 3 minutes.
After they are browned, remove them onto the turnip mash and cover with aluminium foil to keep warm. Set aside. Back into the pot add the two tablespoons of the beef broth to deglaze the bottom of the pot while stirring and scraping the bottom with a spoon. Add the remaining butter and onions. Sauté the onions until they are translucent then pour in the balsamic vinegar. Stir for another minute. In a bowl, mix the arrowroot starch with water and pour into the pot.
Stir and add the remaining beef broth. Allow the sauce to thicken and adjust the taste with salt and pepper. Turn off the heat once a slurry is formed. Dish the mashed potatoes and sausages in serving plates. Spoon the gravy over and serve with steamed green beans.
Nutrition Values: Calories 300, Protein 12g, Net Carbs 3g, Fat 16g

374. Herby Cuban Pork Roast
Cooking Time: 55 minutes
Servings: 8
Ingredients
3 pounds Pork Shoulder
3 tbsp Olive oil
1 tsp Vinegar
Juice of 1 Lime
½ tsp Onion Flakes
1 tsp dried Parsley
1 tsp Cumin seeds
1 tsp Garlic Powder
Salt and Pepper, to taste
1 ½ cups Beef Broth
1 Red Chilli, deseeded and chopped
1 tbsp fresh Cilantro, chopped to garnish
Directions
In a bowl, combine the olive oil, lime juice, vinegar, and spices and herbs. Rub the mixture on the meat. Add the pork inside the Pot and cover with the remaining marinade.
Pour the broth around the pork and seal the lid. Select the Meat/mode and cook on HIGH pressure for 40 minutes. When it goes off, do a quick pressure release. Slice or shred the meat before serving.
Nutrition Values: Calories 305, Protein 32g, Net Carbs 2g, Fat 13g

375. Pork Stew
Cooking Time: 60 minutes
Servings: 4
Ingredients
1 lb Pork Loin, cut into cubed
1 cup Cauliflower Florets
1 cup Broccoli Florets
1 Celery Stalk, chopped
½ Onion, diced
2 Garlic Cloves, minced
14 ounces diced canned Tomatoes
3 cups Beef Broth
1 cup Snap Peas, chopped
Salt and Black Pepper, to taste
1 tsp dried Thyme

1 tbsp Arrowroot mixed with 1 tbsp Water
2 tbsp Coconut Oil
Directions
Melt half of the coconut oil on Sauté. Add the pork and season with salt and pepper. Cook for a few minutes, until browned on all sides. Remove to a plate.
Add the remaining coconut oil and cook the onions for 2 minutes. Then, stir in garlic and celery, and cook for 1 minute. Add in the remaining ingredients, except the arrowroot mixture.
Seal the lid, press Meat/Stew and cook for 15 minutes on HIGH pressure. When it goes off, do a natural pressure release, for 10 minutes. Stir in the arrowroot mixture and set to Sauté. Cook for a few minutes or until slightly thickened. Serve immediately.!
Nutrition Values: Calories 385, Protein 28g, Net Carbs 6.2g, Fat 22g

376. Lemony Pork Belly
Cooking Time: 55 minutes
Servings: 4
Ingredients
2 pounds Pork Belly
1 tbsp Sweetener
2 tbsp Lime Juice
1 Onion, chopped
½ cup Chicken Broth
2 cups Water
Directions
Combine the pork belly and water in your Instant Pot and seal the lid. Press Manual and cook for 25 minutes on HIGH pressure. Meanwhile, place the remaining ingredients in a food processor and pulse until pureed.
When the timer goes off, do a quick pressure release. Remove the pork to a baking dish and pour the puree over. Do not discard the water in the pot. Lower the trivet in the pot. Place the dish on top and seal the lid. Cook for 15 minutes on HIGH pressure. Do a quick pressure release.
Nutrition Values: Calories 453, Protein 25g, Net Carbs 6g, Fat 35g

377. Ham with Collard Greens
Cooking Time: 10 minutes
Servings: 4
Ingredients:
20 oz Collard Greens, chopped
5 tbsp Chicken Bouillon
4 cups Water
½ cup diced Sweet Onion
2 ½ cups diced Ham
Directions:
Place the ham at the bottom of the pot. Add the collard greens and onion. Then, add the chicken cube to the water and dissolve it. Pour the mixture into the pot. Seal the lid, select Steam mode on Low pressure for 5 minutes. Once ready, do a quick pressure release.
Spoon the vegetables and the ham with sauce into a serving platter. Serve with a steak dish.
Nutrition Values: Calories 128, Protein 6.5g, Net Carbs 0g, Fat 3.5g

378. Pork in Mushroom Gravy
Cooking Time: 35 minutes
Servings: 4
Ingredients:
4 Pork Chops
1 tbsp Olive oil
3 cloves Garlic, minced
Salt and Pepper to taste
1 tsp Garlic Powder
1 (10 oz Mushroom Soup
8 oz Mushrooms, sliced
1 small Onion, chopped
1 cup Beef Broth
1 sprig Fresh Thyme
Chopped Parsley to garnish
Directions:
Heat oil on Sauté, and add mushrooms, garlic, and onion. Sauté stirring occasionally until translucent, for 3 minutes. Season pork chops with salt, garlic powder, and pepper.
Add into the pot followed by the thyme and broth. Seal the lid, select Meat/Stew and cook on High pressure for 15 minutes. Once ready, do a natural pressure release for about 10 minutes, then a quick pressure release to let the remaining steam out. Select Sauté and add mushroom soup. Stir until the mixture thickens. Dish the pork and gravy into a serving bowl and garnish with parsley. Serve with a side of creamy squash mash.
Nutrition Values: Calories 227, Protein 15.5g, Net Carbs 0g, Fat 15.5g

379. Pork Tenderloin with Ginger Soy Sauce
Cooking Time: 20 minutes
Servings: 4
Ingredients:
2 lb Pork Tenderloin
½ cup sugar-free Soy Sauce
¼ cup Monk Fruit Sugar
½ cup Water + 2 tbsp Water
3 tbsp grated Ginger
2 cloves Garlic, minced
2 tbsp Sesame Oil
2 tsp Arrowroot Starch
Chopped Scallions to garnish
Sesame Seeds to garnish
Directions:
Add soy sauce, monk fruit sugar, half cup of water, ginger, garlic, and sesame oil; stir. Then, add the pork. Seal the lid, and select Meat/Stew mode on High for 10 minutes. Once ready, do a quick pressure release and remove the pork onto a serving plate.
In a bowl, mix the arrowroot starch with the remaining water until smooth and pour into the pot. Select Sauté mode, stir the sauce frequently and cook until it thickens. Once the sauce is ready, serve the pork with a side endive salad and spoon the sauce all over it.
Nutrition Values: Calories 240, Protein 21g, Net Carbs 3g, Fat 9g

380. Beef Bourguignonne
Cooking Time: 45 minutes
Servings: 4
Ingredients:
2 lb Stewing Beef, cut in chunks
Salt and Pepper to taste
2 ½ tbsp Olive oil
¼ tsp Red Wine Vinegar
¼ cup Pearl Onion
3 tsp Tomato Paste
½ lb Turnips, peeled and halved
2 Carrots, peeled and chopped
1 Onion, sliced
2 cloves Garlic, crushed
1 cup Red Wine
2 cups Beef Broth
1 bunch Thyme
½ cup Cognac
2 tbsp Almond flour
Directions:
Season the beef with salt, pepper, and a light sprinkle of flour. Heat oil on Sauté, and brown the beef on all sides. This can be done in batches but after all the meat should be returned to the pot. Pour the cognac into the pot and stir the mixture to deglaze the bottom of the pot.
Add the thyme, red wine, beef broth, tomato paste, garlic, turnips, onion, and pearl onions. Stir with a spoon. Seal the lid, select Meat/Stew on High for 25 minutes. Once ready, do a quick pressure release to let out the remaining steam.
Use the spoon to remove the thyme, adjust the taste with salt and pepper, and add the vinegar. Stir the sauce and dish in a serving bowl. Serve with a side of cauli rice or low carb bread.
Nutrition Values: Calories 339, Protein 36.3g, Net Carbs 0.1g, Fat 11.7g

381. Beef Burger
Cooking Time: 20 minutes
Servings: 4
Ingredients:
1 lb Ground Beef
1 (1 oz packet Dry Onion Soup Mix
1 cup Water
Assembling:
4 low carb Burger Buns
4 Tomato Slices
4 Cheddar Cheese Slices
4 small leaves Lettuce
Mayonnaise
Mustard
Sugar-Free Ketchup
Directions:
In a bowl, add the beef and onion mix, and combine them well together with your hands.
Make 4 patties with your hands and wrap them in each foil paper. Pour the water into the Instant Pot and fit the steamer rack in it. Place the wrapped patties on the trivet, close the lid, and secure the pressure valve. Select Meat/Stew mode on High pressure for 10 minutes.
Once ready, do a quick pressure release to let out the remaining steam,. Use a set of tongs to remove the wrapped beef onto a flat surface and carefully unwrap them.
Assemble the burger:
In each half of the buns, put a lettuce leaf, then a beef patty, a slice of cheese, and a slice of tomato. Top with the other halves of buns. Serve with some ketchup, mayonnaise, and mustard.
Nutrition Values: Calories 580, Protein 28g, Net Carbs 2g, Fat 42g

382. Pork Carnitas Lettuce Cups
Cooking Time: 30 minutes
Servings: 6
Ingredients:
3 lb Pork Shoulder
2 tbsp + 2 tbsp Olive oil
1 small head Butter Lettuce, dried
2 Limes, cut in wedges
2 Carrots, grated
1 ½ cup Water
1 Onion, chopped
½ tsp Cayenne Pepper
½ tsp Coriander Powder
1 tsp Cumin Powder
1 tsp Garlic Powder
1 tsp White Pepper
2 tsp dried Oregano
1 tsp Red Pepper Flakes
Salt to taste
1 tbsp Cocoa Powder, unsweetened
Directions:
In a bowl, add the onion, cayenne pepper, coriander powder, garlic powder, white pepper, dried oregano, red pepper flakes, salt, and cocoa powder. Mix them well with a spoon.
Sprinkle the spice mixture on the pork and use your hands to rub the spice well onto the meat. Then, wrap the meat in plastic wrap and refrigerate overnight. The next day, turn on the Instant Pot, open the pot, and select Sauté mode.
Pour 2 tablespoons of olive oil in the pot and once is heating, remove the pork from the fridge, remove the wraps and put in the pot. Brown on both sides for 6 minutes and then pour the water on it. Seal the lid, select Meat/ Stew mode on High pressure for 20 minutes.
Once ready, do a quick pressure release. Use a set of tongs to remove the pork onto a cutting board and use two forks to shred it. Empty the pot and wipe clean. Set the pot on Sauté mode and add the remaining olive oil. Once has heated, add the shredded pork to and fry until browns lightly for 5 minutes. Turn off the heat and begin assembling. Arrange double layers of lettuce leaves on a flat surface, make a bed of grated carrots, and spoon the pulled Pork on top.
Nutrition Values: Calories 315, Protein 28.2g, Net Carbs 0g, Fat 18.5g

383. Easy BBQ Ribs
Cooking Time: 40 minutes
Servings: 2 to 3
Ingredients:
½ lb rack Baby Back Ribs

Salt and Pepper to season
½ cup sugar-free Barbecue Sauce
3 tbsp Apple Cider Vinegar
Directions:
Heat oil on Sauté, and season the ribs with salt and pepper. Brown the ribs in the oil for 1 to 2 minutes per side. Pour the barbecue sauce and apple cider vinegar over the ribs and use tongs to turn to be well coated. Seal the lid, set on Steam on High for 30 minutes.
Once the timer goes off, do a natural pressure release for 15 minutes, then a quick pressure release to let out the remaining steam. Remove the ribs onto a serving platter and set the pot on Sauté to simmer until the sauce thickens, for 6 minutes. Use a knife to slice the ribs and pour the sauce all over. Serve the ribs with a generous side of steamed crunchy green beans.
Nutrition Values: Calories 310, Protein 21g, Net Carbs 3g, Fat 10g

384. Braised Pork Neck Bones
Cooking Time: 40 minutes
Servings: 6
Ingredients:
3 lb Pork Neck Bones
3 to 4 tbsp Olive oil
Salt and Black Pepper to taste
2 cloves Garlic, smashed
1 tbsp sugar-free Tomato Paste
1 tsp dried Thyme
1 White Onion, sliced
½ cup Red Wine
1 cup Beef Broth
Directions:
Turn on the Instant Pot, open the lid, and select Sauté mode. Pour in the olive oil and while heats, quickly season the pork neck bones with salt and pepper; brown on all sides. You can work in batches for the best browning result. Each batch should take about 5 minutes.
After, use a set of tongs to remove them onto a plate. Add the onion and sprinkle with some salt as desired. Stir with a spoon and cook the onions until they have softened. Then, add the smashed garlic, thyme, pepper, and tomato paste. Cook them for 2 minutes but with constant stirring to prevent the tomato paste from burning.
Next, pour the red wine into the pot to deglaze the bottom of the pot. Add the pork neck bones back to the pot and pour the beef broth over it. Close the lid, secure the pressure valve, and select Meat/Stew mode on High pressure for 5 to 15 minutes.
Once ready, let the pot sit for 10 minutes before doing a quick pressure release. Open the pot. Dish the pork neck soup into a serving bowl and serve with a good amount of broccoli mash.
Nutrition Values: Calories 106, Protein 13.4g, Net Carbs 0g, Fat 6.5g

385. Pork Roast Sandwich
Cooking Time: 20 minutes
Servings: 4
Ingredients:
2 lb Chuck Roast
¼ cup Monk Fruit Sugar
1 tsp Paprika
1 tsp Garlic Powder
1 White Onion, sliced
3 2 cups Beef Broth
Salt to taste
2 tbsp Apple Cider Vinegar
Assembling:
3 Low Carb Buns, halved
White Cheddar Cheese, grated
Directions:
Place the pork roast on a clean flat surface and sprinkle with paprika, garlic powder, monk fruit sugar, and salt. Use your hands to rub the seasoning on the meat. Add beef broth to it, onions, pork, and apple cider vinegar. Seal the lid, select Meat/Stew and cook on High for 15 minutes.
Once ready, do a quick pressure release, and open the pot. Turn off the pot. Remove the roasts with tongs and place them on a cutting board. Use two forks to shred.
In the buns, add the shredded pork with as much meat as desired, add some cooked onions from the pot, and top with the cheese. Serve warm with cheese.
Nutrition Values: Calories 305, Protein 45g, Net Carbs 0g, Fat 35g

386. Balsamic Pork Tenderloin
Cooking Time: 30 minutes
Servings: 4
Ingredients:
2 lb Pork Tenderloin
2 tbsp Olive oil
¼ cup Monk Fruit Sugar
½ cup Chicken Broth
Salt and Black Pepper to taste
1 clove Garlic, minced
1 tsp Sage Powder
1 tbsp Dijon Mustard
¼ cup Balsamic Vinegar
1 tbsp sugar-free Worcestershire Sauce
½ tbsp Xanthan Gum
4 tbsp Water
Directions:
Season the pork with salt and pepper. Select Sauté mode. Heat oil on Sauté, and brown the pork on both sides for 4 minutes in total. Remove to a plate and set aside.
Add the monk fruit sugar, chicken broth, balsamic vinegar, garlic, Worcestershire sauce, mustard, and sage. Stir the ingredients and return pork to the pot. Seal the lid, select Meat/Stew and cook on High pressure for 10 minutes. Once done, do a quick pressure release.
Remove the pork with tongs onto a plate and wrap in aluminum foil. Next, mix the xanthan gum with water and pour into the pot. Select Sauté mode, stir the mixture and cook to thicken. Then, turn the pot off after the desired thickness is achieved.
Unwrap the pork and use a knife to slice with 3 to 4-inch thickness. Arrange the slices on a serving platter and spoon the sauce all over it. Serve with a sautéed Brussels sprouts and red onion chunks.

Nutrition Values: Calories 154, Protein 23.3g, Net Carbs 2g, Fat 10.1g

387. Tender Greek Pork

Cooking Time: 60 minutes
Servings: 6
Ingredients:
3 lb Pork Roast, cut into pieces
3 tbsp Cavender's Greek Seasoning
1 tsp Onion Powder
¼ cup Beef Broth
¼ cup fresh Lemon Juice
Salt to taste
Directions:
Open the Instant Pot and put the pork chunks in it. In a bowl, add the greek seasoning, onion powder, beef broth, lemon juice, and some more salt as desired. Mix them using a spoon and pour the sauce over the pork in the Instant Pot. Close the lid, secure the pressure valve, and select Meat/Stew mode on High pressure for 45 minutes.
Once ready, do a natural pressure release for 10 minutes then do a quick pressure release to let out any more steam, and open the pot. Use a slotted spoon to remove the pork chunks onto a chopping board and use forks to shred. Add the shredded pork to a salad and serve.
Nutrition Values: Calories 210, Protein 22.9g, Net Carbs 0g, Fat 12.4g

388. Pork in Vegetable Sauce

Cooking Time: 40 minutes
Servings: 4
Ingredients:
2 lb Pork Loin Roast
Salt and Pepper to taste
3 cloves Garlic, minced
1 medium Onion, diced
2 tbsp Butter
3 stalks Celery, chopped
3 Carrots, chopped
1 cup Chicken Broth
2 tbsp sugar-free Worcestershire Sauce
½ tbsp Monk Fruit Sugar
1 tsp Yellow Mustard
2 tsp dried Basil
2 tsp dried Thyme
1 tbsp Arrowroot Starch
¼ cup Water
Directions:
Turn on the Instant Pot, open the lid, and select Sauté mode. Pour the oil in and while heats quickly season the pork with salt and pepper. Put the pork to the oil and sear to golden brown on both sides. This is about 4 minutes.
Then, include the garlic and onions and cook them until they are soft for 4 minutes too.
Top with the celery, carrots, chicken broth, Worcestershire sauce, mustard, thyme, basil, and monk fruit sugar. Use a spoon to stir it. Seal the lid, select Meat/Stew mode on High pressure for 20 minutes. Once ready, do a quick pressure release. Remove the meat from the pot onto a serving platter. Add the arrowroot starch to the water, mix with a spoon, and add to the pot. Select Sauté and cook the sauce to become a slurry with a bit of thickness. Season with salt and pepper and spoon the sauce over the meat in the serving platter. Serve with a side of steamed almond garlicky rapini mix.
Nutrition Values: Calories 326, Protein 25.7g, Net Carbs 0g, Fat 16.1g

389. Creamy Pork with Bacon

Cooking Time: 23 minutes
Servings: 4
Ingredients
⅓ cup Heavy Cream
1 cup Chicken Broth
1 ½ tsp Arrowroot
1 tbsp Water
3 Bacon Slices, chopped
1 tsp Olive oil
1 pound Pork Tenderloin, cut into strips
1 tsp dried Thyme
¼ tsp Garlic Powder
Salt and Pepper, to taste
Directions
Set your Instant Pot to Sauté, add the bacon and cook for 5-6 minutes, until crispy. Remove to a plate lined with paper towel to drain excess oil and set aside. Heat the olive oil in the pot until sizzling. Add the pork strips and season with salt and pepper; cook until browned on all sides, for 6 minutes. Pour the broth over and stir in the spices.
Seal the lid, select Manual and cook on HIGH pressure for 15 minutes. After the beep, do a quick pressure release. Stir in the heavy cream and cook on Sauté for 2 minutes.
Whisk together arrowroot and water, and stir the mixture into the sauce. Adjust the seasoning.
Nutrition Values: Calories 355, Protein 28g, Net Carbs 2g, Fat 25g

390. Pulled Pork in Lettuce Wraps

Cooking Time: 50 minutes
Servings: 4
Ingredients
3 lb Pork Roast
1 tbsp Olive oil
1 head Lettuce, washed, pat dry
1 large avocado, chopped
½ cup mayonnaise
2 cups Water
Spice Mix:
1 tbsp unsweetened Cocoa Powder
Salt to taste
White Pepper to taste
½ tsp Garlic Powder
½ tsp Red Pepper Flakes
2 tsp Oregano
½ tsp Cumin
¼ tsp Coriander Powder
¼ tsp Cayenne Pepper
1 large red Onion, chopped finely
Directions
Mix the spices and rub onto pork. Wrap the pork in plastic wrap, and marinate in the refrigerator overnight. Heat oil on Sauté, and brown the pork on

all sides. Pour the water, seal the lid and cook on High for 50 minutes. Once ready, do a natural pressure release for 20 minutes. Remove to a platter. Press Sauté and simmer the juices down. Shred the pork and set aside. Place a pan over medium heat, heat the olive oil and add the pork. Drizzle some of the cooking liquid on the pork, stir and turn off. Arrange lettuce wraps on a flat surface, fill each wrap with a bit of avocado and mayonnaise and top with pork.
Nutrition Values: Calories 350, Protein 39g, Net Carbs 6g, Fat 15g

391. Coconut Ginger Pork
Cooking Time: 45 minutes
Servings: 4
Ingredients:
3 lb Shoulder Roast
1 tbsp Olive oil
Salt and Black Pepper to season
2 cups Coconut Milk
1 tsp Coriander Powder
1 tsp Cumin Powder
3 tbsp grated Ginger
3 tsp minced Garlic
1 Onion, peeled and quartered
Parsley Leaves (unchopped, to garnish
Directions:
In a bowl, add the coriander, salt, pepper, and cumin. Use a spoon to mix them. Season the pork with the spice mixture. Then, use your hands to rub the spice on the meat.
Turn on the Instant Pot and open the pot. Add the olive oil and pork to it. Add the onions, ginger, garlic, and coconut milk. Seal the lid, select Meat/Stew mode and cook on High pressure for 40 minutes. Once ready, do a quick pressure release. Dish the meat with the sauce into a serving bowl, garnish with the parsley, and serve with a side of keto bread.
Nutrition Values: Calories 267, Protein 38g Net Carbs 0g, Fat 11g

392. Sweet Spicy Pork Chops
Cooking Time: 25 minutes
Servings: 4
Ingredients
4 Pork Chops, Boneless and cubed
6 cloves Garlic, minced
1 Onion, cut in big chunks
2 Zucchinis, chopped in big chunks
2 tbsp Sesame Oil
1 tsp Red Chili Flakes
½ tsp Ginger Juice
½ tsp Orange Zest
1 tbsp Tahini
2 tbsp Monk Fruit Syrup
1 tbsp Plain Vinegar
½ tbsp Arrowroot Powder
1 tsp Sriracha Sauce
1/6 cup Water
Salt and Pepper to taste
Directions
Season the pork with pepper and salt. Heat half of the oil on Sauté. Add the garlic and pork. Brown the pork on all sides. Mix the remaining oil, ginger juice, zest, tahini, flakes, monk syrup and vinegar.
Mix evenly and pour over the pork. Seal the lid and cook on High Pressure for 12 minutes. Once done, quickly release the pressure. Add in zucchinis and onion, seal the lid and cook for 5 minutes on High pressure. Once done, release the pressure quickly. Mix the arrowroot powder with water and pour in the pot. Stir in the sriracha sauce and serve.
Nutrition Values: Calories 231, Protein 15.1g, Net Carbs 0.7g, Fat 8.3g

393. Green Chile Pork Carnitas
Cooking Time: 55 minutes
Servings:
Ingredients
4 lb Pork Shoulder, cut 3 pieces
3 tbsp Olive oil
Salt and Black Pepper to taste
2 Jalapenos, seeded, minced
2 Green Bell peppers, seeded, chopped
2 Poblano Peppers, seeded, minced
1 ½ lb Tomatillos, husked, quartered
4 cloves Garlic, peeled
2 medium Red Onions, chopped
2 tsp Cumin Powder
2 tsp Dried Oregano
2 ½ cups Pork Broth
3 Bay Leaves
Toppings:
Red Onion, chopped
Queso Fresco
Cilantro, roughly chopped
Directions
Season the pork with pepper and salt. Heat oil on Sauté, and brown pork on all sides for 6 minutes. Add bell pepper, peppers, tomatillo, onion, cumin, garlic, oregano, bay leaves and broth.
Stir, close the lid, secure the pressure valve and select Manual mode on High Pressure for 10 minutes. Once done, do a natural pressure release for 15 minutes.
Remove the meat from the pot, shred it in a plate; set aside. Puree the remaining ingredients in the pot using a stick blender. Add the pork back. Set on Sauté and simmer for 5 minutes. Stir twice and serve in keto tacos with the toppings.
Nutrition Values: Calories 690, Protein 27g, Net Carbs 1g, Fat 48g

394. Pork in Peanut Sauce
Cooking Time: 50 minutes
Servings: 4
Ingredients:
3 lb Pork Roast
1 cup Hot Water
1 large Red Bell pepper, seeded and sliced
Salt and Pepper to taste
1 large White Onion, sliced
½ cup sugar-free Soy Sauce
1 tbsp Plain Vinegar
½ cup Peanut Butter
1 tbsp Lime Juice
1 tbsp Garlic Powder

1 tsp Ginger Puree
To Garnish:
Chopped Peanuts
Chopped Green Onions
Lime Wedges
Directions:
Pour soy sauce, vinegar, peanut butter, lime juice, garlic powder, and ginger puree to a bowl. Use a whisk to mix them together and even. Add a few pinches of salt and pepper, and mix it.
Open the Instant Pot and put the pork in it. Pour the hot water and peanut butter mixture over. Close the lid, secure the pressure valve, and select Meat/Stew mode on High pressure for 20 minutes. Once ready, do a quick pressure release.
Use a slotted spoon or a set of tongs to remove the meat onto a cutting board and use two forks to shred it. Return to the sauce and select Sauté mode. Let simmer for about 2 minutes, then turn the Instant Pot off. On a bed of broccoli cauli rice, spoon the meat with some sauce and garnish with the chopped peanuts, green Onions, and the Lemon wedges.
Nutrition Values: Calories 243, Protein 27g, Net Carbs 0g, Fat 6.6g

395. Carrot and Pork Stew
Cooking Time: 45 minutes
Servings: 6
Ingredients:
1 Onion, chopped
2 Tomatoes, chopped
2 Carrots, sliced
½ lb Pork meat, pieces, boiled
2 cups Chicken broth
½ tbsp Garlic paste
½ tbsp Ginger paste
½ tbsp Cumin powder
½ tbsp Cinnamon powder
½ tbsp Chili powder
¼ tbsp Salt
¼ tbsp Turmeric powder
3 tbsp Olive oil
2 Jalapeño peppers, whole
Directions:
Heat oil on Sauté, and sauté onion for 2 minutes. Add in tomatoes, ginger, garlic, salt, chili, and turmeric; stir-fry for 1 minute. Add pork and cook for 10 minutes.
Add carrots and cook until the meat lightly tender, about 4-5 minutes. Next, add the chicken broth and jalapeños. Seal the lid and cook on High pressure for 30 minutes.
When ready, do a quick pressure release and stir in cinnamon and cumin powder.
Nutrition Values: Calories 151, Protein 8g, Net Carbs 1.5g, Fat 5.2g

396. Beef Steak in Balsamic Sauce
Cooking Time: 30 Minutes
Servings: 6
Ingredients:
4 -pounds beef steak
1 small red onion; finely chopped.
1 cup bone broth
1/2 cup heavy cream
1/2 cup button mushrooms; sliced
1 cup balsamic vinegar
2 tablespoon olive oil
4 garlic cloves; finely chopped
1 teaspoon fresh rosemary; finely chopped
2 teaspoon fresh thyme; finely chopped.
1 teaspoon black peppercorns; whole
2 teaspoon sea salt
Directions:
Rinse the meat under cold running water and transfer to a large bowl. Add balsamic vinegar, salt, thyme, peppercorns, and rosemary. Mix to combine and cover with an aluminum foil. Refrigerate for at least 30 minutes
Plug in your instant pot and grease the stainless steel insert with olive oil. Press the *Sauté* button and add mushrooms, garlic, and onions. Cook for 5 minutes, stirring occasionally. Add meat along with marinade and pour in the broth.
Securely lock the lid and press the *Manual* button. Set the timer for 15 minutes and cook on *High* pressure When done; perform a quick pressure release and press the *Sauté* button again. Stir in the heavy cream and cook for 5 more minutes.
Transfer the meat to a serving platter and spoon over the balsamic sauce. Optionally, sprinkle with some finely chopped green onions or fresh parsley
Nutrition Info: Calories: 670; Total Fats: 27.3g; Net Carbs: 2.5g; Protein: 95.8g; Fiber: 0.7g

397. Rosemary Beef Roast Recipe
Cooking Time: 40 Minutes
Servings: 6
Ingredients:
2 -pounds beef chuck roast; cut into large pieces
1 small onion; finely chopped
1 teaspoon balsamic vinegar
1 teaspoon olive oil
1/2 cup heavy cream
1 medium-sized red bell pepper; stripped
1 cup bone broth
3 garlic cloves; crushed
1 teaspoon black pepper; freshly ground.
1 teaspoon dried marjoram; ground.
1 teaspoon fresh rosemary; finely chopped
1/2 teaspoon dried parsley; ground.
1 teaspoon salt
Directions:
Plug in your instant pot and grease the stainless steel insert with olive oil. Press the *Sauté* button and add onions and garlic. Stir-fry for 3-4 minutes, or until translucent
Add meat and generously sprinkle with salt. Cook for 3-4 minutes on each side, or until lightly browned. Now; add all the remaining ingredients and spices. Close the lid and adjust the steam release handle. Press the *Manual* button and set the timer for 25 minutes. Cook on *High* pressure
When you hear the cooker's end signal, perform a quick release of the pressure and open the pot. Transfer all to a serving bowl and garnish with fresh rosemary before serving.

Nutrition Info: Calories: 619; Total Fats: 46.7g; Net Carbs: 3g; Protein: 43.6g; Fiber: 0.8g

398. Instant Lamb Shoulder Hash
Cooking Time: 35 Minutes
Servings: 3
Ingredients:
9-ounce lamb shoulder; chopped into bite-sized pieces
1 large tomato; finely chopped
2 green bell peppers; finely chopped.
2 celery stalks; finely chopped.
1/4 cup almonds; minced
3 large eggs
2 tablespoon olive oil
2 tablespoon butter
1/4 cup beef broth
1/2 teaspoon garlic powder
1/4 teaspoon black pepper; ground.
1 teaspoon salt
Directions:
Plug in the instant pot and grease the inner pot with oil. Add chopped meat and season with salt.
Cook for 5-6 minutes and then add bell peppers and celery stalks. Continue to cook for 10 minutes, stirring occasionally
Now pour in the stock and add tomatoes. Bring it to a boil and simmer for 15 minutes.
When most of the liquid has evaporated, stir in the butter and season with garlic powder and black pepper. Optionally, add some more salt
Gently crack the eggs and continue to cook until completely set.
Nutrition Info: Calories: 465; Total Fats: 32.6g; Net Carbs: 7.9g; Protein: 33.7g; Fiber: 3g

399. Beef Shoulder Roast
Cooking Time: 45 Minutes
Servings: 4
Ingredients:
3 -pounds beef shoulder roast
1 medium-sized yellow bell pepper; chopped
1 tablespoon olive oil
1 cup tomatoes; diced
2 cups beef broth
1 small red onion; finely chopped.
3 garlic cloves; crushed
1 teaspoon dried oregano; ground.
1 teaspoon dried basil; ground.
1 teaspoon fresh rosemary; finely chopped
1 teaspoon red chili powder
1 teaspoon smoked paprika; ground.
2 teaspoon sea salt
Directions:
Place the rinsed meat in a large bowl and generously rub with salt, chili powder, paprika, oregano, and basil, Set aside
Plug in the instant pot and grease the stainless steel insert with olive oil. Press the *Sauté* button and add onions and bell peppers. Stir-fry for 3-4 minutes and add meat
Cook for 5 minutes on each side, or until golden brown.

Add diced tomatoes and pour in the broth. Securely lock the lid and set the steam release handle. Press the *Manual* button and set the timer for 20 minutes. Cook on *High* pressure
When you hear the cooker's end signal, perform a quick pressure release and open the pot. Carefully transfer the meat to a cutting board. Using two forks, shred and return the meat to the pot.
Press the *Sauté* button and cook until sauce thickens. Turn off the pot and stir in the fresh rosemary. Serve warm.
Nutrition Info: Calories: 595; Total Fats: 28.7g; Net Carbs: 5.8g; Protein: 72.9g; Fiber: 2.1g

400. Beef with Greens
Cooking Time: 50 Minutes
Servings: 8
Ingredients:
2 -pounds beef chuck roast; cut into bite-sized pieces
4 garlic cloves; finely chopped
1 cup fresh spinach; chopped
1 small onion; chopped
1 cup fresh kale; chopped
2 cups beef broth
2 tablespoon butter
1/2 teaspoon black pepper; ground.
1/4 teaspoon dried thyme; ground.
1 teaspoon sea salt
Directions:
Combine spinach and kale in a large colander. Rinse thoroughly under cold running water and drain.
Chop into small pieces and set aside
Plug in the instant pot and press the *Sauté* button. Melt 1 tablespoon of the butter in the stainless steel insert and add garlic and onions. Cook for 3-4 minutes, stirring occasionally
Add meat and sprinkle with salt and pepper. Pour in the broth and lock the lid. Set the steam release handle and press the *Manual* button. Set the timer for 20 minutes and cook on *High* pressure
When done, perform a quick pressure release by moving the valve to the *Venting* position. Open the pot and add spinach, kale and the remaining butter. Cook for 5 more minutes, or until the greens are wilted.
Turn off the pot and transfer all to a serving bowl. Optionally, top with sour cream or cream cheese and enjoy!
Nutrition Info: Calories: 458; Total Fats: 34.8g; Net Carbs: 2.2g; Protein: 31.5g; Fiber: 0.5g

401. Fried Beef Roast
Cooking Time: 25 Minutes
Servings: 8
Ingredients:
2 -pounds beef chuck roast; cut into bite-sized pieces
1/2 cup shallots; chopped.
1 tablespoon olive oil
1/2 cup heavy cream
3 garlic cloves; crushed
1/4 cup balsamic vinegar
1 tablespoon dried parsley; finely chopped
1/4 teaspoon dried marjoram; ground.
1 teaspoon black pepper; ground.

1 teaspoon dried oregano; ground.
1 teaspoon salt
Directions:
Rinse the meat under cold running water and pat dry with a kitchen towel. Transfer to a large cutting board and cut into bite-sized pieces. Rub with salt and pepper and set aside
Grease the stainless steel insert of your instant pot with olive oil. Add shallots and garlic. Stir-fry for 2-3 minutes, stirring constantly
Now; add meat chops and cook for 10 minutes
Pour in the heavy cream and balsamic vinegar. Sprinkle with the remaining spices and give it a good stir. Bring it to a boil and cook for 10-15 more minutes, or until the sauce thickens
Transfer to a serving dish and optionally, drizzle with some lemon juice before serving.
Nutrition Info: Calories: 464; Total Fats: 36.1g; Net Carbs: 2.5g; Protein: 30.2g; Fiber: 0.2g

402. Shiitake Beef Sirloin
Cooking Time: 50 Minutes
Servings: 6
Ingredients:
2 -pounds beef sirloin; cut into bite-sized pieces
1 cup pearl onions; chopped.
5 bacon slices; chopped
3 cups beef broth
1 cup heavy cream
1 tablespoon butter
1 cup Shiitake mushrooms; chopped
1 teaspoon fresh sage; chopped.
1 teaspoon black pepper; freshly ground.
1 teaspoon fresh thyme; chopped
1 teaspoon salt
Directions:
Plug in your instant pot and press the *Sauté* button. Add chopped bacon and stir-fry for 2-3 minutes. Remove the bacon from the pot and set aside
Add butter and gently melt, stirring constantly. Add mushrooms and onions. Cook for 5-7 minutes and remove from the pot
Add meat and sprinkle with salt and pepper. Cook for 5 minutes and then pour in the broth. Close the lid and adjust the steam release handle. Press *Manual* button and set the timer for 25 minutes. Cook on *High* pressure
When done; perform a quick pressure release by moving the valve to the *Venting* position
Open the pot and add mushroom mixture, bacon, and heavy cream. Press the *Sauté* button and bring it to a boil. Stir in the sage and thyme. Simmer for 10 more minutes. Turn off the pot and transfer all to a serving dish.
Nutrition Info: Calories: 431; Total Fats: 18.8g; Net Carbs: 5.9g; Protein: 55.1g; Fiber: 1.5g

403. Beef Shank
Cooking Time: 40 Minutes
Servings: 8
Ingredients:
3 -pounds beef shank
1 cup green onions
3 cups beef broth

For the marinade:
1 teaspoon black pepper; ground.
2 garlic cloves; crushed
1/2 teaspoon smoked paprika; ground.
1 cup olive oil
1 tablespoon fresh rosemary; chopped.
2 teaspoon fresh thyme; chopped
1 teaspoon salt
Directions:
In a large bowl, combine all marinade ingredients. Mix until well incorporated and set aside
Rinse the meat under cold running water and pat dry with a kitchen paper. Place in a large Ziploc bag and pour in the marinade. Shake well to coat the meat evenly with the marinade. Refrigerate for 1 hour
Plug in your instant pot and press the *Sauté* button. Drain the meat and place in the stainless steel insert. Cook for 5 minutes on each side, or until golden brown
Pour in the broth and securely lock the lid. Adjust the steam release handle and press the *Manual* button. Set the timer for 20 minutes and cook on *High* pressure
When you hear the cooker's end signal, release the pressure naturally
Open the pot and transfer the meat to a serving plate
Drizzle with some marinade and garnish with green onions.
Nutrition Info: Calories: 369; Total Fats: 14.7g; Net Carbs: 1.5g; Protein: 53.8g; Fiber: 0.7g

404. Spicy Masala Beef Roast
Cooking Time: 40 Minutes
Servings: 4
Ingredients:
2 -pounds beef shoulder roast
1-egg; beaten
1 cup of cherry tomatoes; diced
1 small onion; diced
4 garlic cloves; crushed
1 small red chili pepper; chopped.
2 tablespoon olive oil
2 cups chicken broth
1/4 teaspoon cardamom; ground.
1/4 teaspoon cinnamon; ground.
1/4 teaspoon nutmeg; ground.
1/2 teaspoon black pepper; ground.
1 teaspoon salt
Directions:
Rinse the meat under cold running water and pat dry with a kitchen paper. Cut into bite-sized pieces and set aside
In a large mixing bowl, combine all spices and mix until blend. Add meat and give it a good stir until all well coated.
Plug in your instant pot and grease the stainless steel insert with olive oil. Press the *Sauté* button and add chili pepper, onions, and garlic. Cook for 2-3 minutes, or until onions translucent
Now; add meat and continue to cook for another 10 minutes, stirring occasionally
Pour in the broth and close the lid. Set the steam release handle by moving the valve to the *Sealing*

position. Press the '*Manual* button and set the timer for 15 minutes. Cook on *High* pressure
When done; release the pressure naturally and open the pot. Stir in the tomatoes and simmer for 5 minutes. The liquid should be reduced by half. Poach the egg on top and cook for additional 2 minutes. Transfer to a serving dish and serve immediately
Nutrition Info: Calories: 458; Total Fats: 25g; Net Carbs: 4.2g; Protein: 50.8g; Fiber: 1.2g

405. Chili Lamb Leg Recipe
Cooking Time: 60 Minutes
Servings: 4
Ingredients:
2 -pounds lamb leg; boneless and chopped
2 cups beef stock
2 red chili peppers; chopped
3 tablespoon olive oil
3 garlic cloves; crushed
1/2 teaspoon black pepper; ground.
1 thyme sprig
2 teaspoon chili powder
1 teaspoon salt
Directions:
Rinse the meat thoroughly under cold running water and pat dry with a kitchen towel.
Rub well with oil and garlic. Sprinkle with salt, pepper, and chili powder. Tightly wrap with aluminum foil and refrigerate for 30 minutes
Now plug in the instant pot and remove the meat from the fridge. Place in the pot and add beef stock. Add thyme sprig and chopped chili peppers.
Seal the lid and set the steam release handle to the *Sealing* position. Press the *Manual* button and set the timer for 20 minutes on high pressure
When done; release the pressure naturally and open the lid. Serve hot and enjoy!
Nutrition Info: Calories: 524; Total Fats: 27.4g; Net Carbs: 0.9g; Protein: 65.2g; Fiber: 0.1g

406. Lamb Kebab Recipe
Cooking Time: 25 Minutes
Servings: 5
Ingredients:
1-pound ground lamb tenderloin
1/2 large eggplant; peeled
3 tablespoon butter; softened
1/2 cup diced canned tomatoes; sugar-free
9-ounce ground beef
1/2 cup onions; finely chopped
3 garlic cloves; crushed
3 tablespoon olive oil
1 tablespoon cayenne pepper
1 teaspoon chili powder
1 teaspoon dried oregano
1 teaspoon cumin powder
1 teaspoon salt
Directions:
In a medium-sized bowl, combine together ground lamb, ground beef, onions, garlic, olive oil, salt, cumin oregano, cayenne, and chili powder. Mix well and shape bite-sized balls, Set aside
Arrange balls and eggplant slices on soaked skewers and drizzle with some more olive oil

Plug in the instant pot and press the *Sauté* button. Grease the inner pot with butter and heat up
Add skewers, in two batches, and cook for 4-5 minutes on one side. Turn over and continue to cook until lightly golden brown.
Remove the skewers from the pot and add diced tomatoes. Season with some salt, pepper, and oregano. Stir well and cook for a couple of minutes. Press the *Cancel'* button to turn off the pot. Place skewers on a serving platter and drizzle with the tomato sauce
Nutrition Info: Calories: 419; Total Fats: 25.3g; Net Carbs: 3g; Protein: 41.9g; Fiber: 2.1g

407. Keto Beef Meatballs
Cooking Time: 30 Minutes
Servings: 6
Ingredients:
2 -pounds ground beef
1 small red onion; chopped
3 garlic cloves
1 cup beef broth
1 cup fresh parsley; finely chopped.
1 tablespoon olive oil
1/4 cup feta cheese
1 medium-sized yellow bell pepper; chopped
3 large eggs
1 cup tomatoes; diced
1/4 teaspoon dried thyme; ground.
1/2 teaspoon dried oregano; ground.
1/2 teaspoon red pepper flakes
1 teaspoon sea salt
Directions:
In a large mixing bowl, combine beef, eggs, parsley, and cheese. Add about 1-2 tablespoons of lukewarm water mix with your hands. Add all the spices and mix until well incorporated
Shape balls with the mixture, approximately 1-inch in diameter. Set aside,
Plug in your instant pot and grease the stainless steel insert with olive oil. Press the *Sauté* button and add onions and garlic. Stir-fry for 3-4 minutes, or until the onions translucent. Stir in the tomatoes and pour in the broth. Carefully place the meatballs in the pot and close the lid
Adjust the steam release handle and press the *Manual* button. Set the timer for 10 minutes and cook on *High* pressure
When you hear the cooker's end signal, perform a quick release of the pressure and open the pot.
Transfer the meatballs to a serving bowl and drizzle with the remaining sauce from the pot.
Optionally, brown the meatballs on each side before cooking in your instant pot.
Nutrition Info: Calories: 383; Total Fats: 16.1g; Net Carbs: 4.3g; Protein: 51.7g; Fiber: 1.4g

408. Keto Korean Beef
Cooking Time: 25 Minutes
Servings: 4
Ingredients:
3 pounds' boneless beef chuck roast; cut into 1-inch cubes.
1/2 teaspoon white pepper

3 tablespoons cornstarch
1 teaspoon sesame seeds
2 green onions; thinly sliced.
1/2 cup beef broth
1/3 cup reduced sodium soy sauce.
1/3 cup brown sugar; packed
4 cloves garlic; minced.
1 tablespoon sesame oil
1 tablespoon rice wine vinegar
1 tablespoon freshly grated ginger.
1 teaspoon Sriracha; or more, to taste
1/2 teaspoon onion powder.
Directions:
In a large bowl, whisk together beef broth, soy sauce, brown sugar, garlic, sesame oil, rice wine vinegar, ginger, Sriracha, onion powder and white pepper
Place chuck roast into an Instant Pot. Stir in beef broth mixture until well combined.
Select manual setting; adjust pressure to high, and set time for 15 minutes. When finished cooking, quick-release pressure according to manufacturer's directions
In a small bowl, whisk together cornstarch and 3 tablespoons water; set aside
Select high sauté setting. Stir in cornstarch mixture and cook, stirring frequently, until the sauce has thickened, about 2-3 minutes
Serve immediately, garnished with green onions and sesame seeds, if desired.
Nutrition Info: Calories: 660; Protein: 60g; Carbs: 6g; Fat: 40

409. Mongolian Style Beef
Cooking Time: 30 Minutes
Servings: 4
Ingredients:
1 pound flank steak; sliced across the grain.
1/2 cup brown sugar or 2/3 cups I prefer the version with more sugar.
1 tablespoon cornstarch
1/2 cup lite soy sauce.
1 cup water
1 tablespoons extra virgin olive oil
10 cloves garlic; minced.
1 tablespoon fresh ginger; minced.
1 teaspoon red pepper flakes
Cornstarch Slurry: (Optional.
2 tablespoons cornstarch.
1/2 cup water
Garnish:
1/4 cup green onions; chopped
1 teaspoon sesame seeds
Directions:
Heat up your pressure cooker: press Sauté -> click on the Adjust button -> select More to get the Sauté More function, which means that the food will be sautéed over medium-high heat. Wait for the Instant Pot indicator to read *Hot*.
Add sliced beef to a large ziplock bag, add 1 tablespoon cornstarch and shake well to coat the beef evenly
Add the oil to the hot Instant Pot, once the oil is hot, add the beef and sauté for 2-3 minutes, stirring a few times

Add the rest of the ingredients to the pot: minced garlic, minced ginger, lite soy sauce, brown sugar, water and red pepper flakes. You can add less sugar, based on your taste and preference
Stir well until all the ingredients are combined and coated in sauce
Close lid and pressure cook at High Pressure for 8 minutes + 10 minutes Natural Release. Turn off the heat. Release the remaining pressure. Open the lid.
Make the cornstarch slurry, in a small bowl mix cornstarch with water until fully combined.
With the Instant Pot on the Sauté function, add the slurry to the pot, stir to combine and cook for 2-3 minutes on Sauté, stirring occasionally, until the sauce thickens
Turn off the Instant Pot and let the Mongolian Beef sit for 8-10 minutes before serving, in this time the sauce will settle and thicken more
Serve hot and garnish with fresh chopped green onions and sesame seeds
Nutrition Info: Calories 327 ; Protein: 35g; Carbs: 5g; Fat: 17g

410. Instant Cheddar Beef Hash
Cooking Time: 20 Minutes
Servings: 4
Ingredients:
1-pound ground beef
1 medium-sized green bell pepper; chopped
1 cup cauliflower; chopped.
1 small celery stalk; chopped
1 tablespoon fresh parsley; finely chopped
1 tablespoon olive oil
1 cup cheddar cheese
1/2 teaspoon black pepper; freshly ground.
1/2 teaspoon smoked paprika; ground.
1 teaspoon sea salt
Directions:
Plug the instant pot and press the *Sauté* button. Grease the stainless steel insert with olive oil. Add ground beef and cook for 5 minutes, or until lightly browned
Now; add bell pepper, cauliflower, and parsley. Add about 1/4 cup of water and continue to cook for another 5 minutes, or until vegetables are tender.
Sprinkle all with smoked paprika, salt, and pepper. Add the cheese on top and allow it to melt
Turn off the pot and transfer all to a serving dish, using a large slotted spoon. Optionally, top with sour cream and enjoy immediately
Nutrition Info: Calories: 373; Total Fats: 2.1g; Net Carbs: 3.1g; Protein: 42.4g; Fiber: 1.3g

411. Cheesey Meatballs
Cooking Time: 20 Minutes
Servings: 6
Ingredients:
2 -pounds lean ground beef
1 tablespoon fresh parsley; finely chopped
1 small Jalapeno pepper; chopped.
1 tablespoon butter
1 tablespoon Dijon mustard
3-ounce cheddar cheese
2 large eggs; beaten

2 garlic cloves; crushed
1 cup beef stock
1/4 teaspoon smoked paprika; ground.
1/2 teaspoon black pepper; ground.
1 teaspoon salt
Directions:
In a large mixing bowl, combine ground beef, cheese, eggs, garlic, Jalapeno pepper, parsley, mustard, paprika, salt, and pepper
Mix until well incorporated
Shape the meatballs, about 1 to 1 ½ –inch in diameter and set aside
Plug in the instant pot and add butter to the stainless steel insert. Gently melt over the *Sauté* mode, stirring constantly
Spread the meatballs on the bottom of the pot and slowly pour in the beef stock.
Securely lock the lid and set the steam release the handle by moving the valve to the *Sealing* position. Press the *Manual* button and set the timer for 10 minutes. Cook on *High* pressure
When done, perform a quick release of the pressure and open the pot.
Transfer the meatballs to a serving platter and drizzle with some of the liquid from the pot.
Optionally, garnish with some finely chopped cilantro before serving.
Nutrition Info: Calories: 387; Total Fats: 17.9g; Net Carbs: 0.9g; Protein: 52.2g; Fiber: 0.3g

412. Keto Beef Ragout
Cooking Time: 40 Minutes
Servings: 6
Ingredients:
2 -pounds beef steak; cut into bite-sized pieces
1 small onion; finely chopped
1 small red chili pepper; diced
1 small celery stalk; chopped
4 garlic cloves; crushed
2 cups beef stock
1 tablespoon olive oil
1 cup tomatoes; diced
1 teaspoon dried oregano; ground.
1 bay leaf
1 teaspoon black pepper; ground.
1 teaspoon salt
Directions:
Plug in the instant pot and grease the stainless steel insert with olive oil. Press the *Sauté* button and add onions, celery, garlic, and chili pepper. Stir-fry for 4-5 minutes, or until the onions translucent
Add meat chops and sprinkle with salt, oregano, and pepper. Pour in the beef stock and throw in the bay leaf. Securely lock the lid and adjust the steam release handle. Press the *Manual* button and set the timer for 20 minutes. Cook on *High* pressure. When you hear the cooker's end signal, perform a quick release of the pressure and open the lid
Stir in the tomatoes and press the *Sauté* button. Bring it to a boil and cook for 10 more minutes, stirring occasionally. Remove the bay leaf and transfer all to a serving dish. Optionally, garnish with some finely chopped parsley or top with sour cream.

Nutrition Info: Calories: 322; Total Fats: 12.1g; Net Carbs: 2.6g; Protein: 47.4g; Fiber: 1g

413. Lamb Neck with Broccoli
Cooking Time: 25 Minutes
Servings: 4
Ingredients:
1-pound lamb neck; chopped.
2 small onions; finely chopped.
1-pound broccoli; chopped
1 large tomato; roughly chopped
1 cup cauliflower; chopped into florets
2 tablespoon olive oil
2 celery stalks; finely chopped.
1/2 small sweet potato; finely chopped
1/2 teaspoon black pepper; freshly ground.
1 tablespoon cayenne pepper
2 teaspoon salt
Directions:
Rinse the meat and chop into bite-sized pieces. Place at the bottom of your pot and add vegetables. Sprinkle with olive oil, salt, cayenne pepper, and black pepper. Pour in the stock and seal the lid
Set the steam release handle to the *Sealing* position. Press the *Manual* button and set the timer for 17 minutes on high pressure
When done, release the pressure naturally and open the lid. Give it a good stir and serve immediately
Nutrition Info: Calories: 346; Total Fats: 15.9g; Net Carbs: 10.4g; Protein: 36.5g; Fiber: 5.3g

414. Beef Curry Recipe
Cooking Time: 50 Minutes
Servings: 2
Ingredients:
1 pound. grass-fed beef stew meat in chunks.
1/2 cup bone broth or vegetable broth.
1 ½ tablespoon curry powder.
1 teaspoon sea salt
1/2 teaspoon black pepper
1 teaspoon dried oregano
1/4 teaspoon paprika
2 tablespoon ghee or coconut oil.
1 onion
1,5 large potatoes or sweet potatoes.
2 carrots
5 cloves garlic
1 cup coconut milk
Directions:
Cut the onion, potatoes and carrots in large chunks. Dice the garlic.
Press the *Sauté* button on the instant pot and put the ghee in the instant pot.
Once the ghee is melted, add the onions and garlic and stir for about 2 minutes
Then, add the stew meat to brown all sides for about 5 minutes
Turn off the instant pot and add the remaining ingredients including the carrots, potatoes, coconut milk, broth, herbs and spices
Stir to make sure all the spices are mixed in the liquid. Place the lid in the locked position and make sure the vent is turned to *sealed*. Press the *meat/stew* button and use the +/- buttons to set to 30 minutes.

Once you get to 30 minutes it will automatically start cooking.
When it's done, serve over cauliflower rice or white rice
Nutrition Info: Calories: 363; Protein: 27g; Carbs: 6g; Fat: 25g

415. Lamb loin Stew Recipe
Cooking Time: 30 Minutes
Servings: 3
Ingredients:
1-pound lamb loin; chopped into bite-sized pieces
1 large zucchini; sliced into 1-inch thick slices
1 cup purple cabbage; shredded
1 small chili pepper; finely chopped.
2 cups beef stock
4 garlic cloves; crushed
3 tablespoon olive oil
1 teaspoon oregano
1/2 teaspoon chili powder
1/4 teaspoon dried thyme
1 teaspoon salt
Directions:
Plug in the instant pot and press the *Sauté* button. Heat up the oil and add garlic. Cook for one minute and then add the meat. Season with salt, chili powder, oregano, and thyme. Stir well and continue to cook for 5-6 minutes, stirring occasionally
Now add zucchini and give it a good stir. Stir-fry for 3 minutes
Pour in the stock and add chili pepper and cabbage. Seal the lid and set the steam release handle to the *Sealing* position.
Press the *Manual* button and set the timer for 12 minutes on high pressure
When done, release the pressure naturally and open the lid. Optionally, top with Greek yogurt before serving.
Nutrition Info: Calories: 442; Total Fats: 25.7g; Net Carbs: 4.6g; Protein: 46.2g; Fiber: 1.9g

416. Beef Neck with Fire Roasted Tomatoes
Cooking Time: 30 Minutes
Servings: 4
Ingredients:
12-ounce beef neck; chopped into bite-sized pieces
2 tablespoon black sesame seeds
1 cup beef broth
1 cup onions; finely chopped.
1 small zucchini; cubed
3 tablespoon butter
1/2 cup Parmesan cheese; grated
2 cups fire-roasted tomatoes; diced
1/2 teaspoon chili pepper
1 tablespoon cayenne pepper
1/2 teaspoon cumin powder
1/2 teaspoon salt
Directions:
Plug in the instant pot and heat up the butter on the *Sauté* mode. Add onions and cook until translucent. Now add tomatoes and sesame seeds. Pour in about 3 tablespoons of water and continue to cook for 5 minutes

Finally, add the meat and zucchini. Sprinkle with salt, chili, cayenne, and cumin powder. Stir well and pour in the broth
Seal the lid and set the steam release handle to the *Sealing* position. Press the *Manual* button and set the timer for 15 minutes.
When done, perform a quick pressure release and open the lid. Sprinkle with grated Parmesan and serve
Nutrition Info: Calories: 310; Total Fats: 17.4g; Net Carbs: 5.1g; Protein: 30.2g; Fiber: 17.4g

417. Easy Beef Chili
Cooking Time: 30 Minutes
Servings: 4
Ingredients:
1-pound ground beef
1 small red onion; chopped
1 tablespoon olive oil
1 medium-sized red bell pepper; chopped.
1 cup heavy cream
1/2 cup beef broth
2 cups tomatoes; diced
3 garlic cloves; minced
1 teaspoon garlic powder
1/2 teaspoon smoked paprika
1/2 teaspoon dried rosemary; ground.
1/2 teaspoon chili powder
1 teaspoon kosher salt
Directions:
Plug in the instant pot and press the *Sauté* button. Grease the stainless steel insert with olive oil and add ground beef, onion, and bell pepper. Sprinkle with salt and garlic powder. Using a wooden spatula, stir well and cook for 5 minutes
Add tomatoes and pour in the broth. Securely lock the lid and set the steam release handle. Press the *Manual* button and set the timer for 5 minutes. Cook on *High* pressure
When done, perform a quick pressure release and open the pot. Stir in the heavy cream and sprinkle with chili powder, salt, paprika, and rosemary
Press the *Sauté* button and cook for 10 more minutes. Transfer all to a serving dish and enjoy!
Nutrition Info: Calories: 390; Total Fats: 22.3g; Net Carbs: 7.7g; Protein: 37.3g; Fiber: 2.3g

418. Crispy Lamb Chops
Cooking Time: 30 Minutes
Servings: 4
Ingredients:
4 lamb chops; about 1-pound
1 cup button mushrooms; sliced
4 tablespoon butter
3 garlic cloves; crushed
1/4 cup soy sauce
2 cups vegetable stock
1/2 teaspoon garlic powder
1/2 teaspoon mustard; ground.
1 teaspoon black pepper; ground.
1/2 teaspoon smoked paprika
1 teaspoon salt
Directions:

Place the meat in the pot and pour in the stock. Seal the lid and set the steam release handle to the *Sealing* position. Press the *Manual* button and cook for 15 minutes on high pressure
When done, perform a quick pressure release and open the lid. Remove the chops from the pot and set aside
Remove the liquid and press the *Sauté* button. Heat up the inner pot and then add butter. Add chops and brown for 3-4 minutes on one side. Turn over and continue to cook for another 2-3 minutes. Remove from the pot.
Now add mushrooms and cook until the liquid evaporates. Add garlic and pour in the soy sauce. Season with spices and cook for another 4-5 minutes, stirring constantly
Press the *Cancel'* button and add browned chops. Coat well with the sauce and serve
Nutrition Info: Calories: 331; Total Fats: 20g; Net Carbs: 2.4g; Protein: 33.9g; Fiber: 0.6g

419. Lamb Chops with Vegetables
Cooking Time: 40 Minutes
Servings: 5
Ingredients:
5 lamb chump chops
2 tablespoon oil
1 bell pepper; finely chopped
1 cup onions; finely chopped.
1 cup vegetable stock
1 cup cauliflower; cut into florets
1/2 teaspoon black pepper
2 bay leaves
1 teaspoon sat
Directions:
Grease the bottom of the stainless steel inert with oil and add lamb chops- sprinkle with some salt and pepper and then add the cauliflower. Top with onions and peppers and pour in the stock
Seal the lid and set the steam release handle to the *Sealing* position. Press the *Manual* button and set the timer for 15 minutes on high pressure
When done; perform a quick pressure release and open the lid. Let it sit for a while
Preheat the oven to 400 degrees F
Transfer the meat to a baking dish and add vegetables. Roast in the oven for 10-12 minutes on each side. Remove from the oven and serve
Nutrition Info: Calories: 331; Total Fats: 15.8g; Net Carbs: 3.8g; Protein: 40.3g; Fiber: 1.4g

420. Easy Beef Bourguignon
Preparation Time:40 minutes
Servings: 6
Ingredients:
1 pound beef stew meat, chopped
8 slices bacon, chopped
1 small yellow onion, chopped
1 ½ cups beef broth
Salt and pepper
1 ½ tablespoons olive oil
3 cloves minced garlic
Directions:
Turn the Instant Pot on to the Sauté setting and let it heat up.
Add the oil then season the beef with salt and pepper and add it to the pot.
Cook for 4 to 5 minutes until browned, stirring often.
Add the bacon, onions, and garlic and cook for 4 minutes, stirring.
Stir in the beef broth then season with salt and pepper.
Close and lock the lid on the Instant Pot.
Press the Manual button and adjust the timer to 30 minutes.
When the timer goes off, let the pressure vent naturally.
When the pot has depressurized, open the lid.
Stir well and adjust seasoning to taste. Serve hot.
Nutrition Values:
calories 255 fat 14g ,protein 29g ,carbs 2g ,fiber 0.5g ,net carbs 1.5g

421. Shredded Beef
Preparation Time:1 hour 30 minutes
Servings: 6
Ingredients:
3 pounds boneless beef rump roast
1 ¼ cups beef broth
Salt and pepper
2 tablespoons olive oil
1 teaspoon dried oregano
1 teaspoon dried basil
1 teaspoon dried thyme
Directions:
Turn the Instant Pot on to the Sauté setting and let it heat up.
Add the oil to the pot and season the beef with salt and pepper.
Add the beef and cook for 2 minutes on each side until browned.
Whisk together the remaining ingredients and pour into the pot with the beef.
Close and lock the lid.
Press the Manual button and adjust the timer to 75 minutes.
When the timer goes off, let the pressure vent naturally. When the pot has depressurized, open the lid.
Shred the beef with two forks and stir into the cooking liquid.
Nutrition Values:
calories 455 fat 18.5g ,protein 71.5g ,carbs 0.5g ,fiber 0g ,net carbs 0.5g

422. Braised Beef Short Ribs
Preparation Time:50 minutes
Servings: 8
Ingredients:
2 pounds boneless beef short ribs
1 small yellow onion, chopped
1 tablespoon Worcestershire sauce
Salt and pepper
1 tablespoon olive oil
¼ cup tomato paste
½ cup red wine
Directions:

Turn the Instant Pot on to the Sauté setting and let it heat up.
Add the oil to the pot and season the short ribs with salt and pepper.
Place the ribs in the pot and cook for 2 minutes on each side to brown.
Remove the ribs then add the onions to the pot and cook for 5 minutes.
Stir in the garlic then add the rest of the ingredients, including the ribs.
Close and lock the lid then press the Manual button and adjust the timer to 35 minutes.
When the timer goes off, let the pressure vent for 5 minutes then do a Quick Release by pressing Cancel and switching the steam valve to "venting".
When the pot has depressurized, open the lid.
Remove the ribs to serve.
Nutrition Values:
calories 480 fat 43g ,protein 16.5g ,carbs 3g ,fiber 0.5g ,net carbs 2.5g

423. Classic Meatloaf
Preparation Time:45 minutes
Servings: 8
Ingredients:
2 pounds ground beef (80% lean
1 cup grated parmesan cheese
3 large eggs
Salt and pepper
1 tablespoon minced garlic
1 teaspoon dried oregano
1 cup almond flour
Directions:
Combine the ground beef, almond flour, parmesan cheese, eggs, garlic, and oregano in a bowl.
Mix well by hand then season with salt and pepper.
Place the steamer rack in your Instant Pot and line with foil.
Shape the meat mixture into a loaf and place it on the foil, close and lock the lid.
Press the Manual button and adjust the timer to 35 minutes.
When the timer goes off, do a Quick Release by pressing Cancel and switching the steam valve to "venting".
When the pot has depressurized, open the lid.
Remove the meatloaf to a roasting pan and broil for 5 minutes to brown before slicing to serve.
Nutrition Values:
calories 460 fat 31g ,protein 39.5g ,carbs 3g ,fiber 1.5g

424. Korean BBQ Beef
Preparation Time:25 minutes
Servings: 6
Ingredients:
3 pounds boneless beef chuck roast, cut into chunks
Salt and pepper
3 cloves minced garlic
1 tablespoon fresh grated ginger
1/3 cup soy sauce
2 tablespoons rice wine vinegar
6 tablespoons powdered erythritol
Directions:
Whisk together the soy sauce, powdered erythritol, ginger, garlic, and rice wine vinegar in a bowl.
Season the beef with salt and pepper then place it in the Instant Pot.
Pour the sauce over it then close and lock the lid.
Press the Manual button and adjust the timer to 15 minutes.
When the timer goes off, do a Quick Release by pressing Cancel and switching the steam valve to "venting".
When the pot has depressurized, open the lid. Serve the beef hot.
Nutrition Values:
calories 440 fat 14g ,protein 70g ,carbs 2.5g ,fiber 0.5g ,net carbs 2g

425. Bolognese Sauce
Preparation Time:40 minutes
Servings: 8
Ingredients:
1 small yellow onion, chopped
1 pound ground beef (80% lean
¼ pound chopped bacon
2 (14-ouncecans crushed tomatoes
1 tablespoon olive oil
¼ cup heavy cream
2 tablespoons tomato paste
Directions:
Turn the Instant Pot on to the Sauté setting and let it heat up.
Add the oil to the pot and add the onions – sauté for 4 to 5 minutes.
Stir in the beef and bacon then cook until browned, about 10 minutes.
Stir in the tomato paste and cook 1 minute more than pour in the wine.
Add tomatoes and ½ cup water, bring to a simmer, then close and lock the lid.
Press the Manual button and adjust the timer to 20 minutes.
When the timer goes off, do a Quick Release by pressing Cancel and switching the steam valve to "venting".
When the pot has depressurized, open the lid.
Stir in the heavy cream and adjust the seasoning to taste.
Press the Sauté button and simmer until the sauce has thickened and serve over zucchini noodles.
Nutrition Values:
calories 305 fat 19g ,protein 23g ,carbs 10g ,fiber 3.5g ,net carbs 6.5g

426. Stewed Beef with Mushrooms
Preparation Time:32 minutes
Servings: 6
Ingredients:
2 pounds beef stew meat, chopped
10 ounces sliced mushrooms
3 cups beef broth
Salt and pepper
1 ½ tablespoons olive oil
2 cloves minced garlic
2 tablespoons almond flour
Directions:

Turn the Instant Pot on to the Sauté setting and let it heat up.
Add the oil to the pot and season the beef with salt and pepper.
Add the beef to the pot and cook for 4 to 5 minutes until browned.
Stir in the mushrooms and garlic and cook for 3 to 4 minutes.
Stir in the almond flour and ¼ cup water, scraping up the browned bits.
Add the beef broth then close and lock the lid.
Press the Manual button and adjust the timer to 5 minutes.
When the timer goes off, let the pressure vent for 10 minutes then do a Quick Release by pressing Cancel and switching the steam valve to "venting".
When the pot has depressurized, open the lid.
Stir everything together well then serve hot.
Nutrition Values:
calories 355 fat 15g ,protein 50g ,carbs 3g ,fiber 1g ,net carbs 2g

427. Beef and Chorizo Chili
Preparation Time:25 minutes
Servings: 6
Ingredients:
½ pound diced chorizo sausage
1 small yellow onion, chopped
1 pound ground beef (80% lean
2 cups diced tomatoes
Salt and pepper
1 tablespoon olive oil
3 cloves minced garlic
Directions:
Turn the Instant Pot on to the Sauté setting and let it heat up.
Add the oil to the pot and season the beef with salt and pepper.
Stir in the chorizo and onion and cook for 4 to 5 minutes until the chorizo is browned.
Add the beef and garlic then season with salt and pepper – cook for 3 minutes.
Stir in the tomatoes then close and lock the lid.
Press the Manual button and adjust the timer to 15 minutes.
When the timer goes off, let the pressure vent for 5 minutes then do a Quick Release by pressing Cancel and switching the steam valve to "venting".
When the pot has depressurized, open the lid. Stir well and serve hot.
Nutrition Values:
calories 370 fat 26g ,protein 28.5g ,carbs 4g ,fiber 1g ,net carbs 3g

428. Quick and Easy Taco Meat
Preparation Time:20 minutes
Servings: 8
Ingredients:
1 small yellow onion, diced
2 pounds ground beef (80% lean
2 tablespoons olive oil
1 teaspoon garlic powder
2 teaspoons dried oregano
½ tablespoon chili powder

Directions:
Turn the Instant Pot on to the Sauté setting and let it heat up.
Add the oil to the pot along with the seasonings.
Cook for 5 minutes, stirring often, then stir in the ground beef.
Sauté for 3 to 4 minutes then close and lock the lid.
Press the Manual button and adjust the timer to 10 minutes.
When the timer goes off, let the pressure vent for 10 minutes then do a Quick Release by pressing Cancel and switching the steam valve to "venting".
When the pot has depressurized, open the lid.
Stir everything together and serve hot.
Nutrition Values:
calories 345 fat 23g ,protein 31g ,carbs 1.5g ,fiber 0.5g ,net carbs 1g

429. Balsamic Beef Pot Roast
Preparation Time:45 minutes
Servings: 8
Ingredients:
3 pounds boneless beef chuck roast
1 small yellow onion
2 cups water
Salt and pepper
1 tablespoon olive oil
¼ cup balsamic vinegar
¼ teaspoon xanthan gum
Directions:
Turn the Instant Pot on to the Sauté setting and let it heat up.
Add the oil to the pot and season the beef with salt and pepper.
Place the beef in the pot (you may need to cut it into two piecesand cook for 2 to 3 minutes on each side to brown.
Sprinkle in the onions then pour in the water and balsamic vinegar.
Close and lock the lid then press the Manual button and adjust the timer to 40 minutes.
When the timer goes off, do a Quick Release by pressing Cancel and switching the steam valve to "venting".
When the pot has depressurized, open the lid.
Remove the beef to a bowl and break it up into pieces while you simmer the cooking liquid on the Sauté setting.
Whisk in the xanthan gum and simmer until thickened.
Stir the beef back into the sauce and serve hot.
Nutrition Values:
calories 335 fat 12.5g ,protein 52g ,carbs 1g ,fiber 0.5g ,net carbs 0.5g

430. Zesty Beef Bites
Preparation Time: 25 minutes,
Servings: 4
Ingredients:
1 pound (cubedBeef stew meat
1 tbsp (gratedLime zest
1 cup Beef stock
2 (mincedGarlic cloves
1 tbsp (choppedOregano

2 tbsp Avocado oil
1 tbsp Lime juice
1 tbsp Smoked paprika
Directions:
Let your Instant Pot preheat on Sauté mode.
Add oil, and meat, then sauté for 5 minutes.
Stir in remaining ingredients and mix well
Seal the pot's lid and cook for 10 minutes on manual mode at High.
Allow the pressure to release in 10 minutes naturally then remove the lid.
Serve fresh and enjoy.
Nutrition Values:
Calories 236, Total Fat: 8.4g, Carbs: 2.8g, Protein: 34.5g, Fiber: 1.6g.

431. Cheesy Beef with Tomato Sauce
Preparation Time: 30 minutes,
servings: 6
Ingredients:
2 lb. Cubed beef .
2 cups Shredded cheddar cheese
1 cup Chicken stock
½ cup Okra
3 Chopped spring onions
A pinch of salt and black pepper
1 tbsp Olive oil .
Mustard 2 tbsp.
1 cup Tomato passata
Directions:
Press 'Sauté' on the instant pot and add the oil. When hot, add brown the meat in the oil for 5 minutes.
Mix in the mustard, passata, chicken stock, okra, spring onions, salt, and pepper and seal the lid to cook for 15 minutes at high pressure.
Natural release the pressure for 10 minutes and spread the cheese over the beef mix and set aside for 10 minutes then share into bowls and serve.
Nutrition Values:
Calories 411, fat 19.3, carbs 5, protein 52.4, fiber 1.6

432. Cheesy Garlic Beef Bowls
Preparation Time: 30 minutes,
servings: 6
Ingredients:
2 lb Thinly sliced beef roast .
1 cup Crumbled feta cheese
1 tbsp Chopped parsley .
½ cup Veggie stock
3 cloves Minced garlic
A pinch of salt and black pepper
1 tsp Balsamic vinegar .
2 tbsp Olive oil .
Directions:
Press 'Sauté' on the instant pot and pour in the oil. When hot, brown the garlic and the meat for 5 minutes.
Mix in the vinegar, stock, salt, and pepper, seal the lid and cook for 15 minutes at high pressure.
Natural release the pressure for 10 minutes, share into plates and serve.
Nutrition Values:
Calories 390, fat 19.4, carbs 1.6, protein 9.5, fiber 0.1

433. Creamy Lime Turkey with Tomato Sauce
Preparation Time: 35 minutes,
servings: 4
Ingredients:
1 Skinless and boneless turkey breasts; cubed
1 tbsp Garam masala .
1 cup Greek yogurt
1 tbsp Lime juice .
¼ tsp Grated ginger .
A pinch of salt and black pepper
1 tbsp Avocado oil .
1 cup Tomato passata
Directions:
Press 'Sauté' on the instant pot and add the oil. When hot, mix in the garam masala, turkey, and ginger to brown for 5 minutes.
Mix in the remaining ingredients and seal the lid to cook for 20 minutes at high pressure.
Natural release the pressure for 10 minutes, share the mix and serve.
Nutrition Values:
Calories 20, fat 4.6, carbs 3.6, protein 0.9, fiber 1.1

434. Spicy Garlic Pork and Okra Jumble
Preparation Time: 40 minutes,
servings: 4
Ingredients:
2 lb. Cubed pork sirloin .
1 ½ cups Okra
2 cloves Minced garlic
A pinch of salt and black pepper
1 tbsp Olive oil .
1 tbsp Smoked paprika .
1 cup Tomato passata
Directions:
Press 'Sauté' on the instant pot and add the oil. When hot, brown the garlic, salt, pepper, and the meat for 5 minutes.
Mix in the rest of the ingredients and seal the lid to cook for 25 minutes at high pressure.
Natural release the pressure for 10 minutes, share into bowls and serve.
Nutrition Values:
Calories 66, fat 3.9, carbs 2.7, protein 1.6, fiber 2

435. Lamb in Tomato Sauce with Olives
Preparation Time: 40 minutes,
servings: 4
Ingredients:
1 ½ lb. Lamb shoulder; cubed .
1 cup Beef stock
1 cup Black olives; pitted and sliced
2 Cubed tomatoes
A pinch of salt and black pepper
1 tbsp Avocado oil .
2 tbsp Chopped basil .
1 cup Tomato passata
Directions:
Press 'Sauté' on the instant pot and add the oil. When hot, brown the lamb meat for 5 minutes.

Mix in the passata, beef stock, olives, tomatoes, salt, and sugar then seal the lid to cook for 25 minutes at high pressure.
Natural release the pressure for 10 minutes, dish into bowls and serve topped with basil.
Nutrition Values:
Calories 251, fat 5.6, carbs 4.7, protein 8.3, fiber 2.7

436. Chili Lamb And Zucchini In Tomato Sauce

Preparation Time: 40 minutes,
servings: 4
Ingredients:
1 tbsp Chopped dill .
¼ cup Veggie stock
2 Slice zucchini
1 lb. Lamb shoulder; cubed .
A pinch of salt and black pepper
2 tbsp Olive oil .
1 tsp Sweet paprika .
2 tbsp Tomato passata .
Directions:
Press 'Sauté' on the instant pot and add the oil. When hot, brown the lamb for 5 minutes.
Mix in the remaining ingredients and seal the lid to cook for 25 minutes at high pressure.
Natural release the pressure for 10 minutes, share into bowls and serve.
Nutrition Values:
Calories 292, fat 15.6, carbs 4.5, protein 33.4, fiber 1.5

437. Balsamic Pork Tenderloin

Preparation Time:45 minutes
Servings: 6
Ingredients:
¼ cup water
1 (2-poundboneless pork tenderloin
Salt and pepper
1 tablespoon olive oil
3 tablespoons powdered erythritol
¼ cup balsamic vinegar
Directions:
Turn the Instant Pot on to the Sauté setting and let it heat up.
Meanwhile, whisk together the water, balsamic vinegar, and powdered erythritol.
Add the oil to the pot and the pork tenderloin – season with salt and pepper.
Cook the pork until it is browned on all sides, rotating as needed, about 8 minutes total.
Pour in the sauce then close and lock the lid.
Press the Meat/Stew button and adjust the timer for 35 minutes.
When the timer goes off, let the pressure vent naturally.
When the pot has depressurized, open the lid. Slice the pork to serve.
Nutrition Values:
calories 160 fat 4g ,protein 28g ,carbs 1.5g ,fiber 0g ,net carbs 1.5g

438. Easy Lamb with Gravy

Preparation Time:1hour 40 minutes
Servings: 5
Ingredients:
2 pounds boneless leg of lamb
1 ½ cups water
2 tablespoons coconut flour
Salt and pepper
1 tablespoon olive oil
1 teaspoon dried oregano
½ cup white wine
Directions:
Turn the Instant Pot on to the Sauté setting and let it heat up.
Add the oil to the pot and season the lamb with oregano, salt, and pepper.
Place the lamb in the pot and cook for 2 to 3 minutes on each side to brown.
Pour in the wine and let it simmer for a few minutes then pour in the water.
Add the lamb then close and lock the lid.
Press the Manual button and cook on High Pressure for 90 minutes.
When the timer goes off, let the pressure vent for 20 minutes then do a Quick Release by pressing Cancel and switching the steam valve to "venting".
When the pot has depressurized, open the lid.
Remove the lamb to a cutting board and keep warm.
Press the Sauté button and whisk the coconut flour into the cooking liquid.
Cook for 5 minutes or until thickened the season with salt and pepper.
Serve the gravy with the lamb.
Nutrition Values:
calories 405 fat 17g ,protein 52g ,carbs 4g ,fiber 2g ,net carbs 2g

439. Spicy Pork Carnitas

Preparation Time:45 minutes
Servings: 10
Ingredients:
¼ teaspoon cayenne
5 pounds boneless pork shoulder, cut into large pieces
1 cup water
Salt and pepper
2 teaspoons ground cumin
1 tablespoon chili powder
½ cup orange juice
Directions:
Combine the chili powder, cumin, and cayenne in a small bowl then rub the mixture into the pork.
Place the pork in the Instant Pot then pour in the water and orange juice.
Close and lock the lid then press the Manual button and adjust the timer to 40 minutes.
When the timer goes off, let the pressure vent for 15 minutes then do a Quick Release by pressing Cancel and switching the steam valve to "venting".
When the pot has depressurized, open the lid.
Shred the pork and season with salt and pepper then serve hot.
Nutrition Values:
calories 330 fat 8g ,protein 59.5g ,carbs 2g ,fiber 0.5g ,net carbs 1.5g

440. Braised Lamb Chops

Preparation Time: 12 minutes
Servings: 4
Ingredients:
8 bone-in lamb chops (about 2 pounds
1 small yellow onion, diced
1 cup beef broth
Salt and pepper
1 tablespoon olive oil
¼ cup low-carb tomato sauce
Directions:
Turn the Instant Pot on to the Sauté setting and let it heat up.
Add the oil to the pot and season the lamb with salt and pepper.
Add the lamb to the pot and cook for 1 to 2 minutes on each side to brown.
Remove the lamb chops and add the onion and tomato sauce to the pot.
Cook for 2 minutes then stir in the beef broth.
Add the lamb then close and lock the lid.
Press the Manual button and adjust the timer for 2 minutes.
When the timer goes off, do a Quick Release by pressing Cancel and switching the steam valve to "venting".
When the pot has depressurized, open the lid.
Spoon the lamb and sauce into a serving bowl and serve hot.
Nutrition Values:
calories 350 fat 16g ,protein 47.5g ,carbs 2.5g ,fiber 0.5g ,net carbs 2g

441. Ginger Soy-Glazed Pork Tenderloin

Preparation Time: 15 minutes
Servings: 4
Ingredients:
¼ cup water
1 (1-poundboneless pork tenderloin
1 tablespoon coconut flour
Salt and pepper
2 tablespoons fresh grated ginger
½ cup soy sauce
Directions:
Whisk together the soy sauce, water, and ginger in a bowl.
Season the pork with salt and pepper then add to the Instant Pot.
Close and lock the lid then press the Manual button and adjust the timer to 5 minutes.
When the timer goes off, let the pressure vent for 10 minutes then do a Quick Release by pressing Cancel and switching the steam valve to "venting".
When the pot has depressurized, open the lid.
Remove the pork to a cutting board and cover with foil.
Stir the coconut flour into the cooking liquid then press the Sauté button.
Cook until thickened then slice the pork and pour the glaze over it to serve.
Nutrition Values:
calories 160 fat 4g ,protein 24g ,carbs 7.5g ,fiber 2g ,net carbs 5.5g

442. Herb-Roasted Lamb Shoulder

Preparation Time: 50 minutes
Servings: 6
Ingredients:
1 ½ teaspoons fresh chopped rosemary
2 ½ pounds boneless lamb shoulder
1 cup water
Salt and pepper
1 teaspoon fresh chopped oregano
1 tablespoon fresh chopped thyme
Directions:
Combine the herbs in a small bowl then rub it into the lamb and season with salt and pepper.
Place the lamb in the Instant Pot and add the water.
Close and lock the lid then press the Manual button and set the timer for 40 minutes.
When the timer goes off, let the pressure vent for 10 minutes then do a Quick Release by pressing Cancel and switching the steam valve to "venting".
When the pot has depressurized, open the lid.
Transfer the lamb to a roasting pan and broil for 10 minutes until browned.
Let the lamb rest on a cutting board for 10 minutes before slicing to serve.
Nutrition Values:
calories 360 fat 20g ,protein 42g ,carbs 1.5g ,fiber 0.5g ,net carbs 1g

443. Curried Pork Shoulder

Preparation Time: 1 hour 5 minutes
Servings: 8
Ingredients:
4 pounds boneless pork shoulder, cut into large pieces
1 small yellow onion, chopped
3 ½ cups unsweetened coconut milk
Salt and pepper
2 tablespoons olive oil
1 tablespoon fresh grated ginger
1 tablespoon curry powder
Directions:
Turn the Instant Pot on to the Sauté setting and let it heat up.
Add the olive oil to the pot and season the pork with salt and pepper.
Add the pork to the pot and cook until browned on all sides, about 8 minutes total.
Remove the pork to a cutting board then add the onions and ginger to the pot.
Cook for 3 minutes then add the coconut milk.
Add the pork back to the pot and sprinkle with curry powder.
Close and lock the lid then press the Manual button and cook on High Pressure for 55 minutes.
When the timer goes off, do a Quick Release by pressing Cancel and switching the steam valve to "venting".
When the pot has depressurized, open the lid.
Cut the pork into chunks and stir back into the sauce to serve.
Nutrition Values:

calories 380 fat 13.5g ,protein 59.5g ,carbs 2.5g ,fiber 1g ,net carbs 1.5g

444. Curried Lamb Stew
Preparation Time:1hour 5 minutes
Servings: 4
Ingredients:
1 small yellow onion, chopped
1 ½ pounds boneless lamb shoulder, chopped
2 cups chopped cauliflower
1 ½ cups chicken broth
Salt and pepper
1 tablespoon olive oil
1 tablespoon curry powder
Directions:
Turn the Instant Pot on to the Sauté setting and let it heat up.
Add the oil then stir in the onions and cook for 4 minutes.
Stir in the chopped lamb, cauliflower, chicken broth, and curry powder. Season with salt and pepper.
Close and lock the lid then press the Manual button and adjust the timer to 50 minutes.
When the timer goes off, let the pressure vent naturally.
When the pot has depressurized, open the lid.
Stir well and adjust seasonings to taste before serving.

445. Nutrition Values:
calories 385 fat 17g ,protein 51g ,carbs 5.5g ,fiber 2g ,net carbs 3.5g

446. Smothered Pork Chops
Preparation Time:40 minutes
Servings: 4
Ingredients:
4 (5-ounceboneless pork loin chops
8 ounces sliced mushrooms
Salt and pepper
2 tablespoons olive oil
½ cup heavy cream
1 tablespoon butter
½ teaspoon xanthan gum
Directions:
Turn the Instant Pot on to the Sauté setting and let it heat up.
Add the oil to the pot and season the pork chops with salt and pepper.
Place the pork chops in the pot and brown for 3 minutes on each side then remove to a plate.
Add the mushrooms to the pot and place the pork chops on top.
Close and lock the lid then press the Manual button and cook on High Pressure for 25 minutes.
When the timer goes off, let the pressure vent for 10 minutes then do a Quick Release by pressing Cancel and switching the steam valve to "venting".
When the pot has depressurized, open the lid.
Remove the pork chops to a plate then add the heavy cream and butter to the pot.
Sprinkle with xanthan gum then simmer on the Sauté setting for 5 minutes until thickened.
Stir the gravy then spoon over the pork chops to serve.

Nutrition Values:
calories 350 fat 20.5g ,protein 39g ,carbs 2.5g ,fiber 0.5g ,net carbs 2g

447. Rosemary Garlic Leg of Lamb
Preparation Time:45 minutes
• **Servings: 8 to 10**
Ingredients:
4 pounds boneless leg of lamb
2 tablespoons chopped rosemary
2 cups water
Salt and pepper
2 tablespoons olive oil
1 tablespoon garlic
Directions:
Turn the Instant Pot on to the Sauté setting and let it heat up.
Add the oil then season the lamb with salt and pepper.
Place the lamb in the pot and cook for 2 to 3 minutes on each side to brown.
Remove the lamb and rub the garlic and rosemary into it.
Place the steamer insert in your pot and add the water.
Add the lamb to the steamer insert then close and lock the lid.
Press the Meat/Stew button and adjust the timer to 30 minutes.
When the timer goes off, let the pressure vent naturally.
When the pot has depressurized, open the lid.
Let the lamb rest on a cutting board for 10 minutes before slicing.
Nutrition Values:
calories 365 fat 16g ,protein 51g ,carbs 1g ,fiber 0.5g ,net carbs 0.5g

448. Hungarian Marha Pörkölt
Preparation Time: 30 minutes
Servings 4
Nutrition Values: 487 Calories; 19g Fat; 11.3g Carbs; 65g Protein; 2.7g Sugars
Ingredients
1 tablespoon sesame oil
1 ½ pounds beef stewing meat, cut into bite-sized chunks
1 cup scallions, chopped
2 cloves garlic, minced
Kosher salt, to taste
1/4 teaspoon freshly ground black pepper, or more to taste
2 carrots, sliced
1 jalapeño pepper, minced
4 cups beef bone broth
1 cup tomato purée
2 sprigs thyme
1 teaspoon dried sage, crushed
2 tablespoons sweet Hungarian paprika
1/2 teaspoon mustard seeds
2 bay leaves
1 cup sour cream
Directions

Press the "Sauté" button to preheat your Instant Pot. Then, heat the sesame oil. Sear the beef for 3 to 4 minutes or until it is delicately browned; reserve. Cook the scallions and garlic in pan drippings until tender and fragrant. Now, add the remaining ingredients, except for sour cream.
Secure the lid. Choose the "Soup" mode and High pressure; cook for 20 minutes. Once cooking is complete, use a quick pressure release; carefully remove the lid.
Divide your stew among four soup bowls; serve with a dollop of sour cream and enjoy!

449. Creamy and Saucy Beef Delight
Preparation Time: 30 minutes
Servings 6
Nutrition Values: 485 Calories; 30.9g Fat; 12.8g Carbs; 37.1g Protein; 2.4g Sugars
Ingredients
1 tablespoon lard, at room temperature
1 shallot, diced
1 ½ pounds beef brisket, cut into 2-inch cubes
Sea salt and freshly ground pepper, to taste
1 teaspoon red pepper flakes, crushed
2 garlic cloves, minced
2 sprigs dried rosemary, leaves picked
2 sprigs dried thyme, leaves picked
1 teaspoon caraway seeds
1 ½ tablespoons flaxseed meal
1/2 cup chicken stock
6 ounces wonton noodles
3/4 cup cream cheese
2 tablespoons toasted sesame seeds
Directions
Press the "Sauté" button to preheat your Instant Pot. Now, melt the lard; once hot, sweat the shallot for 2 to 3 minutes.
Toss beef brisket with salt, ground pepper, and red pepper flakes. Add beef to the Instant pot; continue cooking for 3 minutes more or until it is no longer pink.
After that, stir in garlic, rosemary, thyme, and caraway seeds; cook an additional minute, stirring continuously.
Add the flaxseed meal, chicken stock, and wonton noodles. Stir to combine well and seal the lid. Choose the "Meat/Stew" setting and cook at High pressure for 20 minutes.
Once cooking is complete, use a quick release; remove the lid. Divide the beef mixture among 6 serving bowls.
To serve, stir in cream cheese and garnish with toasted sesame seeds. Bon appétit!

450. Sunday Hamburger Pilaf
Preparation Time: 15 minutes
Servings 4
Nutrition Values: 493 Calories; 28.8g Fat; 34.9g Carbs; 42.1g Protein; 3.3g Sugars
Ingredients
1 tablespoon sesame oil
1/2 cup leeks, chopped
1 teaspoon garlic, minced
1 jalapeño pepper, minced
1 (1-inchpiece ginger root, peeled and grated
1 ½ pounds ground chuck
1 cup tomato purée
Sea salt, to taste
1/3 teaspoon ground black pepper, or more to taste
1 teaspoon red pepper flakes
2 cups Arborio rice
1 ½ cups roasted vegetable broth
Directions
Press the "Sauté" button to preheat your Instant Pot. Now, heat the sesame oil and sauté the leeks until tender.
Then, add the garlic, jalapeño and ginger; cook for 1 minute more or until aromatic.
Add the remaining ingredients; stir well to combine.
Secure the lid. Choose the "Manual" mode and High pressure; cook for 7 minutes. Once cooking is complete, use a quick pressure release; carefully remove the lid. Serve immediately.

451. Italian-Style Steak Pepperonata
Preparation Time: 1 hour 10 minutes
Servings 6
Nutrition Values: 309 Calories; 7.4g Fat; 10.8g Carbs; 46.9g Protein; 5.1g Sugars
Ingredients
2 teaspoons lard, at room temperature
2 pounds top round steak, cut into bite-sized chunks
1 red onion, chopped
1 pound mixed bell peppers, deveined and thinly sliced
2 cloves garlic, minced
1 tablespoon Italian seasoning blend
Sea salt and ground black pepper, to taste
1 tablespoon salt-packed capers, rinsed and drained
1/2 cup dry red wine
1 cup water
Directions
Press the "Sauté" button to preheat your Instant Pot. Then, melt the lard. Cook the round steak approximately 5 minutes, stirring periodically; reserve.
Then, sauté the onion for 2 minutes or until translucent.
Stir in the remaining ingredients, including the reserved beef.
Secure the lid. Choose the "Manual" mode and High pressure; cook for 60 minutes. Once cooking is complete, use a natural pressure release; carefully remove the lid. Bon appétit!

452. Wine-Braised Beef Shanks
Preparation Time: 45 minutes + marinating time
Servings 6
Nutrition Values: 329 Calories; 10.5g Fat; 25.8g Carbs; 32g Protein; 2.7g Sugars
Ingredients
1 ½ pounds beef shanks, cut into pieces
1/2 cup port
1 cup wine
2 garlic cloves, crushed
1 teaspoon celery seeds
12 teaspoon dried thyme
1 tablespoon olive oil

1/2 cup leeks, chopped
2 potatoes, diced
2 carrots, chopped
1 1/3 cups vegetable stock
Salt and black pepper, to taste
Directions
Add beef shanks to a bowl; now, add port, red wine, garlic, celery seeds, and dried thyme. Let it marinate overnight.
On an actual day, preheat your Instant Pot on "Sauté" function. Add olive oil; once hot, brown marinated shanks on all sides; reserve.
Now, cook leeks, potatoes and carrots in pan drippings until they have softened. Add vegetable stock, salt, and pepper to taste.
Pour in the reserved marinade and secure the lid. Select the "Meat/Stew" and cook for 35 minutes at High pressure. Once cooking is complete, use a quick release; remove the lid.
Now, press the "Sauté" button to thicken the cooking liquid for 5 to 6 minutes. Taste, adjust the seasonings and serve right away!

453. Holiday Osso Buco

Preparation Time: 30 minutes
Servings 8
Nutrition Values: 302 Calories; 7.2g Fat; 21.7g Carbs; 34.3g Protein; 3g Sugars
Ingredients
2 tablespoons olive oil
1 ½ pounds Osso buco
2 carrots, sliced
1 celery with leaves, diced
1 cup beef bone broth
1/2 cup rose wine
2 garlic cloves, chopped
1 onion, chopped
2 bay leaves
1 sprig dried rosemary
1 teaspoon dried sage, crushed
1/2 teaspoon tarragon
Sea salt and ground black pepper, to taste
Directions
Press the "Sauté" button to preheat your Instant Pot. Now, heat the olive oil. Sear the beef on all sides.
Add the remaining ingredients.
Secure the lid. Choose the "Meat/Stew" mode and High pressure; cook for 25 minutes. Once cooking is complete, use a natural pressure release; carefully remove the lid. Bon appétit!

454. Tagliatelle with Beef Sausage and Cheese

Preparation Time: 10 minutes
Servings 6
Nutrition Values: 596 Calories; 32.6g Fat; 52.1g Carbs; 26.5g Protein; 11.3g Sugars
Ingredients
2 teaspoons canola oil
1 pound beef sausage, sliced
1 ½ pounds tagliatelle pasta
3 cups water
2 cups tomato paste
Sea salt and ground black pepper, to taste
8 ounces Colby cheese, grated
5 ounces Ricotta cheese, crumbled
2 tablespoons fresh chives, roughly chopped
Directions
Press the "Sauté" button to preheat your Instant Pot. Now, heat the oil. Cook the sausages until they are no longer pink; reserve.
Then, stir in the pasta, water, tomato paste, salt, and black pepper.
Secure the lid. Choose the "Manual" mode and High pressure; cook for 4 minutes. Once cooking is complete, use a quick pressure release; carefully remove the lid.
Next, fold in the cheese; seal the lid and let it sit in the residual heat until heated through. Add the reserved sausage and stir; serve garnished with fresh chives. Bon appétit!

455. Balkan-Style Beef Stew

Preparation Time: 35 minutes
Servings 6
Nutrition Values: 403 Calories; 21.3g Fat; 16.4g Carbs; 36.8g Protein; 8.7g Sugars
Ingredients
1 tablespoon olive oil
2 pounds beef sirloin steak, cut into bite-sized chunks
1 cup red onion, chopped
2 garlic cloves, minced
1 pound bell peppers, seeded and sliced
1 cup vegetable broth
4 Italian plum tomatoes, crushed
Salt and ground black pepper, to taste
1 teaspoon paprika
1 egg, beaten
Directions
Press the "Sauté" button to preheat your Instant Pot. Now, heat the oil. Cook the beef until it is no longer pink.
Add onion and cook an additional 2 minutes. Stir in the minced garlic, peppers, broth, tomatoes, salt, black pepper, and paprika.
Secure the lid. Choose the "Soup" mode and High pressure; cook for 20 minutes. Once cooking is complete, use a quick pressure release; carefully remove the lid.
Afterwards, fold in the egg and stir well; seal the lid and let it sit in the residual heat for 8 to 10 minutes. Serve in individual bowls with mashed potatoes. Enjoy!

456. Bacon and Blade Roast Sandwiches

Preparation Time: 1 hour 30 minutes
Servings 8
Nutrition Values: 698 Calories; 40.1g Fat; 36.9g Carbs; 46g Protein; 19g Sugars
Ingredients
2 center-cut bacon slices, chopped
2 1/2 pounds top blade roast
Salt and ground black pepper, to taste
1 teaspoon dried marjoram
1/2 teaspoon dried rosemary
1 teaspoon Juniper berries

1 (12-ounce bottle lager
1 ½ cups unsalted beef stock
8 slices Cheddar cheese
2 tablespoons Dijon mustard
8 burger buns
Directions
Press the "Sauté" button and preheat the Instant Pot. Cook the bacon for 4 minutes or until crisp; reserve. Add beef and sear 8 minutes, turning to brown on all sides.
In the meantime, mix salt, pepper, marjoram, rosemary, Juniper berries, lager, and beef stock. Pour the mixture over the seared top blade roast and seal the lid.
Choose the "Manual" setting and cook for 1 hour 10 minutes at High pressure. Once cooking is complete, use a quick release; remove the lid.
Now, shred the meat and return to the cooking liquid; stir to soak well. Return the reserved bacon to the Instant Pot.
Assemble sandwiches with meat/bacon mixture, cheddar cheese, mustard, and burger buns. Enjoy!

457. Tuscan-Style Cassoulet

Preparation Time: 35 minutes
Servings 6
Nutrition Values: 376 Calories; 19.3g Fat; 18.1g Carbs; 36.3g Protein; 1.6g Sugars
Ingredients
1 tablespoon olive oil
1 ½ pounds beef shoulder, cut into bite-sized chunks
1/2 pound beef chipolata sausages, sliced
1 onion, chopped
2 garlic cloves, minced
1 cup beef stock
1/2 cup tomato purée
1/2 tablespoon ancho chili powder
Sea salt and ground black pepper, to taste
1 tablespoon fresh thyme leaves
1 (15-ounce can white beans, drained and rinsed
1 cup sour cream
Directions
Press the "Sauté" button and preheat the Instant Pot. Heat the oil and sear the meat and sausage until they are delicately browned; reserve.
Then, sauté the onion in pan drippings for 3 to 4 minutes.
Stir in garlic, stock, tomato purée, ancho chili powder, salt, black pepper, thyme leaves and beans.
Secure the lid. Choose the "Bean/Chili" mode and High pressure; cook for 25 minutes. Once cooking is complete, use a quick pressure release; carefully remove the lid.
Garnish each serving with sour cream and serve. Bon appétit!

458. Barbecued Beef Round with Cheese

Preparation Time: 50 minutes
Servings 6
Nutrition Values: 336 Calories; 9.5g Fat; 23.4g Carbs; 37.5g Protein; 17.6g Sugars
Ingredients
2 pounds bottom round
1 cup beef stock
1 cup barbecue sauce
2 tablespoons tamari sauce
1 cup scallions, chopped
2 cloves garlic, minced
2 teaspoons olive oil
1 teaspoon chili powder
1 cup Cheddar cheese, grated
Directions
Place all of the above ingredients, except for Cheddar cheese, in your Instant Pot.
Secure the lid. Choose the "Meat/Stew" mode and High pressure; cook for 45 minutes. Once cooking is complete, use a quick pressure release; carefully remove the lid.
Top with freshly grated cheese and serve immediately. Enjoy!

459. Home-Style Beef Tikka Kebabs

Preparation Time: 30 minutes
Servings 4
Nutrition Values: 590 Calories; 29g Fat; 22.5g Carbs; 58g Protein; 1.8g Sugars
Ingredients
2 tablespoons olive oil
1 ½ pounds lean steak beef, cubed
1/2 cup onion, sliced
2 cloves garlic, minced
2 tablespoons fresh cilantro, chopped
Salt and ground black pepper, to taste
1 teaspoon Aleppo chili flakes
1/2 teaspoon sumac
1/2 teaspoon turmeric powder
1/3 cup chicken stock
1 tablespoon champagne vinegar
1/3 cup mayonnaise
4 tablespoons pickled slaw
4 Bazlama flatbread
Directions
Press the "Sauté" button to heat up the Instant Pot. Now, heat olive oil and brown beef cubes, stirring frequently.
Add onion, garlic, and seasonings to the Instant Pot. Cook an additional 4 minutes or until onion is translucent.
Pour chicken stock and champagne vinegar over the meat. Seal the lid.
Choose the "Meat/Stew" setting and cook for 20 minutes at High pressure. Once cooking is complete, use a quick release; remove the lid.
Assemble sandwiches with mayonnaise, pickled slaw, the meat mixture, and Bazlama bread. Bon appétit!

460. Favorite Tex-Mex Tacos

Preparation Time: 15 minutes
Servings 8
Nutrition Values: 566 Calories; 33.4g Fat; 38.6g Carbs; 30.7g Protein; 6.5g Sugars
Ingredients
1 tablespoon olive oil
1/2 cup shallots, chopped
2 cloves garlic, pressed
2 pounds ground sirloin
1/2 teaspoon ground cumin

1/2 cup roasted vegetable broth
1/2 ketchup
Sea salt, to taste
1/2 teaspoon fresh ground pepper
1 teaspoon paprika
1 can (16-ouncesdiced tomatoes, undrained
2 canned chipotle chili in adobo sauce, drained
12 whole-wheat flour tortillas, warmed
1 head romaine lettuce
1 cup sour cream
Directions
Press the "Sauté" button and preheat the Instant Pot. Heat the oil and cook the shallots and garlic until aromatic.
Now, add the ground sirloin and cook an additional 2 minutes or until it is no longer pink.
Add ground cumin, broth, ketchup, salt, black pepper, paprika, tomatoes, and chili in adobo sauce to your Instant Pot.
Secure the lid. Choose the "Poultry" mode and High pressure; cook for 5 minutes. Once cooking is complete, use a natural pressure release; carefully remove the lid.
Divide beef mixture between tortillas. Garnish with lettuce and sour cream and serve.

461. Traditional Beef Pho Noodle Soup
Preparation Time: 15 minutes
Servings 4
Nutrition Values: 417 Calories; 14g Fat; 27.5g Carbs; 43.1g Protein; 3.6g Sugars
• **Ingredients**
1 tablespoon sesame oil
1 pound round steak, sliced paper thin
4 cups roasted vegetable broth
1 tablespoon brown sugar
Kosher salt and ground black pepper, to taste
2 carrots, trimmed and diced
1 celery stalk, trimmed and diced
1 cinnamon stick
3 star of anise
1/2 (14-ouncepackage rice noodles
1 bunch of cilantro, roughly chopped
2 stalks scallions, diced
Directions
Press the "Sauté" button and preheat the Instant Pot. Heat the oil and sear the round steak for 1 to 2 minutes.
Add the broth, sugar, salt, black pepper, carrots, celery, cinnamon stick, and star anise. Top with rice noodles so they should be on top of the other ingredients.
Secure the lid. Choose the "Manual" mode and High pressure; cook for 3 minutes. Once cooking is complete, use a quick pressure release; carefully remove the lid.
Serve in individual bowls, topped with cilantro and scallions. Enjoy!

462. Ground Beef Taco Bowls
Preparation Time: 15 minutes
Servings 4
Nutrition Values: 409 Calories; 15.7g Fat; 37.5g Carbs; 29.5g Protein; 6.6g Sugars
Ingredients
1 tablespoon peanut oil
1 pound ground chuck
1 cup beef bone broth
1 bell pepper, seeded and chopped
1 red chili pepper, seeded and chopped
1 onion, chopped
1 (1.25-ouncepackage taco seasoning
4 tortilla bowls, baked
1 (15-ouncecan beans, drained and rinsed
2 fresh tomatoes, chopped
Directions
Press the "Sauté" button and preheat the Instant Pot. Heat the oil and cook the ground chuck until it is no longer pink.
Add the broth, bell pepper, chili pepper, onion, and taco seasoning.
Secure the lid. Choose the "Manual" mode and High pressure; cook for 5 minutes. Once cooking is complete, use a quick pressure release; carefully remove the lid.
Divide the mixture between tortilla bowls. Top with beans and tomatoes. Enjoy!

463. Barbeque Chuck Roast
Preparation Time: 45 minutes
Servings 6
Nutrition Values: 252 Calories; 9.9g Fat; 9g Carbs; 30.1g Protein; 5.9g Sugars
Ingredients
2 tablespoons lard, at room temperature
2 pounds chuck roast
4 carrots, sliced
1/2 cup leek, sliced
1 teaspoon garlic, minced
3 teaspoons fresh ginger root, thinly sliced
Salt and pepper, to taste
1 ½ tablespoons fresh parsley leaves, roughly chopped
1 cup barbeque sauce
1/2 cup teriyaki sauce
Directions
Press the "Sauté" button on your Instant Pot. Now, melt the lard until hot.
Sear chuck roast until browned, about 6 minutes per side. Add the other ingredients.
Choose "Manual" setting and cook for 35 minutes at High pressure or until the internal temperature of the chuck roast is at least 145 degrees F.
Once cooking is complete, use a quick release; remove the lid.
Serve with crusty bread and fresh salad of choice. Bon appétit!

464. Beef Pad Thai
Preparation Time: 20 minutes
Servings 6
Nutrition Values: 418 Calories; 24.1g Fat; 5.2g Carbs; 46.1g Protein; 1.2g Sugars
Ingredients
2 tablespoons peanut oil
2 pounds skirt steak, cut into thin 1-inch-long slices

1 small Thai chili, finely chopped
1 cup beef bone broth
1/2 cup shallots, chopped
2 tablespoons oyster sauce
1/4 cup peanuts, finely chopped
Directions
Press the "Sauté" button to preheat your Instant Pot. Heat the oil and sear the beef until it is delicately browned on all sides.
Add Thai chili, broth, shallots, and oyster sauce.
Secure the lid. Choose the "Poultry" mode and High pressure; cook for 15 minutes. Once cooking is complete, use a quick pressure release; carefully remove the lid.
Garnish with chopped peanuts and serve warm.

465. Easy Balsamic Beef
Preparation Time: 50 minutes
Servings 6
Nutrition Values: 282 Calories; 13.3g Fat; 9.1g Carbs; 32.5g Protein; 5.4g Sugars
Ingredients
2 tablespoons sesame oil
2 pounds beef chuck, cut into bite-sized pieces
1/4 cup balsamic vinegar
1/2 teaspoon dried basil
1 teaspoon dried rosemary, crushed
1/2 teaspoon cayenne pepper
1/2 teaspoon ground black pepper
Sea salt, to taste
1 onion, chopped
2 cloves garlic, minced
1 tablespoon cilantro, finely chopped
1/2 cup water
1/2 cup tomato paste
1 jalapeño pepper, finely minced
Directions
Press the "Sauté" button to preheat your Instant Pot. Heat the sesame oil until sizzling.
Once hot, cook the beef for 2 to 3 minutes. Add the remaining ingredients.
Secure the lid. Choose the "Meat/Stew" mode and High pressure; cook for 45 minutes. Once cooking is complete, use a natural pressure release; carefully remove the lid.
Afterwards, thicken the sauce on the "Sauté" function. Serve over hot macaroni and enjoy!

466. Juicy Round Steak
Preparation Time: 55 minutes
Servings 8
Nutrition Values: 363 Calories; 17.9g Fat; 3.1g Carbs; 44.5g Protein; 1.1g Sugars
Ingredients
2 ½ pounds round steak, cut into 1-inch pieces
Kosher salt and freshly ground black pepper, to taste
1/2 teaspoon ground bay leaf
3 tablespoons chickpea flour
1/4 cup olive oil
2 shallots, chopped
2 cloves garlic, minced
1 cup red wine
1/4 cup marinara sauce
1/3 cup bone broth
1 celery with leaves, chopped
Directions
Press the "Sauté" button to preheat your Instant Pot. Toss round steak with salt, pepper, ground bay leaf, and chickpea flour.
Once hot, heat olive oil and cook the beef for 6 minutes, stirring periodically; reserve.
Stir in the shallots and garlic and cook until they are tender and aromatic. Pour in the wine to deglaze the bottom of the pan. Continue to cook until the liquid has reduced by half.
Add the other ingredients, stir, and seal the lid. Choose the "Meat/Stew" setting and cook at High pressure for 45 minutes.
Once cooking is complete, use a natural release; remove the lid. Taste, adjust the seasonings and serve warm.

467. Ground Beef Bulgogi
Preparation Time: 15 minutes
Servings 6
Nutrition Values: 274 Calories; 17.5g Fat; 4.1g Carbs; 25.4g Protein; 0.8g Sugars
Ingredients
2 tablespoons canola oil
1/2 cup leeks, chopped
1 (2-inchknob ginger, grated
2 garlic cloves, finely chopped
1 ½ pounds ground chuck
Sea salt and ground black pepper, to taste
2 cups roasted vegetable broth
1/2 cup sour cream
1 ½ tablespoons flax seed meal
2 tablespoons sesame seeds
Directions
Press the "Sauté" button to preheat your Instant Pot. Heat the oil and sweat the leeks until tender.
Then, add ginger and garlic; continue to sauté an additional 2 minutes or until fragrant.
Add the ground meat and cook for 2 more minutes or until it is no longer pink. Add the salt, black pepper, and broth to the Instant Pot.
Secure the lid. Choose the "Manual" mode and High pressure; cook for 5 minutes. Once cooking is complete, use a natural pressure release; carefully remove the lid.
Lastly, fold in sour cream and flax seed meal; seal the lid again; let it sit until thoroughly heated.
Ladle into individual bowls and top with sesame seeds. Bon appétit!

468. Classic Beef Stroganoff
Preparation Time: 25 minutes
Servings 6
Nutrition Values: 536 Calories; 19.6g Fat; 45g Carbs; 50g Protein; 8.5g Sugars
Ingredients
2 tablespoons sesame oil
1/2 cup shallots, chopped
1 teaspoon minced garlic
1 bell pepper, seeded and chopped
1 ½ pounds stewing meat, cubed
1 celery with leaves, chopped
1 parsnip, chopped

1/2 cup rose wine
1 cup tomato paste
1/2 cup ketchup
1 can (10 ¾-ounce condensed golden mushroom soup
9 ounces fresh button mushrooms, sliced
6 ounces cream cheese
1/4 cup fresh chives, coarsely chopped

Directions
Press the "Sauté" button to preheat your Instant Pot. Heat the oil and sauté the shallots until they have softened.
Stir in the garlic and pepper; continue to sauté until tender and fragrant.
Add meat, celery, parsnip, wine, tomato paste, ketchup, mushroom soup, and mushrooms.
Secure the lid. Choose the "Meat/Stew" mode and High pressure; cook for 20 minutes. Once cooking is complete, use a quick pressure release; carefully remove the lid.
Stir cream cheese into beef mixture; seal the lid and let it sit until melted. Serve garnished with fresh chives. Enjoy!

469. Pepper Jack Beef and Cauliflower Casserole
Preparation Time: 35 minutes
Servings 4
Nutrition Values: 523 Calories; 39.6g Fat; 10.9g Carbs; 30.8g Protein; 5.3g Sugars
Ingredients
1 head cauliflower, chopped into small florets
2 tablespoons olive oil
1/2 cup yellow onion, chopped
2 garlic cloves, minced
1/2 pound ground beef
2 spicy sausages, chopped
2 ripe tomatoes, chopped
1 ½ tablespoons brown sugar
2 tablespoons tamari sauce
Salt and freshly ground black pepper, to your liking
1 teaspoon cayenne pepper
1/2 teaspoon celery seeds
1/2 teaspoon fennel seeds
1 teaspoon dried basil
1/2 teaspoon dried oregano
1 cup Pepper Jack cheese, shredded

Directions
Parboil cauliflower in a lightly salted water for 3 to 5 minutes; remove the cauliflower from the water with a slotted spoon and drain.
Press the "Sauté" button to preheat your Instant Pot. Now, heat the oil and sweat the onions and garlic.
Then, add ground beef and sausage and continue to cook for 4 minutes more or until they are browned.
Stir in the remaining ingredients, except for shredded cheese, and cook for 4 minutes more or until heated through. Add cauliflower florets on top.
Secure the lid and choose the "Manual" mode, High pressure and 6 minutes. Once cooking is complete, use a quick release; remove the lid.
Top with shredded cheese and let it melt for 5 to 6 minutes. Bon appétit!

470. Hayashi Rice Stew
Preparation Time: 30 minutes
Servings 6
Nutrition Values: 368 Calories; 16.1g Fat; 30.9g Carbs; 25.5g Protein; 3g Sugars
Ingredients
1 tablespoon lard, at room temperature
1 ½ pounds ribeye steaks, cut into bite-sized pieces
1/2 cup shallots, chopped
4 cloves garlic, minced
Salt and black pepper, to taste
1/2 teaspoon sweet paprika
1 sprig dried thyme, crushed
1 sprig dried rosemary, crushed
1 carrot, chopped
1 celery stalk, chopped
1/4 cup tomato paste
2 cups beef bone broth
1/3 cup rice wine
1 tablespoon Tonkatsu sauce
1 cup brown rice

Directions
Press the "Sauté" button to preheat your Instant Pot. Now, heat the oil and cook the beef until it is delicately browned.
Add the remaining ingredients; stir to combine.
Secure the lid. Choose the "Bean/Chili" mode and High pressure; cook for 25 minutes. Once cooking is complete, use a natural pressure release; carefully remove the lid. Bon appétit!

VEGETABLES

Healthy Brussels Sprouts with Mushrooms
Preparation Time: 25 Minutes
Servings: 4
Ingredients:
1 lb Brussels sprouts; trimmed and halved
1 lb button mushrooms; sliced
1 medium-sized celery stalk; chopped.
2 garlic cloves; crushed
1 tbsp fresh parsley; finely chopped.
2 tbsp olive oil
1/4 cup Greek yogurt; full-fat
1/2 tsp black pepper; ground
1 tsp ginger; freshly grated
1/4 tsp red chili flakes
1 tsp sea salt
Directions:
Plug in your instant pot and place the Brussels sprouts, mushrooms, and celery in the stainless steel insert. Sprinkle with some salt and pour water enough to cover all
Securely lock the lid and set the steam release handle by turning the valve to the *Sealing* position. Press the *Manual* button and set the timer for 10minutes. Cook on *High* pressure
Meanwhile; in a medium-sized bowl, combine Greek yogurt, garlic, parsley, olive oil, and remaining spices. Mix until well combined and set aside
When you hear the cooker's end signal, perform a quick pressure release by moving the valve to the *Venting* position
Open the pot and stir in the yogurt mixture. Press the *Saute* button and cook for 5 more minutes.
Turn off the pot and transfer all to a serving bowl.
Nutrition Values: Calories: 145; Total Fats: 13.7g; Net Carbs: 10.7g; Protein: 8.5g; Fiber: 5.7g

472. Keto Spinach Pepper Stew
Preparation Time: 15 Minutes
Servings: 4
Ingredients:
1 lb spinach; chopped.
1 cup fresh kale; chopped.
2 medium-sized bell peppers; chopped.
1 cup vegetable stock
2 tbsp butter
1/4 cup cream cheese; full-fat
1/2 tsp dried mint; ground
1/4 tsp black pepper; ground
1/2 tsp red chili flakes
1 tsp salt
Directions:
Plug in the instant pot and press the *Saute* button. Melt the butter in the stainless steel insert and add spinach, kale, and bell peppers. Sprinkle with salt, pepper, and red chili flakes. Stir well and cook for 5 minutes, or until greens are wilted
Pour in the vegetables stock and give it a good stir. Securely lock the lid and set the steam release handle. Press the *Manual* button and set the timer for 8 minutes. Cook on *High* pressure
When you hear the cooker's end signal, perform a quick release of the pressure by moving the valve to the *Venting* position. Open the pot and stir in the cream cheese and mint
Transfer to a serving dish and optionally, add more salt to taste. Serve warm.
Nutrition Values: Calories: 209; Total Fats: 15.3g; Net Carbs: 9.8g; Protein: 7.5g; Fiber: 5g

473. Easy Portobello Mushrooms in Lime Sauce
Preparation Time: 15 Minutes
Servings: 2
Ingredients:
1 lb Portobello mushrooms; thinly sliced
1 small onion; chopped.
4 garlic cloves; minced
1 whole lime; freshly juiced
1 tsp lime zest; freshly grated
1 cup heavy cream
1 tbsp butter
1 tsp fresh ginger; grated
1 tsp apple cider vinegar
1 tsp black peppercorns; freshly ground
1 tsp sea salt
Directions:
In a food processor, combine garlic, onion, lime juice, heavy cream, ginger, apple cider vinegar, and black peppercorns. Process until smooth and creamy, Set aside
Plug in your instant pot and press the *Saute* button. Add butter to the stainless steel insert and stir until melts.
Add sliced mushrooms and cook for 5 minutes, stirring occasionally. Remove the mushrooms to a plate and set aside
Pour the lime sauce in the pot and bring it to a boil- Simmer for 4 - 5 minutes, stirring occasionally. Turn off the pot.
Place the mushrooms on a serving plate and drizzle with lime sauce. Sprinkle with lime zest and serve immediately
Nutrition Values: Calories: 338; Total Fats: 28.1g; Net Carbs: 13.5g; Protein: 8.8g; Fiber: 4.4g

474. Creamy Broccoli Avocado
Preparation Time: 15 Minutes
Servings: 3
Ingredients:
1 ripe avocado; cut into thin slices
1/2 cup fresh basil; chopped.
1 cup broccoli; sliced
1/2 cup fresh arugula; chopped.
1/2 cup heavy cream
1 tsp apple cider vinegar
2 tbsp olive oil
2 tbsp butter
1 small red onion; sliced
2 garlic cloves
1/2 tsp dried rosemary; ground
1/2 tsp dried thyme; ground
1/2 tsp black peppercorns; freshly ground
1 tsp sea salt

Directions:
In a food processor, combine arugula, basil, heavy cream, apple cider vinegar, olive oil, salt, peppercorns, thyme, and rosemary. Blend until all well incorporated, Set aside
Plug in the instant pot and grease the stainless steel insert with olive oil. Add onions and stir-fry for 3 - 4 minutes, or until translucent
Add sliced avocado and broccoli. Sprinkle with pinch of salt and cook for 3 minutes.
Pour in the previously prepared sauce and securely lock the lid. Set the steam release handle and press the *Manual* button. Set the timer for 3 minutes and cook on *High* pressure
When done; perform a quick pressure release and open the pot
Transfer all to a serving dish and serve immediately
Nutrition Values: Calories: 380; Total Fats: 37.7g; Net Carbs: 5.7g; Protein: 3.3g; Fiber: 6.2g

475. Kale Spinach Muffins
Preparation Time: 15 Minutes
Servings: 3
Ingredients:
1 cup fresh spinach; chopped.
1 cup mozzarella cheese
2 garlic cloves; crushed
1 cup fresh kale; chopped.
2 tsp baking powder
1 tbsp olive oil
3 large eggs
1/2 tsp onion powder
1/4 tsp black pepper; ground
1/2 tsp red chili flakes
1 tsp salt
Directions:
Combine spinach and kale in a large colander. Rinse thoroughly under cold running water. Drain well and chop into small pieces.
In a large bowl, combine spinach, kale, eggs, garlic, baking powder, and mozzarella cheese. Sprinkle with salt, onion powder, chili flakes, and black pepper. Mix until well incorporated. Divide the mixture evenly between 6 silicone cups and set aside
Plug in the instant pot and pour 1 cup of water in the stainless steel insert. Set the trivet on the bottom and place the silicone cups on the top
Close the lid and set the steam release handle. Press the *Manual* button and set the timer for 8 minutes. Cook on *High* pressure
When done; perform a quick pressure release and open the pot. transfer the cups to a wire rack and let it chill for 10 minutes before serving.
Optionally, top with Greek yogurt or sour cream.
Nutrition Values: Calories: 160; Total Fats: 11.4g; Net Carbs: 5.4g; Protein: 10.1g; Fiber: 0.7g

476. Button Mushrooms in Tomato Sauce
Preparation Time: 25 Minutes
Servings: 3
Ingredients:
2 cups button mushrooms; sliced
1/2 cup green onions; chopped.
1 cup tomatoes; chopped.
1 cup cream cheese; full-fat
1/2 cup zucchini; chopped.
2 tbsp butter
1 tbsp olive oil
1/2 tsp black peppercorns
1/2 tsp fresh mint; finely chopped.
1/2 tsp dried oregano; ground
1/2 tsp dried rosemary; ground
1 tsp sea salt
Directions:
In a food processor, combine tomatoes, salt, oregano, rosemary, and peppercorns. Blend until smooth and creamy, Set aside
Plug in the instant pot and press the *Saute* butter. Gently stir with a wooden spatula until melts. Add zucchini and green onions. Cook for 5 minutes, stirring occasionally. Remove from the pot and transfer to a large bowl. Cover with a lid and set aside
Add mushrooms and pour in 1 cup of water. Close the lid and set the steam release handle. Press the *Manual* button and set the timer for 3 minutes. Cook on *High* pressure
When done; perform a quick pressure release and open the pot
Stir in the tomato mixture, cream cheese, and reserved vegetables. Press the *Saute* button and continue to cook for 5 more minutes.
Transfer to a serving dish and optionally, drizzle with some balsamic vinegar.
Nutrition Values: Calories: 409; Total Fats: 39.7g; Net Carbs: 6.2g; Protein: 8.6g; Fiber: 2.1g

477. Keto Vegetarian Pizza
Preparation Time: 1 hour 25 Minutes
Servings: 4
Ingredients:
For the base:
1 cup almond flour
1/2 cup sunflower seeds; minced
1/2 cup sesame seeds; minced
1/4 cup flaxseed meal
3 tbsp coconut oil; melted
2 cups hot water
1 ½ tbsp psyllium husk
For the topping:
2 tbsp olive oil
1/2 cup button mushrooms; sliced
1/2 cup mozzarella; sliced
1/2 tsp dried oregano
1 small tomato; sliced
1 tsp salt
Directions:
First, you'll have to prepare the crust. In a large bowl, combine together all dry crust ingredients and mix well. Add coconut oil and pour in two cups of boiling water. Let it sit for one hour
Line a small baking pan with some parchment paper and add half of the crust mixture. Flatten the surface with your hands as evenly as possible and top with half of the toppings. The mixture will give you two small pizzas.
Loosely cover with aluminum foil and set aside

Plug in the instant pot and set the trivet at the bottom of inner pot. Pour in one cup of water and place the pan on top.
Seal the lid and set the steam release handle to the *Sealing* position. Press the *Manual* button and cook for 5 minutes on high pressure
When done; perform a quick pressure release and open the lid. Remove the pan from the pot and repeat the process with the remaining ingredietns. To enjoy Serve it immediately
Nutrition Values: Calories: 233; Total Fats: 19.2g; Net Carbs: 4.3g; Protein: 4.3g; Fiber: 8.5g

478. Cauliflower with Avocado
Preparation Time: 25 Minutes
Servings: 2
Ingredients:
2 cups cauliflower; cut into florets
2 tbsp cream cheese; full-fat
1 ripe avocado; sliced
1/2 cup spinach; chopped.
1/4 cup pine nuts
1 tbsp lemon juice; freshly squeezed
1 tbsp butter
1/4 tsp dried mint; ground
1/4 tsp dried rosemary; ground
1/4 tsp red pepper; ground
1/4 tsp dried thyme; ground
1 tsp sea salt
Directions:
Plug in the instant pot and place the cauliflower in the stainless steel insert. Sprinkle with some salt and pour in water enough to cover all. Close the lid and set the steam release handle. Press the *Manual* button and set the timer for 5 minutes. Cook on *High* pressure
Meanwhile; combine avocado, spinach, cream cheese, pine nuts, lemon juice, and the remaining spices in a food processor. Blend until smooth and creamy
When you hear the cooker's end signal, perform a quick release of the pressure and open the pot. Remove the cauliflower and the liquid from the pot. Clean the stainless steel insert and pat-dry with a kitchen paper
Set the pot and press the *Saute* button. Melt the butter and add cauliflower. Cook for 2 - 3 minutes and add the avocado pesto. Stir well and cook until heated through. Transfer all to a serving dish and enjoy!
Nutrition Values: Calories: 440; Total Fats: 40.7g; Net Carbs: 7.8g; Protein: 7.5g; Fiber: 10.4g

479. Zucchini Eggplant with Cucumber Sauce
Preparation Time: 20 Minutes
Servings: 3
Ingredients:
1 eggplant; sliced
1 small zucchini; sliced
2 garlic cloves; finely chopped.
1 small chili pepper; finely chopped.
1 tbsp olive oil
For the sauce:
1/4 tsp black pepper; ground
1/4 tsp cayenne pepper; ground
1/2 tsp onion powder
1 cucumber; sliced
1/2 cup sour cream
1 tbsp fresh chives; finely chopped.
1/2 tsp salt
Directions:
Combine all sauce ingredients in a food processor and blend until smooth and creamy, Set aside
Plug in the instant pot and press the *Saute* button. Heat up the olive oil and add garlic and chili pepper. Cook for 2 - 3 minutes, stirring constantly
Add eggplant and zucchini. Sprinkle with some salt and cook for 2 minutes on each side
Pour in the vegetable broth and close the lid. Set the steam release handle and press the *Manual* button. Set the timer for 4 minutes and cook on *High* pressure
When done; perform a quick pressure release and open the pot.
Transfer the vegetables to a serving plate and drizzle with cucumber sauce. Optionally, sprinkle with some lemon juice and enjoy!
Nutrition Values: Calories: 188; Total Fats: 13.2g; Net Carbs: 10.3g; Protein: 4.1g; Fiber: 6.6g

480. Broccoli Cauliflower Frittata
Preparation Time: 35 Minutes
Servings: 4
Ingredients:
2 cups cauliflower; chopped.
2 cups Greek yogurt; full-fat
1 cup of broccoli; chopped.
1 cup of Brussels sprouts; halved
1 small onion; sliced
4 large eggs
2 tbsp green onions; finely chopped.
2 tbsp olive oil
1/2 tsp black pepper; freshly ground
1/4 tsp dried thyme; ground
1/2 tsp Italian seasoning
1 tsp salt
Directions:
Line a medium-sized baking sheet with parchment paper and set aside
In a large mixing bowl, combine Greek yogurt, eggs, green onions, salt, pepper, thyme, and Italian seasoning. Whisk until combined and set aside
Plug in the instant pot and grease the stainless steel with olive oil. Press the *Saute* button and add onions. Cook for 3 - 4 minutes, or until translucent
Add cauliflower, broccoli, and Brussels sprouts. Sprinkle with some salt and cook for 2 - 3 minutes. When done; perform a quick pressure release and open the pot. Transfer the vegetables to a prepared baking sheet. Top with Greek yogurt and spread evenly with a spatula
Place it in the oven and bake for 15 minutes at 350 degrees.
Nutrition Values: Calories: 247; Total Fats: 14.4g; Net Carbs: 9.5g; Protein: 19g; Fiber: 3.2g

481. Tofu with Mushrooms
Preparation Time: 25 Minutes

Servings: 4
Ingredients:
1 cup silken tofu; cubed
1 cup tomatoes; diced
1/2 cup shallots; finely chopped.
1 large red bell pepper
2 tbsp olive oil
1/2 cup feta cheese; crumbled
1/2 cup mozzarella cheese
1 cup vegetable stock
1 cup oyster mushrooms; chopped.
1/2 tsp black pepper
1 tsp dried oregano; ground
1/2 tsp dried thyme; ground
1 tsp fresh ginger; grated
1 tsp garlic powder
1 tsp salt
Directions:
Plug in the instant pot and grease the stainless steel insert with olive oil. Press the *Saute* button and add shallots. Cook for 3 - 4 minutes, or until translucent
Add tofu and cook for 5 minutes, stirring occasionally
Remove all from the pot and set aside, covered.
Add mushrooms and red bell pepper. Pour in the vegetable stock and close the lid. Set the steam release handle and press the *Manual* button. Set the timer for 3 minutes and cook on *High* pressure
When done; perform a quick pressure release and open the pot
Stir in the tomatoes, feta cheese, and all the spices. Cook for 3 minutes, stirring occasionally
Now; add tofu and top with mozzarella and cook for 2 more minutes.
Transfer all to a serving dish and serve immediately
Nutrition Values: Calories: 192; Total Fats: 13.2g; Net Carbs: 10.1g; Protein: 8.8g; Fiber: 2g

482. Keto Green Quiche
Preparation Time: 30 Minutes
Servings: 4
Ingredients:
1 cup fresh kale; chopped.
1 small onion; chopped.
1 cup collard greens; chopped.
1 cup spinach; chopped.
2 garlic cloves; finely chopped.
5 large eggs
1/2 cup cream cheese
1/2 cup goat's cheese; crumbled
1/4 cup Parmesan cheese; grated
2 tbsp heavy cream
1 tsp olive oil
1 tsp Italian seasoning
1/2 tsp black pepper; ground
1/2 tsp dried thyme; ground
1/2 tsp salt
Directions:
Combine kale, collard greens, and spinach in a large colander. Rinse thoroughly under cold running water and drain. Chop into small pieces and set aside
In a large bowl, mix cream cheese, goat's cheese, and Parmesan. Whisk in the eggs and heavy cream. Sprinkle with salt, pepper, thyme, and Italian seasoning. Mix until well combined and set aside

Line some parchment paper over a fitting springform pan and grease the walls with some olive oil. Pour half of the cheese mixture in the pan and then add greens. Now; pour in the remaining cheese mixture
Plug in the instant pot and pour in 1 cup of water in the stainless steel insert. Position a trivet on the bottom and place the springform pan on top
Securely lock the lid and adjust the steam release handle. Press the *Manual* button and set the timer for 20 minutes. Cook on *High* pressure
When done; release the pressure naturally and open the pot.
Optionally, sprinkle with some red pepper flakes.
Nutrition Values: Calories: 366; Total Fats: 29.3g; Net Carbs: 6.6g; Protein: 19.7g; Fiber: 1.3g

483. Yummy Greens in Cayenne Sauce
Preparation Time: 15 Minutes
Servings: 3
Ingredients:
1 cup broccoli; sliced
1 tbsp lime juice; freshly squeezed
1 cup sour cream
1 tbsp butter
1 cup cauliflower
2 garlic cloves; peeled
2 large eggs
1/4 tsp dried oregano; ground
1 tsp onion powder
1 tsp cayenne pepper; ground
1 tsp sea salt
Directions:
In a food processor, combine sour cream, garlic, eggs, lime juice, onion powder, cayenne pepper, oregano, and salt. Pulse until well incorporated and set aside
Plug in the instant pot and place the butter in the stainless steel insert. Press the *Saute* button and gently stir until melts
Add broccoli and cauliflower. Sprinkle with a pinch of salt and cook for 5 minutes, stirring occasionally
Remove the vegetables to a bowl and cover with a lid
Now; pour in the blended mixture and close the lid. Adjust the steam release handle and press the *Manual* button. Set the timer for 3 minutes and cook on *High* pressure
When you hear the cooker's end signal, perform a quick pressure release and open the pot.
Drizzle the broccoli and cauliflower with sauce and give it a good stir. Transfer to a serving plate and enjoy!
Nutrition Values: Calories: 272; Total Fats: 23.5g; Net Carbs: 7.1g; Protein: 8.5g; Fiber: 1.9g

484. Steamed Broccoli with Basil
Preparation Time: 20 Minutes
Servings: 3
Ingredients:
1 lb broccoli; chopped.
2 garlic cloves; peeled
1/2 cup fresh basil; chopped.
1/2 cup cottage cheese
1/2 cup avocado; chopped.
1 tbsp olive oil

1 tbsp lemon juice; freshly squeezed
1/4 tsp dried oregano; ground
1/2 tsp red pepper; ground
1/4 tsp dried parsley; ground
1 tsp salt
Directions:
Plug in the instant pot and pour in 1 cup of water in the stainless steel insert.
Place the trivet on the bottom of the pot and set the steam basket on top. Place broccoli in the steam basket and sprinkle with salt and pepper. Close the lid and set the steam release handle by moving the valve to the *Sealing* position. Press the *Steam* button and set the timer for 10 minutes
Meanwhile; combine basil, cottage cheese, avocado, garlic, olive oil, lemon juice, red pepper, parsley, and oregano in a food processor. Pulse until smooth and well incorporated
When you hear the cooker's end signal, release the pressure naturally. Open the pot and transfer the broccoli to a serving plate. Top with basil cream and serve immediately
Nutrition Values: Calories: 187; Total Fats: 10.8g; Net Carbs: 10g; Protein: 10.4g; Fiber: 6g

485. Classic Cauliflower Spread with Thyme
Preparation Time: 25 Minutes
Servings: 6
Ingredients:
1 lb cauliflower; chopped into florets
1/4 cup cream cheese
1/2 cup canned tomatoes; sugar-free
3 tbsp butter
2 tbsp Parmesan cheese
2 chili peppers; diced
2 tbsp apple cider vinegar
1/4 cup heavy cream
1/2 tsp white pepper
2 tsp dried thyme
1/2 red pepper flakes
1 tsp salt
Directions:
Plug in the instant pot and grease the inner pot with butter. Press the *Saute* button and add peppers. Briefly cook, for 2 mintues and then add canned tomatoes. Season with salt and one teaspoon of thyme. Continue to cook for 4 - 5 minuts, stirring occasionally
Now add cauliflower and season with the remaining thyme, pepper flakes, and white pepper. Pour in one cup of water and seal the lid
Set the steam release handle to the *Sealing* position and press the *Manual* button. Cook for 12 minutes on high pressure
When done; perform a quick pressure release and open the lid. Chill for a while and transfer to a food processor along with heavy cream, cream cheese, Parmesan, and cider. Process until smooth.
Transfer to glass jars with tight lids and refrigerate up to a week
Nutrition Values: Calories: 140; Total Fats: 12.1g; Net Carbs: 3.1g; Protein: 4g; Fiber: 2.1g

486. Chessy Cannelloni Eggplant
Preparation Time: 30 Minutes
Servings: 5
Ingredients:
1 small eggplant; sliced lengthwise
1 small chili pepper; sliced
1 onion; finely chopped.
3 tbsp oil
4 tbsp cottage cheese
3 tbsp Feta cheese
2 tbsp sour cream
1 cup cherry tomatoes; whole
1/4 tsp dried thyme
1/2 tsp dried oregano
1 tsp salt
Directions:
In a small bowl, combine together cottage cheese, Feta cheese, and sour cream. Sprinkle with some dried thyme and set aside
Slice eggplants lengthwise into about 1/4-inch-thick slices. Sprinkle with some salt and set aside for ten minutes
Meanwhile; plug in the instant pot and grease the inner pot with oil. Add onions and chili pepper. Sprinkle with some more salt and sauté for 3 - 4 minutes. Now add tomatoes and continue to cook until soft. If necessary, add 2 - 3 tbsp of water. Remove from the pot and set aside
Now rinse well the eggplants and gently squeeze with your hands, Set aside
Line s small baking pan with some parchment paper and add the tomato sauce. Place eggplant slices, one at the time, and spread about two tablespoons of the cheese mixture on each. Gently roll up and secure with toothpicks. Repeat the process with the remaining eggplant slices and loosely cover with some aluminum foil.
Position a trivet at the bottom of the instant pot and place the pan on top. Pour in one cup of water. Seal the lid and set the steam release handle to the *Sealing* position
Press the *Manual* button and set the timer for 13 minutes on high pressure
When done; perform a quick pressure release and open the lid. Remove the pan from the pot and chill for a while
Sprinkle with some Parmesan before serving
Nutrition Values: Calories: 146; Total Fats: 10.9g; Net Carbs: 5.6g; Protein: 4g; Fiber: 4.2g

487. Spinach with Goat's Cheese
Preparation Time: 15 Minutes
Servings: 4
Ingredients:
3 cups spinach; finely chopped.
1 cup kale; finely chopped.
2 small onions; finely chopped.
1 large leek; finely chopped.
1/2 cup fresh goat's cheese
1/2 cup Greek yogurt
2 tbsp Parmesan; freshly grated
2 garlic cloves; crushed
4 tbsp olive oil
1/2 tsp dried mint

1/2 tsp salt
Directions:
Plug in the instant pot and press the *Saute* button.
Grease the inner pot with olive oil and heat up.
Add onions and leeks. Stir-fry for 3 - 4 minutes and then add garlic. Continue to cook for one minute
Now add spinach and kale. Season with salt and mint and continue to cook until wilted
Add goat's cheese and half of the Greek yogurt. Give it a good stir and optionally season with more salt
Continue to cook for 3 minutes
When done; press the *Cancel'* button and divide the mixture between serving plates. Sprinkle with some Parmesan and top with the remaining Greek yogurt. Serve
Nutrition Values: Calories: 216; Total Fats: 17.2g; Net Carbs: 8.7g; Protein: 6.8g; Fiber: 1.9g

488. Simple Stuffed Bell Peppers
Preparation Time: 25 Minutes
Servings: 3
Ingredients:
2 medium-sized yellow bell peppers; halved
1/2 cup mozzarella cheese
1/2 cup tomatoes; diced
2 medium-sized green bell pepper; halved
2 cups button mushrooms; diced
1 cup feta cheese; crumbled
2 tbsp celery leaves; finely chopped.
2 tbsp olive oil
1/2 tsp black pepper; ground
1/2 tsp smoked paprika; ground
1/4 tsp cayenne pepper; ground
1/2 tsp salt
Directions:
Cut the bell peppers in half and remove the stem and seeds, Set aside
In a large mixing bowl, combine button mushrooms, feta cheese, mozzarella cheese, tomatoes, celery, and olive oil. Add all spices and mix until well incorporated. Stuff the bell pepper halves with this mixture. Use some additional oil to brush the peppers from outside
Line some parchment paper over a fitting springform pan and set aside
Plug in the instant pot and pour 1 cup of water in the stainless steel insert. Set the trivet on the bottom and place the stuffed peppers on top
Close the lid and set the steam release handle. Press the *Manual* button and set the timer for 30 minutes. Cook on *High* pressure
When done; perform a quick pressure release and open the pot
Transfer the peppers to a serving plate and sprinkle with some dried oregano or dried rosemary before serving. Optionally, top with Greek yogurt.
Nutrition Values: Calories: 202; Total Fats: 16g; Net Carbs: 7g; Protein: 8.3g; Fiber: 1.7g

489. Bell Pepper Zucchini Salad
Preparation Time: 20 Minutes
Servings: 3
Ingredients:
2 large red bell peppers; cut into strips
1 small red onion; sliced
3 garlic cloves; crushed
1 small zucchini; thinly sliced
1 cup button mushrooms; sliced
1/2 cup feta cheese; cubed
For the marinade:
1/2 tsp black peppercorns
1 bay leaf
2 tbsp lemon juice; freshly squeezed
1/2 cup olive oil
1 tsp coriander seeds
2 fresh thyme sprigs
1 tsp sea salt
Directions:
Combine all marinade ingredients in a large bowl. Mix until combined and bell peppers, zucchini, mushrooms, and garlic. Mix again until all is well coated. Cover with a lid and refrigerate for 20 minutes
Plug in the instant pot and press the *Saute* button. Add vegetables along with marinade and cook for 3 - 4 minutes
Now; pour in 1/2 cup of water and securely lock the lid. Set the steam release handle by moving the valve to the *Sealing* position. Press the *Manual* button and set the timer for 3 minutes. Cook on *High* pressure
When done; release the pressure naturally and open the pot
Transfer to a large bowl and stir in the feta cheese. Optionally, sprinkle with some finely chopped chives or green onions.
Nutrition Values: Calories: 200; Total Fats: 15.1g; Net Carbs: 10.3g; Protein: 6.1g; Fiber: 2.4g

490. Tasty Stuffed Bell Peppers
Preparation Time: 25 Minutes
Servings: 4
Ingredients:
4 red bell peppers
1 small onion; finely chopped.
4 tbsp olive oil
1/4 cup fresh parsley; finely chopped.
3 tbsp butter; melted
1/2 cup feta cheese
2 tbsp sharp cheddar; grated
2 tbsp gorgonzola; crumbled
2 tbsp almond flour
1/2 tsp black pepper; freshly ground
1 tsp dreid celery
1/4 tsp dried rosemary
1/4 tsp salt
Directions:
Rinse peppers and pat dry with a kitchen towel. Place on a cutting board and remove the steam of each pepper. Carefully remove the seeds and rinse well again, Set aside
In a small bowl, combine feta cheese, cheddar, gorgonzola, one tablespoon of olive oil, almond flour, parsley, and onions. Sprinkle with salt, celery, rosemary, and pepper. Mix well and set aside
Take a small baking dish and grease with the remaining oil. Tightly fit peppers in the baking dish and fill each with the cheese mixture

Cover with some aluminum foil and set aside
Plug in the instant pot and position a trivet at the bottom of the inner pot. Pour in one cup of water and place the baking pan
Seal the lid and set the steam release handle. Press the *Manual* button and set the timer for 15 minutes on high pressure
When done; perform a quick pressure release and open the lid. Optionally, top with some Greek yogurt before serving.
Nutrition Values: Calories: 329; Total Fats: 30g; Net Carbs: 9.8g; Protein: 6.5g; Fiber: 2.4g

491. Sauteed Vegetables
Preparation Time: 15 Minutes
Servings: 3
Ingredients:
1 red bell pepper; sliced
1 small onion; sliced
1 small zucchini; cut into cubes
1 green bell pepper; sliced
1/4 cup dried porcini mushrooms
1/4 cup Feta cheese
1/2 cup sour cream
2 tbsp tamari sauce
2 tbsp sesame oil
1/2 tsp dried thyme
1/4 tsp dried oregano
1 tsp pink Himalayan salt
Directions:
Plug in the instant pot and press the *Saute* button. Heat up the sesame oil and add zucchini. Sprinkle with some salt and cook for 5 - 6 minutes, stirring constantly
Now add bell peppers and onions. Sprinkle with tamari sauce and give it a good stir. Optionally, drizzle with some rice vinegar
Season with some more salt, thyme, and oregano. Continue to cook fro 2 - 3 minutes and then add Feta cheese and mushrooms. Pour in about three tablespoons of water and cook for 3 - 4 minutes.
When done; press the *Cancel'* button and stir in the sour cream. To enjoy Serve it immediately
Nutrition Values: Calories: 171; Total Fats: 12g; Net Carbs: 9.2g; Protein: 5.3g; Fiber: 2.8g

492. Zucchini Eggplant Recipe
Preparation Time: 20 Minutes
Servings: 3
Ingredients:
1 medium-sized zucchini; thinly sliced
1 small red onion; thinly sliced
1 medium-sized eggplant; thinly sliced
2 garlic cloves; minced
1 tbsp butter
2 tbsp lemon juice; freshly squeezed
1/2 cup sour cream
1/2 tsp black pepper; ground
1/4 tsp red chili flakes
1 tsp fresh ginger; grated
1 tsp lemon zest; freshly grated
1/2 tsp Himalayan pink salt
Directions:

Plug in your instant pot and place butter in the stainless steel insert. Add zucchini, eggplant, garlic, and onion. Sprinkle with salt and pepper. Cook for 5 minutes, stirring occasionally
Now; pour 1 cup of water and securely lock the lid. Set the steam release handle and press the *Manual* button. Set the timer for 3 minutes and cook on *High* pressure
When done; perform a quick pressure release and stir in the sour cream, ginger, and red chili flakes. Press the *Saute* button and cook for 5 more minutes, stirring occasionally
Transfer all to a serving plate and sprinkle with lemon zest. To enjoy Serve it immediately
Nutrition Values: Calories: 183; Total Fats: 12.4g; Net Carbs: 9.8g; Protein: 4.1g; Fiber: 6.9g

493. Yummy Creamy Spinach Balls
Preparation Time: 20 Minutes
Servings: 5
Ingredients:
7 oz spinach; finely chopped.
1 large tomato; sliced
1 cup cream cheese
1/4 cup Feta cheese
1/4 cup shredded mozzarella
5 large eggs
1/2 cup almond flour
3 tbsp butter; melted
2 tbsp olive oil
2 tbsp heavy cream
1 tsp garlic powder
1/2 tsp dried oregano
1/4 tsp dried thyme
1/2 tsp salt
Directions:
In a large bowl, combine together spinach, cheese, eggs, melted butter, and almond flour. Season with salt, thyme, oregano, and garlic powder
Mix well and shape 10 equal balls. If the mixture is too sticky, add some more almond flour.
Coat a small oven-safe bowl with olive oil and add a layer of sliced tomatoes. Gently place the balls on top and tightly wrap with aluminum foil
Plug in the instant pot and position a trivet at the bottom of the inner pot. Pour in one cup of water and place the bowl on the trivet
Seal the lid and set the steam release handle to the *Sealing* position. Press the *Manual* button and set the timer for 8 minutes on high pressure
When done; perform a quick pressure release and open the lid. Carefully remove the bowl from the pot and chill for a while. Optionally, top with some Greek yogurt before serving.
Nutrition Values: Calories: 420; Total Fats: 39.3g; Net Carbs: 4g; Protein: 13.5g; Fiber: 1.6g

494. Braised Kale Recipe
Cooking Time:20 minutes
Servings:2
Ingredients:
10 oz. kale; chopped.
3 carrots, sliced
1/2 cup chicken stock

5 garlic cloves; chopped.
1 yellow onion, thinly sliced
A splash of balsamic vinegar
1/4 tsp. red pepper flakes
1 tbsp. kale
Salt and black pepper to the taste
Directions:
Set your instant pot on Sauté mode; add ghee and melt it.
Add carrots and onion, stir and sauté for 2 minutes
Add garlic, stir and cook for 1 minute more
Add kale, stock, salt and pepper; then stir well. Seal the Instant Pot lid and cook at High for 7 minutes
Quick release the pressure, open the instant pot lid, add vinegar and pepper flakes, toss to coat, divide among plates and serve.

495. Corn Pudding
Cooking Time: 55 minutes
Servings: 8
Ingredients:
1 (4.5-ouncecan chopped mild green chiles
1/2 cup whole milk
1 (8.5-ouncepackage corn muffin mix
2 ¼ cups water
Vegetable oil
1 (14-ouncecan creamed corn
1/2 tsp. unflavored powdered gelatin
Poblanos & Corn in Cream
Directions:
Generously grease a 6-inch springform pan with oil. In a large bowl, combine the corn muffin mix, creamed corn, chiles, milk, ¼ cup of the water and the gelatin.
Stir well to combine. Pour the batter into the prepared pan. Cover the top with aluminum foil
Pour the remaining 2 cups water into the Instant Pot. Place a steamer rack in the pot. Set the pan on the rack.
Now secure the lid on the pot and close the valve. Now Press "Manual" and set the pot at "High" pressure for 25 minutes. After completing the cooking time, allow the pot to sit undisturbed until the pressure has released
Set the pudding on a wire rack to cool to room temperature. Run a knife around the edges to separate the pudding from the sides of the pan Carefully remove the springform ring. Cut the pudding into wedges. Top with Poblanos & Corn in Cream, if you like.

496. Pinto Bean Stew
Cooking Time: 2 hours
Servings: 8
Ingredients:
1 cup dried pinto beans
3 cups cool water
1 cup finely chopped onions
1 (14.5-ouncecan fire-roasted diced tomatoes; undrained
1/2 cup chopped fresh cilantro
1/2 green bell pepper, finely chopped
4 garlic cloves; minced
3 cups hot water
2 tsp. ground cumin
1 tsp. salt or as your liking
Directions:
In a medium bowl, soak the beans in the hot water for 1 hour. Drain. In your Instant Pot, combine the beans, tomatoes and their juices, onions, cilantro, bell pepper, garlic, cumin and salt. Add the cool water. Now secure the lid on the pot and close the valve. Now Press "Manual" and set the pot at "High" pressure for 30 minutes
After completing the cooking time, allow the pot to stand undisturbed for 10 minutes, then release any remaining pressure
If you'd like, blend with an immersion blender directly in the pot for 10 seconds to mash some of the beans and thicken the broth slightly.

497. Collard Greens
Cooking Time: 20 minutes
Servings: 2
Ingredients:
2 cups frozen collard greens
1/4 cup chopped yellow onion
2 cups water
1 tbsp. extra-virgin olive oil
1 tsp. paprika
1/2 tsp. ground turmeric
1 tsp. minced garlic
1/2 tsp. salt or as your liking
2 tsp. apple cider vinegar
Directions:
In a medium bowl, combine the collard greens, onion, garlic, paprika, turmeric and salt. Toss to combine. Place on a sheet of aluminum foil. Bring the edges of the foil together and crimp tightly to seal
Pour the water into the Instant Pot. Place a steamer rack in the pot. Place the packet on top of the rack. Now secure the lid on the pot and close the valve. Now Press "Manual" and set the pot at "High" pressure for 5 minutes. After completing the cooking time, quick release the pressure
In a medium skillet, heat the olive oil over medium heat until shimmering. Add the steamed vegetables to the pan and cook, stirring, for 2 minutes. Add the vinegar and toss to coat.

498. Mushroom Kale Stroganoff
Cooking Time: 25 minutes
Servings: 5
Ingredients:
1 pound baby bella mushrooms, sliced
1 cup Cashew Sour Cream
3 cups kale leaves; rinsed and torn into bite-size pieces
3 cups dried campanelle pasta; or similar shape
3 ¼ cups Vegetable Stock
1 sweet onion; diced
1 bay leaf
1 tomato; diced
2 garlic cloves; minced
1 tbsp. olive oil
1 tsp. smoked paprika
1/2 tsp. salt or as your liking
Directions:

Select the "Sauté" Low mode on your instant pot. When the display reads "Hot," add the oil and heat until it shimmers.
Add the onion. Sauté for 2 minutes, stirring frequently. Turn off the Instant Pot and add the garlic. Cook for 1 minute, stirring
Add the mushrooms, tomato, paprika, bay leaf and salt. Let sit for 2 to 3 minutes.
Stir in the pasta and stock. Lock the lid and turn the steam release handle to Sealing. Using the Manual function, set the cooker to High Pressure for 3 minutes.
After completing the cooking time, let the pressure release naturally for 5 minutes; quick release any remaining pressure
Remove the lid carefully and remove and discard the bay leaf. If there is excess liquid in the pot, select Sauté Low again and cook for 1 to 2 minutes, stirring frequently, to evaporate some of it.
Turn off the pot and stir in the sour cream and kale. Let sit for 1 to 2 minutes while the kale wilts. Taste and season with more salt, as needed.

499. Tuscan Stew
Cooking Time: 65 minutes
Servings: 6
Ingredients:
2 cups stale sourdough bread cubes
4 cups vegetable broth
1 cup dried cannellini beans
1 (14.5-ouncecan fire-roasted diced tomatoes; undrained
1/2 cup freshly grated Parmesan cheese
1 (12-ouncepackage frozen spinach
1 small onion; chopped
1 cup coarsely chopped carrots
1 cup coarsely chopped celery
2 tbsp. tomato paste
1 tbsp. minced garlic
1 tsp. red pepper flakes
1 tsp. dried thyme
1 tsp. dried rosemary
1 tsp. salt or as your liking
1 tsp. black pepper
Directions:
In your Instant Pot, combine the broth, beans, tomatoes and their juices, spinach, onion, carrots, celery, tomato paste, garlic, red pepper flakes, thyme, salt, black pepper and rosemary. Stir to combine.
Now secure the lid on the pot and close the valve. Now Press "Manual" and set the pot at "High" pressure for 30 minutes. After completing the cooking time, allow the pot to sit undisturbed for 15 minutes, then release any remaining pressure
Now Press "Sauté". Using the back of a spoon, coarsely mash a few of the beans and vegetables to thicken the soup to desired consistency.
When the broth is boiling, add the bread cubes and cook the soup for 5 minutes more, or until the bread is completely soft
Add water, if needed, to create a relatively thick stew. Now Press "Cancel". Ladle the soup into serving bowls and top with the cheese.

500. Hearts Of Palm Soup
Cooking Time: 30 minutes
Servings: 4
Ingredients:
1 (14-ouncecan hearts of palm, drained, liquid reserved and coarsely chopped
¾ cup heavy cream
1/4 cup finely chopped scallions
2 ½ cups chicken broth
1 cup chopped yellow onion
1/2 tsp. freshly grated nutmeg, plus more for garnish
1/2 cup shredded Parmesan cheese, plus more for garnish
1 tbsp. minced garlic
1 tsp. salt or as your liking
1 ½ tsp. black pepper
Directions:
In your Instant Pot, combine the hearts of palm and their liquid, the broth, onion, garlic, salt and pepper. Now secure the lid on the pot and close the valve. Now Press "Manual" and set the pot at "High" pressure for 5 minutes
After completing the cooking time, allow the pot to sit undisturbed for 10 minutes, then release any remaining pressure. Using an immersion blender, puree the soup directly in the pot until smooth
Stir in the cream, cheese and nutmeg. Pulse the soup with the immersion blender until everything is well incorporated. Garnish with the chopped scallions and additional nutmeg and cheese and serve.

501. Asian Coconut Rice and Veggies
Cooking Time: 30 minutes
Servings: 5
Ingredients:
8 ounces white button mushrooms, sliced
1 (14-ouncecan lite coconut milk
1 (8-ouncecan sliced water chestnuts, drained
1 large carrot, sliced
1 small onion; diced
1 cup jasmine rice; rinsed and drained
1 cup water
1 cup chopped bok choy
1 cup sugar snap peas; rinsed
2 garlic cloves; minced
1 tbsp. sesame oil
1/2 tsp. ground ginger
1 tsp. Chinese five-spice
1 tsp. soy sauce
1 tsp. salt or as your liking
Directions:
In the Instant Pot, combine the rice, water, salt and ginger. Lock the lid and turn the steam release handle to Sealing.
Using the Manual function, set the cooker to High Pressure for 4 minutes. After completing the cooking time, let the pressure release naturally for 5 minutes; quick release any remaining pressure
Remove the lid carefully and fluff the rice. Transfer to a bowl and set aside
Select the "Sauté" Low mode on your instant pot. When the display reads "Hot," add the oil and heat until it shimmers

Add the carrot, onion, bok choy, snap peas, garlic, mushrooms and water chestnuts. Sauté for 2 to 3 minutes.
Stir in the coconut milk, five-spice powder, soy sauce and cooked rice. Simmer for 5 to 6 minutes more, stirring occasionally, until the coconut milk is reduced.

502. Moo Goo Gai Pan
Cooking Time: 1 hour 20 minutes
Servings: 4
Ingredients:
For Marinade:
1 garlic clove; minced
½-inch piece fresh ginger, peeled and grated
2 tbsp. lite soy sauce
1 tbsp. sesame oil
2 tbsp. Vegetable Stock
For Stir-Fry:
1 (14-ounceblock firm tofu, pressed for least 1 hour, but overnight is best; chopped into bite-size cubes
1 (8-ouncecan sliced water chestnuts, drained
1 (8-ouncecan bamboo shoots, drained
1 tbsp. cornstarch
⅓ cup water
8 ounces white mushrooms, sliced
1 cup sugar snap peas; rinsed, tough ends removed
1 carrot, sliced into matchsticks
1 garlic clove; minced
1-inch piece fresh ginger, peeled and grated
1 cup Vegetable Stock
2 tbsp. soy sauce
1 tbsp. sesame oil
Hot cooked rice or noodles; for serving; optional
Directions:
To Make Marinade:
In a small bowl, whisk the stock, soy sauce, oil, garlic and ginger. Set aside.
To Make Stir-Fry:
In a shallow dish, combine the tofu cubes and marinade. Cover the dish and let sit for at least 30 minutes.
Select the "Sauté" Low mode on your instant pot. When the display reads "Hot," add the oil and heat until it shimmers
Add the marinated tofu. Cook for 8 to 10 minutes, using tongs to turn the tofu carefully.
Turn off the Instant Pot and add the mushrooms, snap peas, carrot, garlic, ginger, stock, soy sauce, water chestnuts and bamboo shoots. Using a large spoon, stir well
Select the "Sauté" Low mode on your instant pot, again. Cover the pot with a tempered glass lid and simmer for 5 minutes, stirring occasionally
In a small bowl, whisk the cornstarch and water. Add this slurry to the pot. Simmer, uncovered, for 5 minutes more; or until the sauce thickens. Serve over rice or noodles.

503. Sweet Potato and Black Bean Tacos
Cooking Time: 20 minutes
Servings: 5
Ingredients:
1 (15-ouncecan black beans; rinsed and drained
1 canned chipotle pepper in adobo sauce; diced
1 avocado, peeled, pitted and mashed
1/4 cup fresh cilantro, chopped
1/2 sweet onion; diced
1/2 cup Vegetable Stock
1 large sweet potato; diced
1 red bell pepper; diced
1 garlic clove; minced
1 tomato; diced
1 tbsp. freshly squeezed lime juice
2 tbsp. olive oil
2 tsp. adobo sauce from the can
2 tsp. chili powder
1/2 tsp. ground cumin
1/2 tsp. salt as your liking
Zest of 1 lime
Corn or flour tortillas; for serving
Cashew Sour Cream; for serving; optional
Sliced red cabbage; for serving; optional
Sliced jalapeño peppers; for serving; optional
Garden Salsa; for serving; optional
Directions:
Select the "Sauté" Low mode on your instant pot. When the display reads "Hot," add the oil and heat until it shimmers.
Add the onion. Cook for 1 minute, stirring. Add the sweet potato and bell pepper. Cook for 1 minute, stirring so nothing burns. Turn off the Instant Pot and add the garlic. Cook for 30 seconds to 1 minute, stirring.
Add the tomato, black beans, chipotle, adobo sauce, chili powder, salt, cumin, stock and lime juice.
Lock the lid and turn the steam release handle to Sealing. Using the Manual function, set the cooker to High Pressure for 4 minutes
After completing the cooking time, turn off the Instant Pot and let the pressure release naturally for 5 minutes; quick release any remaining pressure
Remove the lid carefully. If there is too much liquid in the inner pot, select Sauté Low again and cook for 1 to 2 minutes, stirring constantly (it gets hot fast!
Stir in the lime zest. Serve in the tortillas, topped with mashed avocado and cilantro and anything else your heart desires.

504. Red Curry Cauliflower
Cooking Time: 12 minutes
Servings: 5
Ingredients:
1 (14-ouncecan full-fat coconut milk
1 (14-ouncecan diced tomatoes and liquid
1 bell pepper, any color, thinly sliced
1 small to medium head cauliflower; cut into bite-size pieces (3 to 4 cups
1/2 to 1 cup water
2 tbsp. red curry paste
1 tsp. garlic powder
1/2 tsp. onion powder
1/4 tsp. chili powder
1 tsp. salt or as your liking
1/2 tsp. ground ginger
Freshly ground black pepper
Cooked rice or other grain; for serving; optional

Directions:
In the Instant Pot, stir together the coconut milk, water, red curry paste, garlic powder, salt, ginger, onion powder and chili powder
Add the bell pepper, cauliflower and tomatoes and stir again. Lock the lid and turn the steam release handle to Sealing. Using the Manual function, set the cooker to High Pressure for 2 minutes.
After completing the cooking time, quick release the pressure
Remove the lid carefully and give the whole thing a good stir. Taste and season with more salt and pepper, as needed. Serve with rice or another grain (if using.

505. Vegetable Salad
Cooking Time: 20 minutes
Servings: 5
Ingredients:
For Dressing:
1/2 cup Vegetable Stock
1/2 cup apple cider vinegar
2 tsp. Dijon mustard
1/2 tsp. garlic powder
1 tsp. salt or as your liking
For Salad:
1 ½ pounds red potatoes, chopped
1/4 cup chopped fresh parsley
2 cups Brussels sprouts, ends trimmed
1 (8-ouncepackage unflavored tempeh; chopped into bite-size pieces
1 small red onion, sliced
2 bay leaves
1 ½ tbsp. olive oil
1 ½ tsp. smoked paprika
1/2 tsp. salt or as your liking
1/4 tsp. garlic powder
Freshly ground black pepper
Directions:
To Make Dressing:
In a medium bowl, whisk the vinegar, stock, mustard, salt and garlic powder until well combined. Set aside.
To Make Salad:
Select the "Sauté" Low mode on your instant pot. When the display reads "Hot," add the oil and heat until it shimmers.
Add the tempeh, paprika, salt and garlic powder. Cook for 5 to 6 minutes, stirring occasionally. Transfer to a bowl and set aside
Now add the potatoes, Brussels sprouts, red onion and bay leaves to the Instant Pot. Pour the dressing over the vegetables.
Lock the lid and turn the steam release handle to Sealing. Using the Manual function, set the cooker to High Pressure for 4 minutes
After completing the cooking time, quick release the pressure
Remove the lid carefully and remove and discard the bay leaves. Stir in the tempeh and parsley.
Taste and season with more salt and pepper, as needed. There will be some liquid left in the bottom, which is perfect for spooning over the salad when it's served

If there's too much liquid for your taste, select Sauté Low again and cook for 2 to 3 minutes more.

506. Cabbage Rolls
Cooking Time: 32 minutes
Servings: 7
Ingredients:
For Tempeh:
1 (8-ouncepackage unflavored tempeh, crumbled
2 garlic cloves; minced
1 bay leaf
1/2 onion; diced
1 tbsp. olive oil
2 tsp. vegan Worcestershire sauce
2 tsp. Montreal steak seasoning
For Deconstructed Cabbage Rolls:
1 head cabbage, thinly sliced
6 ounces tomato paste
1 ½ cups Vegetable Stock
1 cup basmati rice; rinsed and drained
1/4 cup chopped fresh parsley
1 cup water
1/2 tsp. salt as your liking
1/2 tsp. paprika
1/4 tsp. freshly ground black pepper
Pinch cayenne pepper; or more as needed
Directions:
To Make Tempeh:
Select the "Sauté" Low mode on your instant pot. When the display reads "Hot," add the oil and heat until it shimmers.
Add the tempeh, Montreal steak seasoning, Worcestershire sauce, garlic, bay leaf and onion. Cook for 3 to 4 minutes, stirring frequently. Transfer to a bowl and set aside.
To Make Deconstructed Cabbage Rolls:
In the Instant Pot, combine the rice, water and salt. Lock the lid and turn the steam release handle to Sealing.
Using the Manual function, set the cooker to High Pressure for 8 minutes. After completing the cooking time, let the pressure release naturally for 10 minutes; quick release any remaining pressure
Remove the lid carefully and fluff the rice. Add the stock, cabbage, tomato paste, paprika, black pepper and cayenne
Select Sauté Low again and cook for 4 to 5 minutes until the cabbage softens a little. Turn off the Instant Pot, remove and discard the bay leaf and stir in the parsley. Taste and season with more salt and pepper, as needed.

507. Black Eyed Peas
Cooking Time: 55 minutes
Servings: 5
Ingredients:
1 cup dried black-eyed peas; rinsed
3 ¼ cups Vegetable Stock
2 cups cooked brown rice
3 cups chopped kale
1 cup frozen peas
1 red bell pepper; diced
2 tomatoes, chopped
1 sweet onion; diced

1 tbsp. olive oil
1/2 tsp. garlic powder
1/2 tsp. dried thyme
1 tsp. chili powder
1 tsp. vegan Worcestershire sauce
1/2 tsp. salt or as your liking
1/4 tsp. freshly ground black pepper
Directions:
Select the "Sauté" Low mode on your instant pot. When the display reads "Hot," add the oil and heat until it shimmers.
Add the onion and bell pepper. Cook for 2 to 3 minutes, stirring occasionally. Turn off the Instant Pot and add the tomatoes, chili powder, Worcestershire sauce, garlic powder, thyme, salt, pepper, black-eyed peas and stock
Lock the lid and turn the steam release handle to Sealing. Using the Manual function, set the cooker to High Pressure for 20 minutes
After completing the cooking time, let the pressure release naturally for about 20 minutes; quick release any remaining pressure
Remove the lid carefully and stir in the frozen peas, rice and kale. Give them a minute or two to warm and enjoy.

508. Mucho Burritos
Cooking Time: 20 minutes
Servings: 7
Ingredients:
2 canned chipotle peppers in adobo sauce
2 cups Cilantro Lime Brown Rice
¼ cup Vegetable Stock
1 bell pepper, any color, sliced
1 small onion, sliced
8 burrito-size tortillas
2 cups Poblano Cheeze Sauce
1 (14-ouncecontainer firm tofu, pressed for at least 1 hour; or overnight if possible and crumbled
1 (16-ouncecan chili beans, drained but not rinsed
1 tbsp. roasted walnut oil
1/2 tsp. garlic powder
1/2 tsp. freshly squeezed lime juice
2 tsp. adobo sauce from the can
1 tsp. ground cumin
1/2 tsp. salt or as your liking
Pinch freshly ground black pepper
Garden Salsa; or store-bought salsa of choice; for filling
Cashew Sour Cream, for filling; optional
Sliced avocado, for filling; optional
Directions:
Select the "Sauté" Low mode on your instant pot. When the display reads "Hot," add the oil and heat until it shimmers.
Add the tofu crumbles, chipotle peppers, adobo sauce, cumin, salt, garlic powder, lime juice and pepper. Cook for 2 to 3 minutes
Add the bell pepper and onion. Cook for 2 minutes more. If you need additional liquid, add 1 to 2 tbsp. of water.
Add the stock and simmer, stirring occasionally, for 4 to 5 minutes until the liquid is cooked out. Turn off the Instant Pot

To build your burritos, layer the tortillas with rice, tofu mixture, chili beans, salsa, poblano cheeze sauce and other fillings, as desired.

509. Barbecue Chickpea Tacos
Cooking Time: 1 hour 20 minutes
Servings: 5
Ingredients:
1 cup dried chickpeas; rinsed
2 cups pineapple chunks
8 taco shells
⅓ cup packed light brown sugar
⅓ cup soy sauce
2 cups plus 3 tbsp. water
3 tbsp. cornstarch
2 tbsp. hot chili oil
3 tbsp. gochujang (Korean hot pepper paste
1/2 tsp. garlic powder
1 tsp. sriracha; or more as needed
2 tsp. rice wine vinegar
1/2 tsp. onion powder
Directions:
In the Instant Pot, combine the chickpeas with enough water to cover.
Lock the lid and turn the steam release handle to Sealing. Using the Manual function, set the cooker to High Pressure for 45 minutes
After completing the cooking time, let the pressure release naturally for 15 minutes; quick release any remaining pressure.
Remove the lid carefully and pour the contents into a colander to drain. Return the chickpeas to the inner pot.
In a small bowl, whisk the cornstarch and 3 tbsp. of water. Set aside. Select the "Sauté" Low mode on your instant pot
To the chickpeas, add the gochujang, brown sugar, soy sauce, chili oil, vinegar, onion powder and garlic powder
Cook until it starts to bubble. Stir in the cornstarch slurry. Simmer for 4 to 5 minutes more, stirring frequently, until the sauce thickens and the chickpeas are nice and coated
In a medium bowl, stir together the pineapple and sriracha. Taste before adding more sauce. Fill the taco shells with the chickpeas and top with the pineapple.

510. Asian Gobi Masala
Cooking Time: 12 minutes
Servings: 5
Ingredients:
1 garlic clove; minced
1 head cauliflower, chopped
1 white onion; diced
1 cup water
1 tbsp. ground coriander
1 tbsp. olive oil
1 tsp. cumin seeds
1/2 tsp. garam masala
1 tsp. ground cumin
1/2 tsp. salt or as your liking
Hot cooked rice; for serving; optional
Directions:

Select the "Sauté" Low mode on your instant pot. When the display reads "Hot," add the oil and heat until it shimmers.
Add the cumin seeds. Cook for 30 seconds, stirring nearly constantly. Add the onion. Cook for 2 to 3 minutes, still stirring.
Turn off the Instant Pot and add the garlic. Cook for about 30 seconds, stirring frequently
Add the cauliflower, coriander, cumin, garam masala, salt and water. Lock the lid and turn the steam release handle to Sealing. Using the Manual function, set the cooker to High Pressure for 1 minute
After completing the cooking time, quick release the pressure
Remove the lid carefully and serve with hot rice.

511. Sloppy Janes
Cooking Time: 20 minutes
Servings: 5
Ingredients:
1 (15-ouncecan vegan refried beans
1 (8-ouncepackage unflavored tempeh
1 (10-ouncecan diced tomatoes with green chilies, with liquid
1/4 cup quick cook oats
6 buns or rolls; for serving
1/2 cup Vegetable Stock
2 tbsp. vegan Worcestershire sauce
1 tbsp. Dijon mustard
1 tbsp. olive oil
1 tsp. smoked paprika
1/2 tsp. salt or as your liking
1/2 tsp. garlic powder
2 pinches chili powder
Freshly ground black pepper
Vegan cheese; for serving
Barbecue sauce; for serving
Sliced onion; for serving
Sliced bell pepper; for serving
Pickles; for serving
Directions:
Select the "Sauté" Low mode on your instant pot. When the display reads "Hot," add the oil and heat until it shimmers.
Crumble in the tempeh and add the paprika and salt. Cook for 4 to 5 minutes, stirring occasionally. Turn off the Instant Pot
Add the refried beans, tomatoes and green chilies, stock, Worcestershire sauce, mustard, garlic powder and chili powder and season to taste with pepper
Lock the lid and turn the steam release handle to Sealing. Using the Manual function, set the cooker to High Pressure for 2 minutes.
After completing the cooking time, quick release the pressure
Remove the lid carefully and stir in the oats. There will likely be too much liquid; if so, select Sauté Medium and cook, uncovered, for 2 to 3 minutes; or until the extra liquid evaporates. Serve on buns, topped as desired.

512. Polenta and Kale
Cooking Time: 45 minutes
Servings: 5
Ingredients:
1 quart Vegetable Stock
2 bunches kale, stemmed, leaves chopped
4 garlic cloves; minced
1 cup polenta
1 tbsp. olive oil
2 tbsp. nutritional yeast
3 tbsp. vegan butter
1 tsp. salt as your liking
Freshly ground black pepper
Directions:
Select the "Sauté" Low mode on your instant pot. When the display reads "Hot," add the oil and heat until it shimmers.
Add the kale, garlic and ½ tsp. of salt. Cook for about 2 minutes, stirring frequently so nothing burns, until the kale is soft and the garlic is fragrant. Note: You can always turn off the Instant Pot if it gets too hot. Transfer the garlicky kale to a bowl and set aside
In the Instant Pot, combine the polenta, stock and remaining ½ tsp. of salt.
Lock the lid and turn the steam release handle to Sealing. Using the Manual function, set the cooker to High Pressure for 20 minutes
After completing the cooking time, let the pressure release naturally for 15 minutes; quick release any remaining pressure
Remove the lid carefully and stir well. Add the nutritional yeast and butter along with any additional salt and pepper. Serve in bowls topped with the kale.

513. Corn Chowder
Cooking Time: 30 minutes
Servings: 4
Ingredients:
4 slices bacon; chopped
2 cups diced potatoes; cut into ½-inch cubes
1 cup chopped yellow onions
3 cups chicken broth
1/2 cup heavy cream
2 cups corn kernels
1 tbsp. minced garlic
1/2 tsp. dried thyme
1/2 tsp. freshly grated nutmeg
1 tsp. salt or as your liking
1 tsp. black pepper
Directions:
In your Instant Pot, combine the broth, corn, potatoes, onions, bacon, garlic, salt, pepper and thyme. Stir to combine
Now secure the lid on the pot and close the valve.
Now Press "Manual" and set the pot at "High" pressure for 5 minutes
After completing the cooking time, allow the pot to sit undisturbed for 5 minutes, then release any remaining pressure.
Using an immersion blender, puree some of the soup to thicken slightly, leaving some chunks of potato and corn intact. Stir in the nutmeg and cream and serve.

514. Vegetable Soup
Cooking Time: 33 minutes
Servings: 4

Ingredients:
2 cups cauliflower florets cut into 3-inch pieces
1 cup potatoes cut into 2-inch pieces
1 large onion; chopped into 2-inch pieces
2 cups water
1 cup chopped tomatoes
1 ½ tsp. Sambhar Spice Mix
1 tsp. ground turmeric
1 tsp. salt or as your liking
Directions:
In your Instant Pot, combine the cauliflower, onion, carrots, tomatoes, spice mix, salt and turmeric. Stir to combine
Now secure the lid on the pot and close the valve.
Now Press "Manual" and set the pot at "Low" pressure for 3 minutes
After completing the cooking time, allow the pot to sit undisturbed for 10 minutes, then release any remaining pressure. Gradually stir in the water to thin the soup to the desired consistency.

515. Chickpea Kale Korma
Cooking Time: 1 hour 20 minutes
Servings: 5
Ingredients:
3 garlic cloves, peeled
2 Roma tomatoes, quartered
½-inch piece fresh ginger, peeled
1 (14-ouncecan lite coconut milk
1/2 cup cashews, soaked in water overnight, drained and rinsed well
1 cup dried chickpeas; rinsed
1 to 2 cups water
1 tsp. curry powder
1/2 tsp. ground cardamom
1 tsp. garam masala
1/2 tsp. ground cumin
1/2 tsp. ground coriander
1/2 tsp. ground turmeric
1/2 tsp. onion powder
1 tsp. salt or as your liking
1/4 tsp. freshly ground black pepper
1 bunch kale, leaves torn from stems and rinsed
Hot cooked rice; for serving; optional
Directions:
In the Instant Pot, combine the chickpeas and enough water to cover. Lock the lid and turn the steam release handle to Sealing.
Using the Manual function, set the cooker to High Pressure for 45 minutes. After completing the cooking time, let the pressure release naturally for 15 minutes; quick release any remaining pressure
Remove the lid carefully. Drain the chickpeas and return them to the Instant Pot
In a high-speed blender or food processor, combine the cashews, tomatoes, garlic and ginger. Blend until smooth
Add the coconut milk and pulse a few more times to combine. Add this purée to the chickpeas along with the garam masala, curry powder, salt, cumin, coriander, cardamom, turmeric, onion powder, pepper and kale

Select the "Sauté" Low mode on your instant pot. Simmer for 8 to 10 minutes until the kale and beans have absorbed the flavor. Serve with rice, if desired.

516. Butternut Mac N Cheese
Cooking Time: 20 minutes
Servings: 6
Ingredients:
1 cup raw cashews; soaked in water for at least 3 to 4 hours; or overnight, drained and rinsed well
4 ½ cups water; divided
1 (16-ouncebox pasta
1 cup nondairy milk; or more as needed
2 cups cooked cubed butternut squash
⅓ cup nutritional yeast
2 tbsp. freshly squeezed lemon juice
⅛ tsp. ground nutmeg
1 tsp. Dijon mustard
2 tsp. salt or as your liking
Freshly ground black pepper
Directions:
In a high-speed blender or food processor, combine the cashews, squash, nutritional yeast, lemon juice, mustard, salt, nutmeg and 2 cups of water.
Blend until smooth (the longer you soaked the cashews, the quicker this will be. Pour the cashew mixture into your Instant Pot
Pour the remaining 2 ½ cups of water into the blender and swish it around to capture any remaining cashew mixture
Add that to the Instant Pot as well, along with the pasta. Lock the lid and turn the steam release handle to Sealing. Using the Manual function, set the cooker to Low Pressure for 2 minutes.
After completing the cooking time, turn off the Instant Pot and let the pressure release naturally for 8 minutes; quick release any remaining pressure
Remove the lid carefully and stir in the milk, adding as much as needed to make it nice and creamy. Taste and season with more salt and pepper, as needed.

517. Layered Casserole
Cooking Time: 25 minutes
Servings: 5
Ingredients:
2 cups mashed sweet potatoes
1 ¼ cups Red Hot Enchilada Sauce; or 1 (10-ouncecan; divided
1 (15-ouncecan black beans; rinsed and drained
1 (10-ouncecan diced tomatoes with green chilies, drained
1/2 cup sliced scallion, green and light green parts; divided
1/2 cup water
1/4 cup frozen sweet corn
1 tbsp. freshly squeezed lime juice
1 tsp. chili powder
1/2 tsp. garlic powder
1/2 tsp. onion powder
9 taco-size, gluten-free corn tortillas
Nonstick cooking spray; for preparing the springform pan
Vegan cheese shreds; for topping; optional
Sliced avocado; for serving

Poblano Cheeze Sauce; for serving
Cashew Sour Cream; for serving
Directions:
Lightly coat the bottom and sides of a 7-inch springform pan with nonstick spray and set aside. In a medium bowl, stir together the mashed sweet potatoes, 1 cup of enchilada sauce, the lime juice, chili powder, garlic powder and onion powder.
In another medium bowl, stir together the black beans, tomatoes and green chilies, ¼ cup of scallion, the corn and 3 tbsp. of enchilada sauce
To build the casserole, spread the remaining 1 tbsp. of enchilada sauce on the bottom of the prepared pan. Add a layer of tortillas, torn as needed to get full coverage. Don't be afraid to overlap. Layer on one-third of the sweet potato mixture.
Using a slotted spoon, top the sweet potato later with one-third of the black bean mixture. Repeat the tortilla layer, sweet potato layer and black bean layer two more times. Top with the remaining ¼ cup of scallion. If using vegan cheese shreds, add them now
Spray a piece of aluminum foil with nonstick spray and cover the pan tightly.
Pour the water into the Instant Pot and place a trivet into the inner pot.
Set the covered casserole on top of the trivet. Lock the lid and turn the steam release handle to Sealing. Using the Manual function, set the cooker to High Pressure for 8 minutes.
After completing the cooking time, let the pressure release naturally for 5 minutes; quick release any remaining pressure
Remove the lid carefully and the trivet and casserole from the Instant Pot. Set aside on a heat-resistant surface
Remove the foil and let cool for at least 5 minutes before releasing the sides of the pan. Plate and add desired toppings before serving.

518. Vegetable Stock
Cooking Time: 35 minutes
Servings: 9
Ingredients:
1 cup mushrooms
8 cups water
8 whole peppercorns
3 celery stalks
1 bay leaf
3 carrots
1 large onion
Directions:
In the Instant Pot, combine the celery, carrots, onion, mushrooms, peppercorns, bay leaf and water, making sure the veggies are completely covered by water.
Lock the lid and turn the steam release handle to Sealing. Using the Manual function, set the cooker to High Pressure for 15 minutes
After completing the cooking time, let the pressure release naturally for 15 minutes; quick release any remaining pressure
Remove the lid carefully. Strain the stock through a fine-mesh strainer into a large heatproof container.
Use immediately or refrigerate in an airtight container for 3 to 4 days; or keep frozen for up to a year.

519. Kimchi Pasta
Cooking Time: 10 minutes
Servings: 5
Ingredients:
8 ounces dried small pasta
1 ¼ cups kimchi, with any larger pieces chopped
1/2 cup Cashew Sour Cream
2⅓ cups Vegetable Stock
2 garlic cloves; minced
1/2 red onion, sliced
1 tsp. salt or as your liking
Directions:
In the Instant Pot, combine the pasta, stock, garlic, red onion and salt.
Lock the lid and turn the steam release handle to Sealing. Using the Manual function, set the cooker to High Pressure for 1 minute
After completing the cooking time, quick release the pressure. Remove the lid carefully. Select the "Sauté" Low mode on your instant pot. Stir in the kimchi. Simmer for 3 to 4 minutes. Stir in the sour cream and serve!

520. Tomato Basil Pasta
Cooking Time: 5 minutes
Servings: 2
Ingredients:
2 cups dried campanelle or similar pasta
12 fresh sweet basil leaves
2 tomatoes; cut into large dice
1 ¾ cups Vegetable Stock
1/2 tsp. salt or as your liking
2 pinches red pepper flakes
1/2 tsp. dried oregano
1/2 tsp. garlic powder
Freshly ground black pepper
Directions:
In the Instant Pot, stir together the pasta, stock and salt. Drop the tomatoes on top "do not stir".
Lock the lid and turn the steam release handle to Sealing. Using the Manual function, set the cooker to High Pressure for 2 minutes
After completing the cooking time, quick release the pressure
Remove the lid carefully and stir in the red pepper flakes; oregano and garlic powder.
If there's more than a few tbsp. of liquid in the bottom, select Sauté Low and cook for 2 to 3 minutes until it evaporates
When ready to serve, chiffonade the basil and stir it in. Taste and season with more salt and pepper, as needed.

521. Vegetarian Quinoa Chili
Servings: 12
Preparation time: 15 minutes
Cook time: 5 minutes
Total time: 20 minutes
Ingredients:
4 cups of vegetable broth
2 cups of canned

2 crushed tomatoes
2 cups of onion, diced
2-4 cloves garlic, minced
1 green bell pepper, diced
1 red bell pepper, diced
1 cup of corn (frozen or canned
1 can of spicy chili beans in sauce (15 oz.
1 cup of canned/cooked black beans, drained and rinsed
3 tablespoons of chili powder
2 tablespoons of cumin
1 teaspoon of dried oregano
½ teaspoon of smoked paprika, plus extra to taste
½ teaspoon of salt and pepper to taste
½ cup o quinoa
½ cup of dried red lentils
Chopped red onion, fresh Pico de gallo or salsa, sliced avocado, fresh cilantro, chopped green onion, jalapeños or bell peppers, sour cream or Greek yogurt, shredded cheddar cheese (skip if veganand corn chips

Directions:
Chop up the veggies. Add the veggie broth and crushed tomatoes with the lentils, quinoa, chili beans (pinto beans in chili sauceand black beans.
Add the onion, garlic, peppers, corn, dried spices and give everything a good mix. Close and lock the lid in place and ensure that the valve is in sealing position.
Select Manual function to cook on High Pressure for about 5 minutes. When the time is up, use a quick pressure release.
Carefully open the lid and adjust seasoning (spices and saltto taste. Add all your desired toppings.
Serve and enjoy!

522. Kerala Mixed Vegetable Curry
Preparation time: 10 minutes
Cook time: 4 minutes
Total time: 14 minutes
Ingredients:
1 tbsp. of coconut oil
½ tsp. of black mustard seeds
30 curry leaves
4 cups of assorted vegetables, cut lengthwise (2-inch long pieces
½ cup of grated coconut
⅔ cup of water
1 Serrano pepper or green chili, slit in half but still intact
1 tsp. of salt, adjust to taste
½ tsp. of ground cumin
¼ tsp. of turmeric
½ cup of yogurt (regular or dairy-free coconut yogurt
Directions:
Press the Sauté function on your Instant Pot and add the coconut oil.
When the oil melts, add the mustard seeds and curry leaves.
Once the mustard seeds start to pop, add the rest of the ingredients to your Instant Pot except for the yogurt.
Close and lock the lid in place and ensure that the valve is in sealing position.
Select Manual function to cook on High Pressure for about 4 minutes.
When the time is up, use a quick pressure release.
Carefully open the lid and stir in the yogurt.
Serve immediately and enjoy!

523. Creamy Vegan Tomato Soup
Preparation time: 10 minutes
Cook time: 20 minutes
Total time: 30 minutes
Servings: 3
Ingredients:
¼ cup of extra virgin olive oil
1 large yellow onion, diced
2 (28-oz.cans crushed tomatoes
6 cups of vegetable stock
1 tsp. of salt
¼ tsp. of black pepper
½ cup of fresh basil
1 ½ cup of whole raw cashews
Directions:
Press the Sauté function on your Instant Pot and add olive oil.
Once hot, add the onions and cook for about 4 minutes until translucent. Add the rest of the ingredients to the pot.
Clos and lock the lid in place and ensure that the valve is in sealing position. Select the Soup function to cook for about 20 minutes.
When the time is up, use a natural pressure release for about 10 minutes, then quick release any remaining pressure.
Carefully open the lid and transfer the soup to a standing blender. Blend on high for about 5 minutes until smooth and creamy.
Sprinkle with vegan parmesan cheese and toast in the oven on 375°F for about 5 minutes.
Serve and enjoy!

524. Portobello Pot Roast
Preparation time: 10 minutes
Cook time: 4 hours
Total time: 4 hours 10 minutes
Ingredients:
lbs. of Yukon gold potatoes, cut into bite-sized pieces
1 lb. of baby belle mushrooms
2 large carrots, peeled and cut into bite-sized pieces
2 cups frozen pearl onions
4 cloves garlic, peeled and minced
3 sprigs fresh thyme
3 cups of vegetable stock, divided
½ cup of dry red or white wine
3 tbsp. of tomato paste
2 tbsp. of (vegetarianWorcestershire
2 tbsp. of cornstarch
Kosher salt and freshly-cracked black pepper
Finely-chopped fresh parsley, optional for garnish
Directions:
Add the potatoes, mushrooms, carrots, onions into the bowl of your Instant Pot.
Add the garlic, thyme, 2.5 cups of vegetable stock, wine and Worcestershire and toss everything to combine.

Close and lock the lid in place and ensure that the valve is in sealing position. Press the Manual function to cook on High Pressure for about 20 minutes. When the time is up, use a natural pressure release for about 15 minutes. Carefully open the lid. In another bowl, whisk together the remaining ½ cup of vegetable stock and cornstarch until combined. Add the mixture to the roast mixture, and toss everything to combine. Cook the contents for additional 2 minutes until the sauce thickens. Serve, garnished with fresh parsley if desired and enjoy!

525. Vegan Green Chile Stew
Preparation time: 30 minutes
Cook time: 38 minutes
Total time: 1 hour 8 minutes
Servings: 10 -12
Ingredients:
Meat Ingredients:
½ package of butler soy curls rehydrated
1 teaspoon of chili powder
1 teaspoon of ground cumin
1 teaspoon of garlic powder
1 teaspoon of onion powder
Broth Ingredients:
1 yellow onion, diced
2 carrots, diced
2 stalks celery, diced
4-5 cloves garlic
2 cups of vegetable broth
2 cups of water
1 teaspoon of oregano
1 cup of dried rinsed, pinto beans
Stew Ingredients:
3 Yukon gold potatoes, cubed
15 oz. can of fire roasted tomatoes
24 oz. package select new Mexico green chilies
¼ cup of lime juice
¼ teaspoon of salt
¼ teaspoon of ground pepper
Directions:
Sauce your 'meat' on Sauté function. Add the garlic powder, onion powder, chili powder, cumin and stir frequently until lightly browned.
Add a little veggie broth to prevent it from sticking. Transfer it from your pot and set aside. Cook the onion, carrots, and celery on Sauté function until soft and translucent.
Scrape up any browned bits on bottom of pot. Add the minced garlic and stir for about 1 minute. Cancel the Sauté function.
Add the veggie broth, water, oregano, and dried Beans. Close and lock the lid in place and ensure that the valve is in sealing position.
Select Manual function to cook on High Pressure for about 30 minutes. When the time is up, use a natural pressure release for 10 minutes.
Carefully open the lid and stir in broth and add potatoes, chilies, tomatoes, and the "meat" you kept aside. Close and secure the lid in place.
Select Manual function to cook on High Pressure for about 8 minutes. When the time is up, do a quick pressure release.
Carefully open the lid and stir in lime juice, masa flour until your desired thickness is achieved.
Serve and enjoy!

526. Buttery Garlic Mashed Potatoes
Preparation time: 10 minutes
Cook time: 6 minutes
Total time: 16 minutes
Ingredients:
3 pounds (1.5kgof red and Yukon Gold potatoes, peeled, halved or quartered
4 garlic cloves, peeled
1 ½ cups (375mllow sodium chicken stock
3 tbsp. of butter or ghee
¾ cup of heavy cream
Salt and freshly ground black pepper
Minced fresh thyme, for garnish (optional
Directions:
Add the potatoes, garlic, salt, black pepper, chicken stock, and butter or ghee into the bottom of your Instant Pot.
Close and lock the lid in place and ensure that the valve is in sealing position.
Select Manual function to cook on High Pressure for about 6 minutes.
When the timer beeps, press the "Keep Warm/Cancel" setting, carefully turn the valve to "Venting", to release the pressure.
Carefully remove the lid and mash the potatoes right in the pot with a potato masher.
Add the heavy cream, and mash until your desired consistency is achieved.
Adjust the seasoning with more salt and pepper.
Serve warm, topped with additional butter or ghee and fresh thyme.

527. Vegetarian Pasta Rigatoni Bolognese
Preparation time: 5 minutes
Cook time: 20 minutes
Total time: 25 minutes
Servings: 6
Ingredients:
3 tablespoons of olive oil
½ cup of onion, finely chopped
½ cup of celery, finely chopped
½ cup of carrots, finely chopped
½ cup of bell peppers, finely chopped
1 tablespoon of garlic, minced
2 cups of fresh mushrooms, chopped
1 cup of water
1 oz. dried porcini mushrooms, chopped
1 (28 oz.can crushed tomatoes
½ teaspoon of black pepper
1 teaspoon of salt (or to taste
¼ teaspoon of dried thyme
1 teaspoon of dried oregano
1 teaspoon of dried basil
1 teaspoon of sugar
1 tablespoon of balsamic vinegar
1 tablespoon of tomato paste
½ teaspoon of crushed red pepper flakes (or to taste
12 oz. rigatoni pasta
1 cup of whole milk

1 cup of red wine
4 oz. mascarpone cheese
¼ cup of parmesan cheese, finely grated
3 tablespoons of fresh parsley, chopped
Directions:
Press 'Sauté' setting on your Instant Pot and add the olive oil.
Add the onions, celery, carrots, bell peppers and garlic and cook for about 3 minutes, stirring frequently. Add the fresh mushrooms and cook for about 2 minutes.
Press the Cancel function and deglaze the pot with 2 tablespoons of water. Add in dried porcini mushrooms, crushed tomatoes, black pepper, salt, thyme and oregano.
Add the basil, sugar, balsamic vinegar, tomato paste, crushed red pepper, pasta, milk, wine and water and give everything a good stir to combine.
Close and lock the lid in place and ensure that the valve is in sealing position. Select Manual function to cook on High Pressure for about 7 minutes.
When the time is up, use a quick pressure release. Carefully open the lid and stir in mascarpone cheese. Allow the pasta to sit for a couple of minutes to thicken up. Sprinkle each serving with Parmesan and fresh parsley.
Serve and enjoy!

528. Lentil Bolognese Sauce
Preparation time: 15 minutes
Cook time: 20 minutes
Total time: 45 minutes
Servings: 6
Ingredients:
2 tablespoons of extra-virgin olive oil
1 cup of minced onion
1 stalk celery, finely chopped
2 carrots, finely chopped
1 cup of finely chopped Crimini mushrooms
4 cloves garlic, minced
2 tablespoons of tomato paste
1/3 cup of red wine
1 cup of dried lentils rinsed
One 28 oz. can crushed tomatoes
¾ cup of water
1 bay leaf
1 teaspoon of dried thyme
2 teaspoons of dried oregano
Dash red pepper flakes
1 tablespoon of balsamic vinegar
Coarse salt and black pepper to taste
1 lb. of Barilla Gluten Free Penne cooked
Pecorino Romano cheese grated or shaved
Fresh basil chopped (optional)
Directions:
Press the Sauté setting on your Instant Pot and add the olive oil.
Add the onion, celery, and carrots and season with salt and pepper. Sauté the onions for about 5 minutes, or until the onions and the vegetables are soft.
Add the mushrooms and garlic. Sauté for about 4 to 5 minutes, or until the mushrooms are soft and the garlic is fragrant.
Add the tomato paste and give everything a good stir to incorporate and brown for about 2 to 3 minutes.
Add the red wine and stir. Scrape up any browned bits that stuck to the bottom of your pot.
Add the lentils, tomatoes, water, and spices into the bottom of your Instant Pot. Close and lock the lid in place and ensure that the valve is in sealing position. Select Manual function to cook on High Pressure for about 20 minutes. When the time is up, use a natural pressure release for about 10 minutes.
Cook your pasta when the Lentil Bolognese sauce is done cooking. Carefully open the lid and stir in the balsamic vinegar, taste and adjust seasoning with salt and pepper.
Serve over cooked pasta and top with grated cheese and fresh basil.

529. Vegan Butter Chicken with Soy Curls & Chickpeas
Preparation time: 11 minutes
Cooking time: 33 minutes
Total time: 44 minutes
Calories: 380 kcal
Servings: 5
Ingredients:
½ tsp. cayenne
4 big ripe tomatoes
3 cloves of garlic
½ inch cube of ginger
1 cup of water
1 tsp. graham masala
½ tsp. paprika or Kashmiri chili powder
¾ tsp. salt
1 cup of soy curls (dry, not rehydrated
1 cup of cooked chickpeas
Cashew cream made with ¼ cup of soaked cashews blended with ½ cup of water
½ tsp. or more graham masala
½ tsp. or more sugar or sweetener
½ moderately hot green chili finely chopped, or use 2 tbsp finely chopped green bell pepper
½ tsp. minced or finely chopped ginger
¼ cup of cilantro for garnish
1 hot or mild green chili
1 tsp. kasoori methi - dried fenugreek leaves or add a ¼ tsp ground mustard
Directions:
Mix together tomatoes, garlic, ginger, chili and blend with water until smooth.
Add the pureed tomato mixture to the Instant Pot or pressure cooker. Put soy curls, chickpeas, spices and salt.
Close and lock the lid in place and ensure that the valve is in sealing position. Press the manual key to cook on high pressure for about 10 minutes.
When the time is up, use a natural pressure release for about 10 minutes. Carefully open the lid once the pressure has been released.
Set the Instant Pot on sauté and put the cashew cream, graham masala, sweetener and fenugreek leaves and mix in. Bring to a boil, taste and adjust salt, heat, sweet.

You may put more cayenne and salt if needed. Fold in the chopped green chili, ginger and cilantro and press cancel on the Instant Pot.
You may also put some vegan butter or oil for additional buttery flavor.
Serve immediately and enjoy!

530. Maple Bourbon Sweet Potato Chili
Preparation time: 10 minutes
Cooking time: 23 minutes
Total time: 33 minutes
Calories: 220 kcal
Servings: 5
Ingredients:
4 cloves garlic, minced
1 tbsp. cooking oil
1 small yellow onion, thinly sliced
2 (14oz. cans kidney beans, drained and rinsed
A few fresh springs of cilantro
4 ½ cups of sweet potatoes, peeled and cut into 1/2" pieces
2 cups vegetable broth
1 ½ tbsp. chili powder
½ tsp. paprika
1/3 tsp. cayenne pepper
1 (15oz. can minced tomatoes
¼ cup of bourbon
2 tbsp. maple syrup
salt and pepper, to taste
2 green onions, minced
3 small corn tortillas, toasted and sliced (optional
2 tsp. cumin
Directions:
Set your Instant Pot to sauté, put oil, and let it heat up for 40 seconds.
Add the onions and heat up for about 5 minutes, stir it periodically, until onions are fragrant. Add the garlic and heat for another 40 seconds.
Add the shredded sweet potatoes, chili powder, cumin, and Paprika, and cayenne pepper, stir until vegetables are well coated.
Add the vegetable broth, beans, tomatoes, maple syrup, and bourbon. Close and lock the lid in place and ensure that the valve is in sealing position.
Press the manual setting to cook on high pressure for about 15 minutes. When the time is up, use a natural pressure release for about 12 minutes.
Carefully open the lid and check to make sure the sweet potatoes are tender.
If you are making use of tortillas, lightly oil a cast iron skillet and pan sauté the tortillas on each side for 3 minutes.
Carefully remove from heat and let cool before shredding into thin strips. Add your desired optional toppings: cilantro, green onions, and toasted tortillas.
Serve and enjoy!

531. Walnut Lentil Tacos
Preparation time: 5 minutes
Cooking time: 10 minutes
Total time: 15 minutes
Servings: 11-12 tacos
Ingredients:
½ tsp. garlic powder
1 white onion, diced
1 ½ tbsp. olive oil
1 cup of dried brown lentils
2 garlic clove, minced
1 tbsp. chili powder
¼ tsp. onion powder
1/3 tsp. red pepper flakes
1 ½ tsp. ground cumin
½ tsp. kosher salt
1/3 tsp. freshly ground pepper
2 ½ cups of vegetable broth
1/2 tsp. paprika
1 14 oz. can fire-roasted diced tomatoes
¾ cup of chopped walnuts
1/3 tsp. oregano
Taco toppings of choice: shredded lettuce, tomato, jalapenos, flour or corn tortillas
Directions:
Switch the Instant Pot on and press the Sauté button.
Add the olive oil, onion and garlic clove and sauté until onion cooked through and stir occasionally for about 4 minutes.
Add the spices and stir together. Press cancel and put the vegetable broth, tomatoes, walnuts and lentils and stir to mix well.
Close and lock the lid in place and ensure that the valve is in sealing position.
Press the manual button to cook on high pressure for about 10 minutes.
When the time is up, use a natural pressure release for about 4 minutes.
Carefully open the lid and stir lentils, seasoning to taste if needed. Add your desired topping.
Serve immediately and enjoy!

532. Cilantro Lime Quinoa
Preparation time: 6 minutes
Cooking time: 10 minutes
Total time: 16 minutes
Calories: 97 kcal
Servings: 5
Ingredients:
2 tbsp. lime juice
1 cup of quinoa rinsed and drained (any color
salt to taste
zest of one lime
½ cup of chopped cilantro
1 ¼ cups of vegetable broth
Directions:
Add the quinoa and 1 ¼ cup vegetable broth to the Instant Pot.
Close and lock the lid in place and ensure that the valve is in sealing position.
Press the manual key to cook on high pressure for about 5 minutes.
When the time is up, use a natural pressure release for about 7 minutes.
Carefully open the lid and pour the lime juice, lime zest, and cilantro. Taste and add salt to taste.
Serve and enjoy!

533. Black Bean Chili
Preparation time: 10 minutes

Cook time: 5 minutes
Total time: 15 minutes
Ingredients:
2 tsp. of olive oil
1 medium yellow onion, diced (about 2 cups
1 red, yellow, or orange bell pepper, diced
1 tsp. of dried oregano
2 medium cloves garlic, minced
2 tbsp. of chili powder
2 tsp. of ground cumin
2 (15 oz.cans or 3 cups of cooked black beans, drained
1 (15 oz.can crushed tomatoes
1 medium jalapeno pepper, seeded and minced
1 tsp. of kosher salt
1 cup of water
Topping ideas: Cashew sour cream, Diced avocado, Cilantro, Diced red onion
Directions:
Set the Instant Pot to "Sauté" function and add the olive oil.
When hot, add the onions, bell pepper, and oregano. Cook, stirring frequently for about 7 minutes or until tender.
Add the garlic, chili powder, and cumin and sauté, stirring constantly, for 1 minute. Add the beans, tomatoes, jalapeño, salt, and water.
Give everything a good stir to combine. Secure the lid in place and ensure that the valve is in sealing position.
Select Manual, High Pressure for 5 minutes. When the timer beeps, do a quick pressure release.
Carefully open the lid and scoop into individual plates.
Serve with your desired topping and enjoy!

534. Vegan Lentil Chili
Preparation time: 10 minutes
Cooking time: 22 minutes
Total time: 32 minutes
Servings: 5
Ingredients:
1 tsp. dried oregano
1 onion, chopped
4 cloves minced garlic
2 carrots, chopped
2 jalapeños, chopped
1 ½ tbsp. chili powder
½ tsp. ground coriander
½ tsp. salt
½ cup of chopped fresh cilantro
1 14 oz. can crushed tomatoes
1 30 oz. can fire roasted diced tomatoes
1 tbsp. olive oil
2 cups of brown or green lentils.
4 ½ cups of vegetable broth
1 tsp. fresh lime juice
1 tbsp. of cumin
Directions:
Add the olive oil in the Instant Pot, hit the sauté button on the Instant Pot and heat the oil for sometimes.
Add the onion, garlic, carrots and jalapeños and heat until soft, about 4 minutes. Put the spices and remaining ingredients except for lime juice and cilantro.
Close and lock the lid in place and ensure that the valve is in sealing position. Press the manual function to cook on high pressure for about 15 minutes.
When the time is up, use a natural pressure release for about 10 minutes. Carefully open the lid once the pressure has been released. Pour lime juice and cilantro.
Serve immediately and enjoy!

535. Spaghetti Squash
Preparation time: 10 minutes
Cook time: 15 minutes
Total time: 25 minutes
Ingredients:
1 whole spaghetti squash
1 cup of water
Directions:
Pour 1 cup water into the bottom of your Instant Pot. Add the trivet and place the squash. Secure the lid in place and ensure that the valve is in sealing position. Select Manual, High Pressure for 15 minutes. When the timer beeps, do a quick pressure release.
Carefully open the lid and check for doneness of squash. Cook for a couple of minutes if middle isn't cooked through. Peel shell, remove seeds, and shred squash.
Serve and enjoy!

536. Mushroom Risotto
Preparation time: 12 minutes
Cooking time: 20 minutes
Total time: 32 minutes
Calories: 370 kcal
Servings: 5
Ingredients:
1 ½ tbsp. olive oil
2 ½ tbsp. vegan butter, divided
1 medium onion, diced
4 cloves garlic, minced
10 oz. cremini mushrooms dry brushed & minced
¾ tsp. dried thyme
1 ½ cups of Arborio rice
½ cup of dry white wine
4 cups of vegetable broth, low sodium
1 ¼ tsp. sea salt, more to taste
Fresh ground pepper to taste
1 cup of frozen peas, thawed
4 tbsp. Vegan Parmesan Cheese (optional
Directions:
Switch on the Sauté mode of your Instant Pot and put the oil and butter. Heat the oil; put the onions and sauté about 3 minutes.
Add the garlic and thyme and sauté for a minute. You can now put the mushrooms and sauté for about 4 minutes until soft.
Add the rice and stir to coat well. Pour the wine and cook until the liquid mostly cooks down. About 2 minutes. Add the broth, salt, and pepper.
Close and lock the lid in place and ensure that the valve is in sealing position. Press the manual setting to cook on high pressure for about 6 minutes.

When the time is up, use a natural pressure release for about 6 minutes. The risotto will look soupy when you first remove the lid.
Just stir for sometimes and it will thicken up. Add the peas, butter, and vegan parmesan. If you need some seasoning, you may add it.
Top with fresh-cut parsley, crushed red pepper flakes, and fresh cracked pepper.
Serve and enjoy!

537. Vegan Potato Curry
Preparation time: 12 minutes
Cooking time: 45 minutes
Total time: 57 minutes
Calories: 270 kcal
Servings: 5
Ingredients:
1 420ml can coconut milk, full fat or light
1 medium yellow onion, chopped
4 large cloves of garlic, chopped finely
950g and about 5 heaping cups baby potatoes
2 tbsp. curry powder or curry paste
500mls and around 2 cups water
3 tbsp. arrowroot powder.
1 tbsp. sugar
Salt and pepper to taste
1 tsp. chili pepper flakes or a small fresh chili chopped
400g and 2 heaping cups fresh green beans, chopped into small sizes
Directions:
Turn your Instant Pot to sauté mode. Once hot, add a few drops of water and cook the onions until soft. Add the garlic and cook for one minute. Press the keep warm/cancel button. Add everything else to the Instant Pot except the green beans and arrowroot. Close and lock the lid in place and ensure that the valve is in sealing position. Press the manual key to cook on High Pressure for about 20 minutes.
When the time is up, use a natural pressure release for about 16 minutes. Add the arrowroot into a small bowl and pour a few tablespoons of water to make it thick.
Pour it into the Instant Pot stirring continuously. Add salt and pepper to taste then add the green beans. Cook for about 5 minutes until they are soft and the gravy has thickened.
Serve immediately and enjoy!

538. Mashed Potatoes with Fried Onions and Bacon
Preparation time: 5 minutes
Cook time: 25 minutes
Total time: 30 minutes
Ingredients:
2 ½ lb. Yukon potatoes, small
Enough water to cover
2 tbsp. of olive oil
4 garlic cloves
1 cup of plant milk, (We like soy
1 ½ tsp. of salt
¼ cup of nutritional yeast
1 cup of canned fried onions (We like the ones from Trader Joe's

½ package, veggie bacon, diced (about ½ cup - 1 cup
Directions:
Wash the potatoes and add them into the bowl of your Instant Pot. Add about 3 cups of water enough to cover.
Secure the lid in place and ensure that the valve is in sealing position. Select Manual, High Pressure for 8 minutes.
When the timer beeps, do a natural pressure release for about 10 minutes, then quick release any remaining pressure.
Carefully open the lid and drain the potatoes. Turn the Instant Pot to sauté and add the olive oil. Add the bacon and garlic and sauté.
Add the 1 cup of milk, salt, and stir. Add the potatoes and mash them with a wooden spoon. Add the fried onions and give everything a good stir to mix.
Serve and enjoy!

539. Vegan Alfredo Sauce
Preparation time: 10 minutes
Cook time: 3 minutes
Total time: 13 minutes
Servings: 6
Calories: 110 kcal
Ingredients:
2 tbsp. of olive oil
8 cloves garlic, minced
6 cups of cauliflower florets (fresh or frozen
¾ cup of raw cashews
3 cups of vegetable broth
½ - 1 tsp. of salt, to taste
1 lb. (16 ouncescooked fettuccine pasta (whole grain or gluten free if desired
Optional: steamed broccoli, kale or green peas
Directions:
Turn the Instant Pot to Sauté button and add the olive oil.
Add the minced garlic and sauté for about 1 to 2 minutes or until fragrant. Press the Cancel function. Add the cauliflower, cashews and vegetable broth. Secure the lid in place and ensure that the valve is in sealing position.
Select Manual, High Pressure for 3 minutes. When the timer beeps, do a natural pressure release. Carefully open the lid and transfer to a blender. Add salt and blend until smooth. Pour over pasta and give everything a good stir.
Add a few tablespoons of water if the sauce is too thick until the desired consistency is achieved.
Serve with steamed broccoli, kale or peas if desired.

540. Carrot Ginger Soup
Preparation time: 15 minutes
Cooking time: 17 minutes
Total time: 32 minutes
Calories: 270 kcal
Servings: 5
Ingredients:
2 tbsp. grape seed oil or preferred oil
1 medium onion, diced
4 cloves garlic , minced
tbsp. fresh ginger, grated
1 tsp. dried thyme

½ tsp. ground coriander
½ tsp. crushed red pepper
2 bay leaves
2 lb. carrots (about 6 large, rough chopped
4 cups of vegetable broth, low sodium
1 tsp. sea salt, more to taste
Fresh cracked pepper to taste (optional
1 cup of canned coconut milk , full-fat
2 tbsp. lime juice (sub lemon

Directions:

Switch on the sauté mode of your Instant Pot and add the oil.

When the oil has heated, add the onions and sauté for about 3 minutes. Add the garlic and ginger, sauté for 2 minutes.

Add the thyme, coriander and crushed red pepper. Sauté for 50 seconds. Cancel the sauté function and put the broth, carrots, bay leaves, salt, and cracked pepper.

Close and lock the lid in place and ensure that the valve is in sealing position. Press the manual button to cook on high pressure for about 6 minutes.

When the time is up, use a natural pressure release for about 3 minutes. Set the steam release handle to the venting position.

Carefully open the lid and remove the bay leaves and put the coconut milk and lime juice. Using a regular blender, blend until smooth.

Taste for seasoning and put more if you desire. If for any reason, the soup is too thick for your taste, you can add a small amount of vegetable broth to thin it out.

Serve immediately and enjoy!

GRAINS & BEANS

541. Chicken & Wild Rice Soup
Cooking Time: 56 minutes
Servings: 4
Ingredients:
1 lb. chicken breasts, skinless, boneless, cut in half
4 carrots, peeled, chopped
2 egg yolks
4 cups chicken broth, divided
1 bay leaf
1 cup water
1 large zucchini, chopped
¾ cup wild rice-brown rice blend
½ teaspoon thyme, dried
1 tablespoon butter
2 tablespoons garlic-infused olive oil
1 small leek, green parts, sliced
3 tablespoons lemon juice
Sea salt and black pepper to taste
Parmesan cheese, grated for garnish
Italian parsley, fresh, chopped for garnish
Directions:
Set your instant pot to the sauté mode, add the oil and heat it. Sauté the leek, in oil, seasoned with salt and pepper for 6-minutes. Place the chicken breasts on a cutting board to rest for a few minutes
Shred the chicken and add to the instant pot and brown meat on all sides for 5-minutes. Transfer chicken and leek to a bowl. Whisk the egg yolks, and pour in ½ a cup of chicken broth, whisking to temper the yolks. Add the yolk mixture to the instant pot along with the rest of the ingredients and stir. Return the shredded chicken and leeks to the instant pot and secure the lid. Set on Manual setting on high with a cook time of 45-minutes. Divide among serving bowls, and garnish with grated parmesan and fresh, chopped Italian parsley. Serve hot!
Nutrition Values:
Calories: 227Fat: 1gFiber: 2gCarbs: 24gProtein: 16g

542. Quinoa Beef Pot
Cooking Time: 20 minutes
Servings: 1
Ingredients:
2 tablespoons of any quinoa, rinsed
2 tablespoons cheddar cheese, diced
2 tablespoons baby spinach, fresh, chopped
2 tablespoons beef, shredded. cooked
1 tablespoon ghee, melted
Grated peel of ½ a lime and a dash of its juice
1 fluid ounce of water
Sea salt and black pepper to taste
Directions:
Before cooking, rinse the quinoa under running water, until it is clear. Pour the quinoa, salt, water, and lime zest into the instant pot. Close the instant pot lid, and press the Manual button, and set it for 1-minute of pressure cooking. When the cooking is done, release the pressure naturally for 10-minutes. Add some lime juice, ghee, shredded beef, pepper, cheese, spinach and mix. You can serve it at room temperature or you may decide to serve it at room temperature or place it in the fridge to cool before serving.
Nutrition Values:
Calories: 636Fat: 61gCarbs: 9gProtein: 14g

543. Keto Clam Chowder
Cooking Time: 20 minutes
Servings: 2
Ingredients:
4 tablespoons of clams
The juice contained from the clam jar in addition to water
2 tablespoons bacon, diced
4 tablespoons heavy cream
2 tablespoons of flour
2 tablespoons ghee
2 tablespoons butter
4 tablespoons sour cream
1 pinch of cayenne pepper, crushed
1 pinch of thyme, dried
1 bay leaf
4 tablespoons white wine
4 tablespoons onion, finely chopped
Directions:
Set your instant pot to the sauté mode, add the ghee and heat it. Add the bacon, without the lid. When the bacon begins to release fat and starts to sizzle, add the salt, pepper, onion, and cook for 5-minutes and stir. Add the wine into the instant pot once the onion has dried and stir. Allow the wine to evaporate almost completely, add the thyme, bay leaf, and cayenne pepper.
Close the lid on the instant pot and set to Manual on high for a 5-minute cook time. Release the pressure naturally for 10-minutes. Prepare the roux that will thicken the clam chowder in a pan over a low flame. Mix in the flour with butter, stirring constantly with a wooden spoon until it thickens. Add the roux, heavy cream, sour cream, add drain the clams and set them in a bowl. Set the instant pot on sauté mode and cook the ingredients for 5-minutes, stirring constantly. Then add the clams back in and stir well. Divide into serving bowls. Serve warm!
Nutrition Values:
Calories: 580Fat: 47gCarbs: 12gProtein: 25g

544. Stuffed Cuttlefish
Cooking Time: 20 minutes
Servings: 3
Ingredients:
3 small cuttlefish, cleaned
2 tablespoons of shallot, chopped
1 tablespoon of tomato sauce
2 tablespoons of olive oil
1 pinch of parsley, dried
2 tablespoons of flour
2 bay leaves
2 tablespoons water
For the Dip:
1 tablespoon anise seeds
1 pinch of chili powder
2 tablespoons of mayonnaise
Directions:

Add all the ingredients in a mixer, except the sauce, bay leaves, water, and cuttlefish. Make the mixture homogenous. Take the cuttlefish and fill with the mixture. Put the sauce on the bottom of the instant pot, add some salt, bay leaves. Add the cuttlefish and water. Close the lid to instant pot, set to the Manual setting for 10-minutes cook time. In the meantime, prepare the dip by combining the ingredients in a small bowl. Release the pressure use the quick-release. Divide among serving plates, drizzle the sauce over fish and serve with dip. Serve warm!
Nutrition Values:
Calories: 590Fat: 47.92 gCarbs: 10gProtein: 27g

545. Saffron Chicken
Cooking Time: 14 minutes
Servings: 2
Ingredients:
1 lb. chicken, skinless, boneless, cut into small strips
3 tablespoons olive oil
2 tablespoons flour
1 teaspoon saffron
1 pinch of sea salt
1 teaspoon rosemary needles
2 tablespoons of cocoa butter
2 tablespoons of white onion, diced
4 tablespoons water
2 teaspoons of triple tomato concentrate
Directions:
Cover the chicken strips with the flour. Set your instant pot to the sauté mode, add the oil to pot and heat it. Brown the chicken strips on all sides for 5-minutes. Add water, salt and saffron and stir. Close the lid and set to Manual setting on high with a cook time of 14-minutes. Release the pressure naturally for 10-minutes. Remove the chicken from pot, set to sauté mode to reduce the sauce. Smear the cocoa butter over the chicken. Divide among serving plates, and drizzle with sauce. Serve warm!
Nutrition Values:
Calories: 713Fat: 63gCarbs: 9gProtein: 36g

546. Sesame Meatball Stew
Cooking Time: 30 minutes
Servings: 2
Ingredients:
For the Meatballs:
1 tablespoon cheddar cheese, grated
2 tablespoons of zucchini, grated
1 small egg
1 pinch of fresh basil, chopped
2 tablespoons olive oil
1 tablespoon of sesame seeds
4 tablespoons flour
4 tablespoons mozzarella cheese
Dash of salt
1 tablespoon parsley, dried
For the Stew:
1 clove of garlic, minced
4 tablespoons tomato sauce
½ small onion, finely chopped
Directions:
Grate the zucchini, and add a little salt in a bowl, and flour, mix. Add the egg and grated cheddar cheese and mix well. Cut the mozzarella into cubes. Take a little of the zucchini dough and form a meatball, add three cubes of mozzarella into the middle. Add the sesame seeds, parsley in a small bowl. Roll the zucchini meatball in the sesame seeds.
Prepare a baking sheet with baking paper and place the meatballs on top of it. Sprinkle the meatballs with olive oil and bake at 400° Fahrenheit for 20-minutes. Pour the tomato sauce, garlic, and onion into your instant pot. Add the meatballs and stir. Set to the Meat/Stew setting for 10-minutes. Release the pressure naturally for 10-minutes. Divide among serving plates, drizzle with sauce. Serve warm!
Nutrition Values:
Calories: 696Fat: 140gCarbs: 15gProtein: 18g

547. Burrito with Chili Colorado
Cooking Time: 40 minutes
Servings: 2
Ingredients:
4 tablespoons of scaled cheese
1 cup of water
4 teaspoons meat broth
4 tablespoons of enchilada sauce
1 cup roasted beef chops, boneless, cubed
For the Tortillas:
2 tablespoons of ghee
1 pinch of baking powder
4 tablespoons of water
4 tablespoons of coconut flour
1 egg white
Directions:
First to prepare your tortillas: Add the egg whites, coconut flour, baking powder, ghee, and water in a mixing bowl. Mix well. Heat a skillet (the size that you want your tortillas to beon low heat. Wait until the skillet is hot, spray it with cooking spray, and drop some of the mix into the center. Tilt the skillet to spread the batter as thin as possible. Allow it to cook for a few minutes, until it starts to rise/bubble then flip it over to the other side. Flip and cook for an additional minute. Repeat the process until you have used up all the batter.
Prepare the stuffing: In your instant pot add the beef, half of the enchilada sauce, broth, and water, stir. Press the Manual setting and set for a cook time of 30-minutes. Release the pressure naturally for 10-minutes. Place the tortillas on an aluminum coated baking pan adding some beef to center of tortilla, fold the ends upwards and roll into a burrito. Repeat with other tortillas, sprinkle tops with the remaining enchilada sauce, and cheese shavings. Grill until cheese bubbles for about 4-minutes.
Nutrition Values:
Calories: 502Fat: 67g Carbs: 8.96gProtein: 33.82g

548. Sour Dumplings
Cooking Time: 45 minutes
Servings: 4
Ingredients:
½ cup sour cream
1 cup broth

4 tablespoons coconut oil
4 tablespoons tomato paste
Salt and black pepper to taste
4 tablespoons of coconut flour
2 cloves of garlic, minced
1 small onion, minced
2 eggs
2 strips of bacon, minced
1 lb. ground pork
Directions:
In a mixing bowl mix the bacon, egg, onion, flour, seasonings, and garlic. Shape into small balls and place on a flat surface. Set your instant pot to the sauté mode, add the coconut oil and heat it. Place the meatballs into the pot, evenly spaced. Cook for 5-minutes, browning all sides of meatballs. Once they are browned remove them and set them on a plate. Add broth to pot, add meatballs back into pot. Close the lid and set pot on Manual setting for 7-minutes. After cook time is complete, release the pressure using the quick-release. Remove the meatballs from pot. Set instant pot back on to sauté mode. Add the sour cream, salt and pepper and stir the pots contents. Allow the to heat for 2-minutes. Add the meatballs back into the sauce and stir. Remove meatballs and sauce and place in bowls. Serve warm.
Nutrition Values:
Calories: 608Fat: 45gCarbs: 12g Protein: 41g

549. Sausage Radish Cakes
Cooking Time: 42 minutes
Servings: 2
Ingredients:
½ cup Chinese radish, peeled and chopped, cooked
1 teaspoon ginger, chopped
2 tablespoons of olive oil
½ cup of sausage, drained, minced
4 tablespoons coconut flour
1 cup water
1 cup chicken broth
2 tablespoons spring onions, chopped
Pinch of salt
Directions:
Set your instant pot to the sauté mode, add the oil and heat it. Add the ginger, spring onions, and chopped sausage and cook for 5-minutes stirring often. Add the chopped Chinese radishes, and brown for 2-minutes. In a bowl mix the flour and water. Add mixture from instant pot into mixing bowl with flour and water. Add mix into a small oven-dish. Add trivet to instant pot, add the water. Place the oven-dish onto the trivet, set instant pot to Steam for 35-minutes. Release the pressure naturally for 10-minutes. Remove the steamed radish cake from instant pot. Allow for it to cool and refrigerate for a few hours. Serve room temperature.
Nutrition Values:
Calories: 692Fat: 60gCarbs: 10g Protein: 26g

550. Seafood Jambalaya
Cooking Time: 45 minutes
Servings: 4
Ingredients:
4-ounces cod, chopped
4-ounces shrimp, peeled, deveined
1 cup brown rice, cooked
1 cup chicken broth
½ teaspoon cumin, ground
1 tablespoon parsley, chopped
Sea salt and black pepper to taste
1 lb. Roma tomatoes, peeled, crushed
1 cup Russet potatoes, chopped
¼ cup yellow onion, diced
½ teaspoon cayenne pepper
2 teaspoons paprika, ground
¼ cup carrots, chopped
6 ½-ounces of crab meat
Directions:
Combine all ingredients in your instant pot, and cook on Meat/Stew setting for 45-minutes. Divide into serving bowls, garnish with fresh chopped parsley. Serve hot!
Nutrition Values:
Calories: 137Fat: 2gCarbs: 13gProtein: 20g

551. Shredded Pork Fajitas
Cooking Time: 40 minutes
Servings: 4
Ingredients:
1lb. stewing pork, chopped
8 whole-wheat fajitas
½ small onion, sliced
1 green pepper, diced
1 jalapeno, minced
1 tablespoon olive oil
½ teaspoon cumin, ground
Sea salt and black pepper to taste
2 cloves garlic, minced
Directions:
Combine all the ingredients in your instant pot, except the fajitas. Cook on Manual setting for 40-minutes on high. Release the pressure naturally for 10-minutes. Remove the pork to a cutting board and shred it with two forks, then add back to the instant pot and stir. Place fajitas on serving plates and top with pork mix from instant pot and roll up. Serve warm!
Nutrition Values:
Calories: 238Fat: 17gCarbs: 18gProtein: 21g

552. Sausage Gumbo
Cooking Time: 35 minutes
Servings: 6
Ingredients:
8-ounces, Andouille sausage, whole
4 cups pork stock
1 cup of brown rice, cooked
1 tablespoon thyme, fresh, chopped
½ teaspoon ginger, ground
½ teaspoon cumin, ground
½ teaspoon cayenne pepper, ground
1 teaspoon paprika, ground
Sea salt and black pepper to taste
2 cups Roma tomatoes, peeled and diced
¼ cup yellow onion, sliced
Directions:

Combine all the ingredients in your instant pot, except the brown rice. Cook on Manual setting on high for a cook time of 35-minutes. Release the pressure naturally for 10-minutes. Add in the cooked brown rice and mix well. Spoon into serving bowls, topped with fresh chopped thyme for garnish. Serve warm!
Nutrition Values:
Calories: 118 Fat: 4g Carbs: 13g Protein: 10g

553. Pork Fried Whole Grain Rice
Cooking Time: 45 minutes
Servings: 4
Ingredients:
1lb. stewing pork, diced
1 tablespoon green onion, chopped
2 eggs, scrambled
½ teaspoon ginger, ground
½ teaspoon cumin, ground
1 clove garlic, minced
1 teaspoon rice vinegar
2 cups whole grain rice, cooked
¼ cup green beans, diced
¼ cup carrots, diced
¼ cup yellow onion, diced
Directions:
Add all the ingredients to your instant pot, except for eggs and green onion. Cook on Manual setting for 45-minutes. Release the pressure naturally for 10-minutes. Stir in the scrambled eggs and green onions. Divide among serving dishes. Serve warm!
Nutrition Values:
Calories: 218 Fat: 16g Carbs: 24g Protein: 21g

554. Bacon Wrapped Jalapenos
Cooking Time: 32 minutes
Servings: 4
Ingredients:
12 large jalapenos
6 slices of bacon
½ teaspoon salt
½ tablespoon olive oil
½ red bell pepper, diced
½ cup brown rice, cooked
Directions:
Slice the tops off the jalapenos, then take a spoon to remove and scoop out the seeds. Set the hollowed jalapenos aside. In a mixing bowl, combine the cooked brown rice, olive oil, bell pepper, and salt. Stuff the mixture into each jalapeno. Slice each piece of bacon in half longways, and wrap one slice around each jalapeno, use toothpick to hold in place. Place the wrapped jalapenos gently inside your instant pot. Cook on Manual setting for 32-minutes. Release the pressure naturally for 15-minutes. Divide among serving plates. Serve warm!
Nutrition Values:
Calories: 187 Fat: 18g Carbs: 12g Protein: 14g

555. Shredded Beef Tacos
Cooking Time: 35 minutes
Servings: 2
Ingredients:
6-ounces beef tenderloin, chopped
4 taco shells
1 jalapeno, diced
½ red bell pepper, sliced
1 tsp. red wine vinegar
½ tsp. cumin, ground
2 cloves garlic, minced
Salt and black pepper to taste
Directions:
Combine all your ingredients in your instant pot, except for the taco shells. Set your instant pot to the Manual setting on a high cook time of 35-minutes. Once the cook time is completed, release the pressure naturally for 10-minutes. Shred the beef with a pair of forks. Scoop the mixture into the taco shells and serve warm.
Nutrition Values:
Calories: 299 Fat: 21g Carbs: 13g Protein: 22g

556. Beef Stuffed Eggplant
Cooking Time: 35 minutes
Servings: 4
Ingredients:
1 tablespoon olive oil
¼ cup yellow onion, diced
½ cup brown rice
½ tablespoon mint, fresh, chopped
1 tablespoon basil, fresh, chopped
Sea salt and black pepper to taste
8-ounces lean ground beef, browned
1 eggplant, cut in half vertically and horizontally (4-pieces
Directions:
Scoop out the insides of the eggplant using a spoon. Leave each piece with a ½-inch thick wall. Dice the removed fruit. Combine the diced eggplant with the remaining ingredients (except the olive oil in a mixing bowl. Fill each eggplant slice with the mixture. Place the stuffed eggplants into your instant pot, and drizzle with olive oil over each piece. Set to Manual setting for a cook time of 35-minutes. When cooking is completed, release the pressure naturally for 10-minutes. Divide among serving plates. Serve warm!
Nutrition Values:
Calories: 284 Fat: 12g Carbs: 26g Protein: 22g

557. Spicy Fire Chicken with Rice
Cooking Time: 45 minutes
Servings: 2
Ingredients:
8-ounces chicken breasts, skinless, boneless, chopped
1 red chili, diced
1 teaspoon crushed red pepper
½ teaspoon paprika, ground
Salt and black pepper to taste
½ tablespoon olive oil
2 cups brown rice, cooked
Directions:
Combine all your ingredients in your instant pot except for the rice. Stir and set to Meat/Stew setting for 45-minutes. When the cooking is completed, release the pressure naturally for 15-minutes. Serve on top of a bed of rice the spicy fire chicken. Serve warm.
2. Nutrition Values:

Calories: 288Fat: 7.5gCarbs: 13gProtein: 40g

558. Spiced Apple & Walnut Chicken
Cooking Time: 40 minutes
Servings: 2
Ingredients:
8-ounces chicken breast, skinless, boneless, chopped
¼ cup walnuts, chopped
½ teaspoon nutmeg, ground
½ teaspoon ginger, ground
1 small apple, peeled and diced
1 tablespoon ghee
Salt and black pepper to taste
2 cups brown rice, cooked
Directions:
Set your instant pot to the sauté mode, and add the ghee and heat it. Add the chicken to instant pot and cook for 5-minutes, browning all sides of meat. Add the remaining ingredients to pot, except cooked brown rice. Set the setting to Manual for a cook time of 35-minutes. When the cook time has completed, release the pressure naturally for 10-minutes. Serve on a bed of brown rice. Serve warm!
Nutrition Values:
Calories: 296Fat: 8gCarbs: 18g bProtein: 49g

559. Pulled Chicken in Soft Whole Wheat Tacos
Cooking Time: 38 minutes
Servings: 6
Ingredients:
1 lb. chicken breast, skinless, boneless, cubed
½ cup chicken broth
2 tablespoons cilantro, chopped, fresh
½ teaspoon cayenne pepper, ground
Salt and black pepper to taste
½ teaspoon cumin
2 Roma tomatoes, peeled, diced
¼ red onion, diced
½ green bell pepper, sliced
½ red bell pepper, sliced
¼ yellow onion, diced
½ teaspoon mustard powder, ground
1 tablespoon coconut oil
Directions:
Set your instant pot to the sauté mode, add the coconut oil and heat it up. Add the chicken and cook for 5-minutes, stir. Add bell peppers, onion and cook for an additional 3-minutes. Add the remaining ingredients to instant pot, except the soft tacos. Secure the lid of instant pot in place, and set to Manual setting for 30-minutes on high cook time. When the cook time is complete, release the pressure naturally for 10-minutes. Spoon the chicken mix on top of soft tacos. Serve warm!
Nutrition Values:
Calories: 158Fat: 3.5g Carbs: 17gProtein: 25g

560. Pesto Chicken & Whole Wheat Pasta
Cooking Time: 35 minutes
Servings: 2
Ingredients:
2 cups whole wheat pasta, cooked
2 chicken breasts, skinless, boneless
2 tablespoons pesto sauce
2 cloves garlic, minced
Sal and black pepper to taste
½ cup of parsley, fresh, chopped for garnish
Directions:
Mix the seasonings together, then run them into each chicken breast. Place the chicken breasts inside instant pot, add a tablespoon of pesto on top of each piece of chicken. Set to Manual setting on high cook time of 35-minutes. When the cooking is completed, release the pressure naturally for 10-minutes. Serve on top of a bed of whole wheat pasta. Garnish with fresh chopped pasta. Serve warm!
Nutrition Values:
Calories: 258Fat: 6gCarbs: 10gProtein: 44g

561. Pasta & Brown Turkey Sauce
Cooking Time: 35 minutes
Servings: 4
Ingredients:
1 cup cooked turkey, shredded
¼ cup cashew cream
½ cup baby portabella mushrooms, chopped
¼ cup carrots, chopped
¼ cup yellow onion, diced
1 clove garlic, minced
2 cups whole wheat pasta, cooked
1 teaspoon rosemary, fresh, chopped
Directions:
Combine all the ingredients, except for the pasta in your instant pot. Set to manual setting on a low cook time of 35-minutes. Once the cook time is completed, release the pressure naturally for 10-minutes. Serve over a bed of whole wheat pasta, and garnish with fresh, chopped rosemary. Serve warm!
Nutrition Values:
Calories: 218Fat: 7gCarbs: 12gProtein: 34g

562. Orange Chicken Drumsticks & Rice
Cooking Time: 40 minutes
Servings: 4
Ingredients:
1 lb. of chicken drumsticks
1 tablespoon olive oil
½ tablespoon basil, fresh, chopped
½ tablespoon parsley, fresh, chopped
1 orange, thin round slices
1 teaspoon rosemary, fresh, chopped for garnish
1 clove garlic, minced
Salt and black pepper to taste
2 cups brown rice
Directions:
Toss the drumsticks, seasonings (except rosemary, and oil and coat drumsticks in mix. Place the drumsticks into your instant pot, and evenly distribute the orange slices evenly around them. Cook on Manual setting on high for a cook time of 40-minutes. Serve on a bed of rice, and garnish with fresh, chopped rosemary. Serve warm!
Nutrition Values:
Calories: 256Fat: 1gCarbs: 9gProtein: 38g

563. Mediterranean Mint & Basil Chicken & Rice

Cooking Time: 40 minutes
Servings: 2
Ingredients:
2 chicken breasts, skinless, boneless, cubed
2 teaspoons mint, fresh, chopped for garnish
1 cup arugula, fresh, chopped
½ red bell pepper, sliced
1 tablespoon basil, chopped
½ yellow onion, diced
Salt and black pepper to taste
2 cups brown rice, cooked
Directions:
Add all your ingredients into your instant pot, except for the arugula and rice. Cook on Manual setting on a high cook time of 40-minutes. When the cook time is completed, release the pressure naturally for 10-minutes. Add the arugula to pot and stir in with chicken mixture. Serve on top of a bed of rice, add fresh, chopped mint as garnish. Serve warm!
Nutrition Values:
Calories: 211Fat: 5gCarbs: 12gProtein: 43g

564. Mango Citrus Chicken & Rice

Cooking Time: 40 minutes
Servings: 2
Ingredients:
2 chicken breasts, skinless, boneless, chopped
1 cup long-grain rice
1 cup mango, fresh, chopped
1 tablespoon orange juice, fresh squeezed
1 clove garlic, minced
½ teaspoon crushed red pepper
Salt and black pepper to taste
1 tablespoon olive oil
1 cup arugula, fresh
¼ cup yellow onion, diced
2 teaspoons mint, fresh, chopped for garnish
Directions:
Combine all the ingredients, except for mango and rice in your instant pot. Set to Manual setting for a high cook time of 40-minutes. When the cook time is completed, release the pressure naturally for 15-minutes. Gently stir in the mango to the instant pot. Serve over a bed of rice, garnish with fresh, chopped mint. Serve warm!
Nutrition Values:
Calories: 295Fat: 12gCarbs: 26gProtein: 40g

565. Lemon, Capers, Chicken & Chinese Black Rice

Cooking Time: 35 minutes
Servings: 2
Ingredients:
2 chicken breasts, boneless, skinless
4 thin slices lemon
1 sprig of rosemary
1 tablespoon capers
2 garlic cloves, minced
½ tablespoon olive oil
2 cups Chinese black rice, cooked
Salt and black pepper to taste
Directions:
Coat the chicken breasts evenly with salt, pepper, and olive oil. Place the chicken breasts into your instant pot, sprinkle with minced garlic, and capers. Lay a sprig of rosemary in the middle of instant pot, and place two lemon slices on each chicken breast. Cook on Manual setting for a high cook time of 35-minutes. When the cook time is completed, release the pressure naturally for 10-minutes. Serve over a bed of Chinese black rice. Serve warm!
Nutrition Values:
Calories: 278 Fat: 8gCarbs: 12gProtein: 39g

566. Jerk Chicken Strips & Wild Rice

Cooking Time: 40 minutes
Servings: 2
Ingredients:
2 chicken breasts, boneless, skinless, cut into slices or strips
2 cups wild rice, cooked
½ tablespoon olive oil
½ tablespoon red wine vinegar
1 small habanero chili, ground into a paste
¼ teaspoon nutmeg, ground
¼ teaspoon ginger, ground
½ teaspoon cumin, ground
½ teaspoon cayenne pepper, ground
Salt and black pepper to taste
2 tablespoons cilantro, fresh, chopped for garnish
Directions:
Combine all the ingredients in your instant pot, except for the wild rice. Set to Manual setting and cook on high for a cook time of 40-minutes. When the cook time is completed, release the pressure naturally for 15-minutes. Serve over a bed of wild rice, and garnish with fresh, chopped cilantro.
Nutrition Values:
Calories: 235Fat: 7.5gCarbs: 9gProtein: 40g

567. Greek Chicken & Sprouted Rice

Cooking Time: 35 minutes
Servings: 2
Ingredients:
2 chicken breasts, boneless, skinless
2 cups sprouted rice, cooked
½ red bell pepper, chopped
2 tablespoons Kalamata olives, chopped
¼ cup artichoke hearts, chopped
1 teaspoon basil, fresh, chopped
1 teaspoon oregano, fresh, chopped
Salt and black pepper to taste
½ tablespoon olive oil
2 teaspoons of parsley, fresh, chopped for garnish
Directions:
Coat the chicken breasts evenly with the olive oil and seasonings. Place them into your instant pot, and pour the remaining ingredients over them, except the sprouted rice. Set the instant pot to the Manual setting on high with a cook time of 35-minutes. When the cook time is completed, release the pressure using the quick-release. Serve alongside the sprouted

rice, and garnish with fresh, chopped parsley. Serve warm!
Nutrition Values:
Calories: 275Fat: 8gCarbs: 18gProtein: 41g

568. Chicken Fried Wild Rice
Cooking Time: 25 minutes
Servings: 4
Ingredients:
2 cups wild rice, cooked
1 cup cooked chicken breast, chopped
1 clove garlic, minced
1 teaspoon rice vinegar
1 tablespoon green onion, chopped
¼ cup scrambled eggs
¼ cup green beans, chopped
½ red bell pepper, diced
¼ cup carrots, diced
Salt and black pepper to taste
2 teaspoons cilantro, fresh chopped for garnish
Directions:
Combine all the ingredients in your instant pot, except for the wild rice. Set the instant pot to Manual on a high cook time of 25-minutes. When the cook time is completed, release the pressure using the quick-release. Add the wild rice into the instant pot and stir to blend. Divide among serving plates, and top with fresh, chopped parsley for garnish. Serve warm!
Nutrition Values:
Calories: 112Fat: 6gCarbs: 22gProtein: 21g

569. Stuffed Bell Peppers
Cooking Time: 40 minutes
Servings: 4
Ingredients:
4 green bell peppers
1 cup of brown rice
¼ cup eggplant, diced
1 tablespoon olive oil
½ tablespoon basil, fresh, chopped
1 teaspoon paprika, ground
1 clove garlic, minced
Salt and black pepper to taste
¼ cup butternut squash, diced
Directions:
Slice the tops off the bell peppers and scoop out the seeds, and discard. Dice the tops that were sliced off. In a bowl combine chopped bell pepper tops with other ingredients. Stuff each bell pepper as much as you can with the filling mixture. Place each bell pepper inside of your instant pot. Pour about ½ an inch of water in bottom of pot. Set to Manual setting for a cook time of 40-minutes. When the cook time is completed, release the pressure naturally for 15-minutes. Divide among serving bowls. Serve warm!
Nutrition Values:
Calories: 71Fat: 1gCarbs: 13gProtein: 4g

570. Chipotle Tacos
Cooking Time: 22 minutes
Servings: 2
Ingredients:
½ cup black beans, cooked
2 tablespoons chili sauce
½ cup water
½ teaspoon salt
½ teaspoon cinnamon powder
¼ cup sweet corn kernels
4 tacos
4 leaves of spinach, finely, chopped
Directions:
Combine all your ingredients into your instant pot, except the tacos. Close the lid and set to Manual setting for 22-minutes. When the cook time is completed, release the pressure naturally for 10-minutes. Fill the tacos with the mixture in instant pot mixture and garnish with some finely chopped spinach. Serve warm!
Nutrition Values:
Calories: 202Fat: 5gCarbs: 8gProtein: 11g

571. Breakfast Burritos
Cooking Time: 24 minutes
Servings: 4
Ingredients:
½ cup lentils
1 teaspoon coconut oil
2 avocados, chopped
Salt and black pepper to taste
¼ cup mushrooms, diced
1 green bell pepper, chopped
¼ cup sundried tomatoes, chopped
2 garlic cloves, minced
½ cup tomato puree
4 whole wheat tortillas
½ cup yellow onions, diced
Directions:
Set your instant pot to the sautė mode, add the onions to instant pot and sautė for 4-minutes. Add the rest of the ingredients, except the tortillas, and set to Manual setting on a cook time of 20-minutes. When the cook time is complete, release the pressure naturally for 10-minutes. Serve the mixture in tortillas. Serve warm!
Nutrition Values:
Calories: 232Fat: 11gCarbs: 14gProtein: 29g

572. Wild Mushroom Rice
Cooking Time: 13 minutes
Servings: 2
Ingredients:
1 cup long grain rice
½ cup vegetable stock
½ cup water
1 teaspoon salt
½ cup Portobello mushrooms, diced
2 onions, finely chopped
1 teaspoon olive oil
Directions:
Set your instant pot to sautė mode, add the oil and heat it. Sautė the mushrooms, and onions for 3-minutes. Add the rice and stir for about 30-seconds. Add remaining ingredients, set instant pot to the rice setting for a cook-time of 10-minutes. Release the pressure naturally for 10-minutes. Serve the rice in a large bowl. Serve warm!
Nutrition Values:
Calories: 163Fat: 6gCarbs: 9gProtein: 11g

573. Spinach Casserole
Cooking Time: 23 minutes
Servings: 4
Ingredients:
1/8 cup whole wheat pastry flour
1 cube vegetable bouillon
4 tablespoons olive oil
1 tablespoon vegetarian gravy (chicken flavor
1 tablespoon nutritional yeast
4 tablespoons barbecue sauce (hickory
1 tablespoon light miso paste
1 lb. firm tofu (crumbled
½ lb. mushrooms, sliced
1 teaspoon paprika
1 cup corn kernels
8 whole black peppercorns
1 bay leaf
1 garlic clove, crushed
1 tablespoon tamari
¾ cup red onion, diced
1 yellow onion, chopped
1 bunch parsley, fresh, chopped
1 celery stalk, chopped
1 cup spinach, chopped
2 cups Wehani rice, cooked
Directions:
Set your instant pot to sauté mode, add the oil and heat it up. Add the mushrooms, garlic, and onions, cook for 3-minutes. Set the instant pot to Manual setting on high with a cook time of 20-minutes. Add the gravy mix, tofu, paprika, yeast, tamari and barbeque sauce and mix well. Release the pressure naturally for 10-minutes. Add in the spinach and cooked rice, and corn, stir well. Divide up into serving bowls. Serve warm!
Nutrition Values:
Calories: 232Fat: 8gCarbs: 14gProtein: 10g

574. Mexican Rice
Cooking Time: 30 minutes
Servings: 6
Ingredients:
2 cups brown basmati rice
1 small jalapeno
3 cloves garlic, minced
Salt and black pepper to taste
2 cups water
½ white onion, chopped
½ cup tomato paste
2 tablespoons olive oil
Directions:
Set the instant pot to the sauté mode, add the oil and heat it. Add the onion, rice, garlic and some salt. Sauté for 4-minutes or until fragrant. Mix the water and tomato paste in a bowl until they are well combined, pour mix into instant pot, throw in whole jalapeno. Set to Manual setting on high cook time of 22-minutes. When the cook time is completed, release the pressure naturally for 15-minutes. Using a fork, fluff the rice then serve hot!
Nutrition Values:
Calories: 253Fat: 1.8gCarbs: 53.7gProtein: 5.9g

575. Rice Pilaf
Cooking Time: 15 minutes
Servings: 4
Ingredients:
2 ½ cups wild rice
2 ½ cups chicken stock
1 cup leftover cooked, meat, chopped
1 tablespoon oyster sauce
Green onions, chopped for garnish
1 tablespoon rice wine
1 tablespoon olive oil
1 lb. white mushrooms, halved
2 carrots, chopped
2 tablespoon soy sauce
3 cups kale, chopped
1 lb. green beans, chopped
Directions:
Rinse the rice with tap water about three times. Drain excess water. Combine the rice with stock in your instant pot, along with rest of ingredients except kale and green onions. Set your pot to manual setting for 15-minutes. When cooking is completed, release the pressure using the quick-release. Gently stir in the chopped kale. Divide among serving bowls, and garnish with chopped green onions. Serve warm!
Nutrition Values:
Calories: 417Fat: 5.6gCarbs: 32gProtein: 24g

576. Red Beans Over Sprouted Brown Rice
Cooking Time: 53 minutes
Servings: 8
Ingredients:
1 lb. dry red kidney beans
1 red bell pepper, diced
1 yellow onion, diced
1 ½ lb. smoked ham, cubed
Salt and black pepper to taste
6 cups water, divided
3 garlic cloves, minced
3 stalks celery, chopped
2 tablespoons olive oil
2 bay leaves
¼ teaspoon cayenne pepper
½ teaspoon thyme, dried
2 cups sprouted brown rice
Directions:
Add two cups of water, and two cups of sprouted brown rice to your instant pot. Set it to the rice setting for 10-minutes. When rice is cooked remove from instant pot and place in large bowl. Clean instant pot. Set the instant pot to the sauté mode, add the oil and heat it. Add the onion, celery, pepper, and cook for 5-minutes. Add the garlic and meat and cook for an additional 3-minutes, stir well.
Rinse the kidney beans and drain. Add all the ingredients into pot, except the cooked rice in bowl. Set the instant pot to Manual setting on high with a cook time of 45-minutes. Release the pressure naturally for 15-minutes. Mash the beans into a creamy gravy and serve over a bed of sprouted rice. Serve warm!
Nutrition Values:
Calories: 369Fat: 11gCarbs: 32gProtein: 27g

577. Israeli Couscous

Cooking Time: 5 minutes
Servings: 10
Ingredients:
1 (16-ounce package of Israeli couscous
2 tablespoons butter
2 ½ cups chicken broth
Salt and black pepper to taste
Directions:
Set your instant pot to the sauté mode, add the butter and heat it. Add the broth and couscous, stir to combine. Close the lid and set to Manual setting on high with a cook time of 5-minutes. When the cook time is completed, release the pressure using quick-release. Fluff the couscous with a fork, season with salt and pepper. Serve as a side dish. Serve warm!
Nutrition Values:
Calories: 201Fat: 2gCarbs: 30gProtein: 9g

578. Wild Rice & Black Beans

Cooking Time: 28 minutes
Servings: 4
Ingredients:
2 cups wild rice
5 cups water
1 cup onion, diced
4 cloves garlic, minced
2 limes
1 teaspoon salt
1 avocado
2 cups dry black beans
Directions:
In your instant pot add the wild rice, onions, garlic, black beans, pour in water and sprinkle with salt. Set to the Manual setting on high for a cook time of 28-minutes. When the cook time is completed, release the pressure using quick-release. Divide into serving bowls, squeeze a lime wedge over bowl, and serve with a couple of avocado slices for garnish. Serve warm!
Nutrition Values:
Calories: 691Fat: 4gCarbs: 36.5gProtein: 28.6g

579. Perfect Brown Rice

Cooking Time: 22 minutes
Servings: 12
Ingredients:
2 cups brown rice
½ teaspoon salt
2 ½ cups of fish broth
Coriander, fresh, chopped for garnish
Directions:
Add the rice to your instant pot and pour the fish broth over it and add salt. Seal the lid of instant pot, and set it to Manual setting on high with a cook time of 22-minutes. When the cook time is completed, release the pressure naturally for 10-minutes. Add rice to a large serving bowl, and garnish with fresh, chopped coriander. Serve warm!
Nutrition Values:
Calories: 245Fat: 2.3gCarbs: 48.5gProtein: 6.8g

580. Lentil & Wild Rice Pilaf

Cooking Time: 14 minutes
Servings: 4
Ingredients:
¼ cup black/wild rice
¼ cup brown rice
½ cup black or green lentils
1 stalk celery, finely chopped
1 cup mushrooms, sliced
½ onion, finely chopped
3 cloves garlic, minced
1 bay leaf
2 cups vegetable broth
¼ teaspoon red pepper flakes
½ teaspoon ground black pepper
1 teaspoon fennel seeds
1 teaspoon coriander, dried
1 teaspoon Italian seasoning blend
Directions:
Combine the rice and lentils in a mixing bowl and allow to soak for 30-minutes. Drain and then rinse thoroughly. Set the instant pot to the sauté mode, add veggies with a bit of water and cook for 5-minutes. Add the rice and lentils, vegetable broth, spices into the instant pot. Close the lid and set to Manual on high for 9-minutes. When the cook time is completed, release the pressure using the quick-release. Stir the pilaf and serve with steamed or fresh veggies. Serve warm!
Nutrition Values:
Calories: 211Fat: 2.6gCarbs: 35.5gProtein: 12g

581. Mung Bean Dahl

Cooking Time: 25 minutes
Servings: 6
Ingredients:
½ cup mung beans, dry
2 teaspoons curry powder
2 cups vegetable stock
½ teaspoon onion powder
¼ teaspoon garlic powder
Salt and black pepper to taste
1 cup spinach, chopped finely
Directions:
Add the stock, curry powder, mung beans, onion and garlic powder into instant pot with some salt. Secure the pot lid in place, and set on Manual setting for a cook time of 25-minutes. When the cook time is completed, release the pressure naturally for 10-minutes. Using a fork, smash about the beans and stir to thicken sauce. Add the spinach and stir allowing it cook within the residual heat. Serve warm!
Nutrition Values:
Calories: 203Fat: 7gFiber: 1gCarbs: 6gProtein: 8g

582. Red Bean & Lentil Chili

Cooking Time: 38 minutes
Servings: 6
Ingredients:
½ cup red beans, dried, soaked in water overnight
½ cup brown lentils, soaked in water overnight
1 teaspoon cumin powder
½ teaspoon coriander powder
1 ½ teaspoons chili powder
1 teaspoon smoked paprika
5 cloves garlic, minced

1 green bell pepper, chopped
1 cup carrot, chopped
½ cup yellow onion, chopped
1 cup frozen corn
¼ cup tomato paste
ounce can of tomatoes, diced
2 tablespoons soy sauce
½ teaspoon cayenne pepper
½ teaspoon allspice
½ teaspoon oregano, dried
1 ½ cups water

Directions:
Soak the beans and lentils in water overnight. When you are ready to cook your chili, rinse and drain the beans and lentils in a fine mesh strainer, then set aside for now. Get all your veggies prepped and measure out all your spices for your chili. Set your instant pot on the sauté mode, and allow it to heat up for 2-minutes. Add the onion, bell pepper, carrot, and garlic and sauté for 5-minutes, stir occasionally. Add in the smoked paprika, coriander powder, chili powder, dried oregano, cumin powder, cayenne, allspice, soy sauce, diced tomatoes, salt, tomato paste, lentils and red beans, stir to combine ingredients. Cook and stir for about a minute then add in the water and stir once more. Secure the lid to pot in place, set it to Manual setting on high with a cook time of 30-minutes. When the cooking is completed, release the pressure using natural release of 15-minutes. Add the corn and stir. Divide among serving bowls, and serve hot!

Nutrition Values:
Calories: 206Fat: 8gFiber: 2gCarbs: 9gProtein: 25g

583. Falafel
Cooking Time: 5 minutes
Servings: 6
Ingredients:
1 cup chickpeas, cooked
1 tablespoon lemon juice
2 teaspoons water
3 tablespoons tahini
4-ounces shallots
1 teaspoon garlic powder
3 garlic cloves
1 teaspoon chili flakes
1 teaspoon paprika
½ cup parsley, chopped
1 tablespoon sesame seeds
½ teaspoon coriander
1 teaspoon cumin
½ teaspoon sea salt
1 teaspoon salt

Directions:
Place the chickpeas, coriander, cumin, parsley, salt, chili flakes, paprika, garlic powder, and water into a blender. Blend the mix until it is a smooth mass. Slice garlic cloves and shallot and add to the chickpea mixture. Continue to blend for another minute. Combine the sea salt and sesame seeds in a mixing bowl, and stir.
Make medium-sized balls with chickpea mixture, and coat them with sesame seed mix. Pour olive oil into instant pot and set it to sauté mode. Allow oil to heat up for a few minutes, then toss in the falafel to cook for a 5-minutes. Once they have formed a crust transfer them to a paper towel to remove the excess oil. Combine the tahini, sliced garlic, and lemon juice together and whisk. Drizzle tahini sauce over cooked falafel. Serve warm!

Nutrition Values:
Calories: 296Fat: 13gFiber: 1gCarbs: 9gProtein: 26g

584. Chickpea Curry
Cooking Time: 11 minutes
Servings: 6
Ingredients:
2 cans (15-ounceof chickpeas, rinsed and drained
1 packed cup kale, chopped
2 tablespoons cilantro leaves, for garnish
1 lime juiced
1 tablespoon honey
1 cup vegetable broth
1 cup okra, frozen, sliced
1 cup corn, frozen
1 (14.5-ouncecan tomatoes, crushed, with juice
1 tablespoon curry powder
2 cloves garlic, minced
1 green bell pepper, diced
2 tablespoons olive oil

Directions:
Set your instant pot to the sauté setting, add the oil and heat it. Add onion and stir, cook for 4-minutes. Add the bell pepper and garlic and cook for an additional 2 minutes. Add the curry powder and stir, cooking for another 30 seconds. Add the corn, okra, kale, broth, honey, tomatoes and juice, stir. Select the Manual setting on high with a cook time of 5-minutes. Once the cook time is completed, release the pressure naturally in 10-minutes. Divide into serving dishes, and garnish with cilantro leaves. Serve hot!

Nutrition Values:
Calories: 232Fat: 10gFiber: 1gCarbs: 23gProtein: 37g

585. Lentil Sloppy Joe's
Cooking Time: 30 minutes
Servings: 6
Ingredients:
2 cups green lentils
3 cups veggie broth
1 red bell pepper, stemmed and chopped
1 yellow onion, chopped
1 (14-ouncecan of tomatoes, crushed
1 tablespoon dark brown sugar
1 tablespoon Dijon mustard
2 tablespoons soy sauce
1 tablespoon olive oil
Salt and black pepper to taste

Directions:
Set your instant pot to the sauté mode, add the oil and heat it. Add the pepper and onion, cook for 3-minutes or until they have softened. Pour in the broth, then add in soy sauce, mustard, lentils, tomatoes, brown sugar, and pepper. Stir until the sugar has dissolved. Close and seal the pot lid. Select Manual setting on high for a cook time of 27-minutes. When the cook time is completed, release the

pressure naturally for 15-minutes. Stir before serving on hamburger buns. Serve hot!
Nutrition Values:
Calories: 208Fat: 17gFiber: 1gCarbs: 8gProtein: 27g

586. Lentil and Wild Rice Pilaf
Cooking Time: 14 minutes
Servings: 6
Ingredients:
¼ cup black or green lentils, soak for 30 minutes before cooking
¼ cup black/wild rice, soak for 30 minutes before cooking
¼ cup brown rice, soak for 30 minutes before cooking
3 cloves garlic, minced
½ onion, finely chopped
1 stalk celery, finely chopped
1 cup mushrooms, sliced
2 cups vegetable broth
¼ teaspoon red pepper flakes
Salt and black pepper to taste
1 teaspoon fennel seeds
1 teaspoon coriander, dried
1 tablespoon Italian seasoning
1 bay leaf
Directions:
Combine the lentils and rice in a bowl, and allow them to soak for 30-minutes. Drain then rinse well. Set your instant pot to the sauté mode. Sauté veggies in pot for about 5-minutes, add a bit of water to prevent the veggies from burning. Add the rice and lentils, vegetable broth, and spices into pot. Close the lid and set to Manual on high pressure with a cook time of 9-minutes. When the cook time is completed, release the pressure naturally for 10-minutes. Serve dish with fresh or steamed veggies. Serve warm!
Nutrition Values:
Calories: 187Fat: 11gFiber: 1gCarbs: 7gProtein: 23g

587. Instant Pot Hummus
Cooking Time: 18 minutes
Servings: 6
Ingredients:
1 cup soaked chickpeas
6 cups water
1 bay leaf
4 garlic cloves, crushed
¼ cup parsley, chopped
2 tablespoons tahini
Dash of paprika
¼ teaspoon cumin
¼ teaspoon salt
Directions:
Soak your chickpeas in water overnight. When you are ready to make the hummus, rinse them and place them into instant pot. Pour in 6 cups of water to pot, add garlic cloves, and bay leaf. Seal the lid of pot shut, and set to Manual on high for a cook time of 18-minutes. When the cook time is completed, release the pressure naturally for 10-minutes. When it is safe to do so, once the pressure has come down, then drain the chickpeas, saving 1 cup of cooking liquid. Remove the bay leaf, before pureeing the chickpeas.

Add the tahini, lemon juice, cumin, and ½ cup of cooking liquid to start. Keep pureeing, and if the mixture is not creamy enough, add a bit more liquid. Add salt and puree once more when you reach the right creaminess. Serve with a sprinkle of paprika and fresh, chopped parsley as garnish. Serve at room temperature!
Nutrition Values:
Calories: 153Fat: 4gFiber: 2gCarbs: 8.2gProtein: 21g

588. Stewed Chickpeas
Cooking Time: 27 minutes
Servings: 4
Ingredients:
2 (14-ouncecans of chickpeas, rinsed and drained
1 ½ tablespoon smoked paprika
3 small onions, chopped
¼ teaspoon allspice
½ teaspoon sea salt
½ teaspoon cumin
1 jar (24-ouncestomatoes, strained
2/3 cup dates, pitted, chopped
3 tablespoons water, or as needed
Directions:
Set your instant pot to the sauté mode, add water as needed to prevent sticking. Cook for about 7-minutes, occasionally stirring. Add the tomatoes, dates, chickpeas, and stir until combined. Cover and lock the pot lid in place and set to Manual on high for a cook time of 20-minutes. When cook time is over, release the pressure using quick-release. Serve over cooked whole-grain, such as millet, quinoa, and brown rice.
Nutrition Values:
Calories: 192Fat: 16gFiber: 1gCarbs: 6.2gProtein: 24g

589. Rainbow Beans
Cooking Time: 20 minutes
Servings: 6
Ingredients:
1 cup chicken stock
1 cup black beans, cooked
½ cup red beans, cooked
½ cup green beans, chopped
½ cup white beans, cooked
1 red sweet pepper, chopped, seeded
1 yellow sweet pepper, chopped, seeded
1 red onion, chopped
3 tablespoons sour cream
1 teaspoon turmeric
3 tablespoons tomato paste
Salt as needed
Directions:
Add the water and chicken stock into your instant pot. Add the red, white, and black beans. Add the chopped veggies to instant pot. Sprinkle mixture with turmeric, tomato paste, sour cream, and salt. Mix gently and close the lid. Set to the Stew mode and cook for a 20-minute cook time. When the cooking is completed, transfer to serving bowls. Serve hot!
Nutrition Values:
Calories: 205Fat: 17gFiber: 1gCarbs: 8.2gProtein: 27g

590. Northern White Bean Dip
Cooking Time: 13 minutes
Servings: 2
Ingredients:
¾ cup Great Northern white beans, soaked overnight
Pinch of red pepper flakes
1 ½ teaspoons chili powder
2 teaspoons cumin, ground
3 tablespoons cilantro, minced
3 tablespoons lemon juice
2 garlic cloves
1/3 cup extra virgin olive oil
Salt and black pepper to taste
Water as needed
Directions:
Drain the beans before putting them in the instant pot. Cover beans with 1-inch of fresh water, close the pot lid and seal. Select Manual setting on high with a cook time of 13-minutes. When the cook time is completed, release the pressure naturally for 10-minutes. Once the pressure is gone, drain the beans and run under cold water. In a food processor, chop up the garlic. Add the rest of the ingredients (except cilantroand puree till smooth. Serve with cilantro on top as a garnish. Serve at room temperature!
Nutrition Values:
Calories: 203Fat: 11gFiber: 2gCarbs: 19gProtein: 36g

591. Greek-Style Gigantes Beans with Feta
Cooking Time: 25 minutes
Servings: 8
Ingredients:
3 cups Gigantes white beans, dried
8 cups water
1 teaspoon oregano, dried
1 can (about 28-ouncescrushed tomatoes
1 large yellow onion, finely diced
1 garlic, clove, peeled
¼ cup extra virgin olive oil
1 teaspoon salt
¼ teaspoon black pepper
¼ cup flat-leaf parsley, fresh, chopped, for garnish
½ cup feta cheese, crumbled, for garnish or topping
Directions:
Combine the beans, salt, and water in the instant pot. Allow the beans to soak in the water for 12 hours before cooking. Secure the lid in place when you are ready to cook. Select the Bean/Chili setting and set the cook time for 15-minutes at high pressure. When the cook time is completed, release the pressure naturally for 15-minutes. Remove lid and ladle out 1 cup of cooking liquid and set aside. Wearing oven-mitts, lift the inner pot out of instant pot and drain the beans in a colander. Return the now empty pot to the instant pot housing for it. Now, select sauté mode, and heat the ¼ cup olive oil in the pot. Add the garlic, onion, celery and sauté for 15-minutes. Add the drained beans, and reserved cup of cooking liquid, tomatoes, oregano, pepper, and stir well.
Close and lock the lid, and reset the instant pot to Bean/Chili setting and set the cook time for 5-minutes on high. Let the pressure release using quick-release. Ladle the beans into a serving dish and garnish or top with feta cheese, parsley, and remaining olive oil, and serve warm!
Nutrition Values:
Calories: 215Fat: 18gFiber: 2gCarbs: 7.4gProtein: 28g

592. Chili Con Carne
Cooking Time: 10 minutes
Servings: 6
Ingredients:
1 can (28-ouncesground and peeled tomatoes
1 teaspoon oregano, dry
1 tablespoon Worcestershire sauce
1 tablespoon chili powder
1 ½ cups onion, large, diced
1 ½ teaspoons cumin, ground
1 ½ lbs. ground beef
1 can (14-ounceblack beans, rinsed and drained
1 can (14-ouncekidney beans, rinsed and drained
3 tablespoons extra virgin olive oil
2 tablespoons garlic, minced
1-2 jalapenos, stems and seeds removed, finely diced
Salt and black pepper to taste
1 cup sweet red bell pepper, large, diced
½ cup water
Directions:
Press the sauté button, allow pot to heat, add in oil. Add the ground beef, and break it up using a wooden spoon, cook for 5-minutes or until beef is browned. Remove excess fat, add the onions, bell pepper, jalapenos, and sauté for 3-minutes. Add the garlic, chili powder, oregano, cumin, salt and pepper, and sauté for 1-minute. Add the beans, water, tomatoes, and Worcestershire sauce and stir to combine. Close and secure the lid. Select Manual setting on high with a cook time of 10-minutes. When the cook time is completed, release the pressure using the quick-release. Serve hot!
Nutrition Values:
Calories: 204Fat: 22gFiber: 2gCarbs: 17gProtein: 26g

593. Smokey Sweet Black-Eyed Peas & Greens
Cooking Time: 13 minutes
Servings: 6
Ingredients:
1 ½ teaspoon chili powder
2 teaspoons smoked paprika
1 ½ cups black-eyed peas, dried and soaked overnight
1 cup red pepper, diced
1 onion, thinly sliced
1 teaspoon oil
4 dates, chopped fine
1 cup water or vegetable stock
1 (15-ouncecan of fire roasted tomatoes with green chilies
2 cups greens, chopped, kale or Swiss chard
Salt to taste
Directions:
Set your instant pot to the sauté mode, add the oil and heat it. Add the onions, and cook for 3-minutes. Add the garlic and peppers and sauté for another 2-

minutes. Add the smoked paprika and chili powder along with the peas and dates. Stir to coat them with spices. Add water, stirring to combine. Close and lock lid of pot, select Manual setting on high with a cook time of 3-minutes. When the cook time is completed, release the pressure naturally for 5-minutes. Add the tomatoes and greens and lock the lid, setting for an additional 5-minutes of cook time. Serve warm!
Nutrition Values:
Calories: 207Fat: 5gFiber: 8gCarbs: 22gProtein: 29g

594. Tex Mex Pinto Beans
Cooking Time: 42 minutes
Servings: 6
Ingredients:
¼ cup cilantro, chopped
1 jalapeno, diced
1 onion, chopped
1 packet taco seasoning
½ cup Salsa Verde
1 clove garlic, diced
5 cups chicken broth
20 ounces package pinto beans with ham
Directions:
Rinse and sort out the dried beans, then place them into your instant pot. Add the broth to the pot. Add onion, garlic, jalapeno, and stir. Add taco seasoning and stir to combine, then close the lid and secure it. Select the Manual setting on high for a cook time of 42-minutes. When the cook time is completed, release the pressure naturally for about 15-minutes. Drain the excess liquid from the pot. Stir in the Salsa Verde, ham seasoning, and cilantro. Add salt to taste. Serve tacos, over rice, or a side dish. Serve hot!
Nutrition Values:
Calories: 232Fat: 21gFiber: 3gCarbs: 22gProtein: 27g

595. Instant Pot Charros
Cooking Time: 56 minutes
Servings: 8
Ingredients:
1 lb. pinto beans dried, rinsed and picked over
½ lb. double smoked bacon
½ lb. Mexican Chorizo raw,
Mexican chorizo sausage, not the dried Spanish chorizo
1 large onion, chopped
1 large jalapeno, seeded and finely chopped
4 cloves garlic
1 can of tomatoes and chilies
3 cups chicken stock
2 cups Mexican beer
2 chipotle chilies canned in adobo, minced
1 teaspoon salt
2 bay leaves
1 tablespoon Epazote, crushed
1 tablespoon Mexican oregano
2 tablespoons cumin
1 tablespoon olive oil
1 cup cilantro, fresh, chopped, for garnish
Directions:
Set your instant pot to the sauté mode, add the oil and heat it up. Add the bacon and fry until it starts to brown for about 5-minutes. Remove the chorizo meat from the casing and add it to pot to brown. Cook for another 4-minutes or until meat is cooked. Add the onion, add cook for another 5-minutes. Add the jalapenos, cumin, garlic, oregano, Epazote and cook for one more minute. Now add in the pinto beans, bay leaves, chipotle chilies, beer, salt, chicken stock, and give it a nice stir. Close the lid and set to cook for 45-minutes on Manual high with a cook time of 45-minutes. When the cook time is completed, release the pressure naturally for 15-minutes. Remove the lid and stir the beans, and set to sauté mode, cooking for an additional 5-minutes. Serve hot! Top with cilantro for garnish.
Nutrition Values:
Calories: 243Fat: 20gFiber: 2gCarbs: 21gProtein: 31g

596. Three Bean Salad
Cooking Time: 15 minutes
Servings: 4
Ingredients:
1 cup chickpeas/garbanzo beans, soaked or quick-soaked
1 cup Borlotti or cranberry beans, soaked or quick-soaked
1 ½ cups of green beans, fresh or frozen
1 bay leaf
1 clove of garlic, lightly crushed
For the dressing:
2 celery stalks, chopped finely
½ red onion, chopped finely
4 tablespoon olive oil
1 teaspoon Truvia
5 tablespoon apple cider vinegar
1 bunch parsley, finely chopped
Salt and pepper to taste
Directions:
Wrap the green beans inside some aluminum foil. Add 4 cups of fresh water to your instant pot, then add the soaked or rinsed chickpeas, garlic clove, and bay leaf. Add the steamer basket with the soaked Borlotti beans. Finally, add the packet of tin foil wrapped green beans. Use a second trivet to keep your packet suspended above the Borlotti. Close and lock the pot lid, and set to Manual on high for a cook time of 15-minutes.
When the cook time is completed, release the pressure naturally for 10-minutes. While the beans are cooking prepare dressing. Slice the onion nice and fine, add to a bowl with vinegar and Truvia, mix and set aside. Remove and open the packet of green beans. Pour the beans from the steamer basket and into a strainer. Rinse beans under cold water. Slice the green beans and place in with other beans and mix well. In a serving bowl add the beans along with dressing and mix well. Add salt and pepper to taste. Serve chilled!
Nutrition Values:
Calories: 198Fat: 18gFiber: 3gCarbs: 19g Protein: 29g

597. Beans Stew
Cooking Time: 67 minutes
Servings: 8
Ingredients:

1 lb. red beans, dry—water as needed
2 carrots, chopped
2 tablespoons vegetable oils
¼ cup cilantro leaves, chopped
1 small onion, diced
2 green onions, chopped
1 tomato, chopped
Salt and black pepper to taste
2 carrots, chopped
Water as needed
Directions:
Add the beans to your instant pot and set to Manual on high for a cook time of 35-minutes. When the cook time is completed, release the pressure naturally for 10-minutes. Add carrots, and salt and pepper to taste, cover instant pot again, setting for a cook time of 30-additional minutes. Meanwhile heat a pan with vegetable oil over medium high heat, add onion, stir for 2-minutes. Add tomatoes, green onions, some salt and pepper and stir again, cook for an additional 3-minutes, then remove from heat. Release the pressure naturally for 10-minutes. Divide among serving plates, and garnish with fresh, chopped cilantro. Serve warm!
Nutrition Values:
Calories: 211Fat: 23g Fiber: 1gCarbs: 26g Protein: 29g

598. Classic Chili Lime Black Beans
Cooking Time:50 minutes
Servings:4
Ingredients:
2 cups black beans, soaked for 8 hours and drained
4 garlic cloves; minced.
3 cups water
1 tsp. smoked paprika
2 tsp. red palm oil
1 tbsp. chili powder
1 yellow onion; chopped.
Salt to the taste
Juice from 1 lime
Directions:
Set your instant pot on Sauté mode; add oil and heat it up
Add garlic and onion, stir and cook for 2 minutes
Add beans, chili powder, paprika, salt and water; then stir well. close the lid and cook on High for 40 minutes.
Release the pressure naturally, open the instant pot lid, add lime juice and more salt; then stir well. divide into bowls and serve

599. Instant Wheat Berry Salad
Cooking Time:45 minutes
Servings:6
Ingredients:
1 ½ cups wheat berries
1 tbsp. extra-virgin olive oil
4 cups water
Salt and black pepper to the taste
For the salad:
1 tbsp. balsamic vinegar
1 tbsp. olive oil
2 green onions; chopped.
2 oz. feta cheese; crumbled.
1/2 cup Kalamata olives; pitted and chopped.
1 handful basil leaves; chopped.
1 handful parsley leaves; chopped.
1 cup cherry tomatoes, cut into halves
Directions:
Set your instant pot on Sauté mode; add 1 tablespoon oil and heat it up.
Add wheat berries; stir and cook for 5 minutes
Add water, salt and pepper to the taste, close the lid and cook on High for 30 minutes.
Release the pressure naturally for 10 minutes, then release remaining pressure by turning the valve to 'Venting', open the instant pot lid, drain wheat berries and put them in a salad bowl
Add salt and pepper, 1 tablespoon oil, balsamic vinegar, tomatoes, green onions, olives, cheese, basil and parsley, toss to coat and serve right away

600. Pasta & Cranberry Beans
Cooking Time:30 minutes
Servings:8
Ingredients:
26 oz. canned tomatoes; chopped.
3 tsp. basil; dried
1/2 tsp. smoked paprika
2 tsp. oregano; dried
2 cups dried cranberry beans; soaked for 8 hours and drained.
7 garlic cloves; minced.
6 cups water
2 celery ribs; chopped.
1 yellow onion; chopped.
2 cups small pasta
3 tbsp. nutritional yeast
1 tsp. rosemary; chopped.
1/4 tsp. red pepper flakes
Salt and black pepper to the taste
10 oz. kale leaves
Directions:
Set your instant pot on Sauté mode; add onion, celery, garlic, pepper flakes, rosemary and a pinch of salt, stir and brown for 2 minutes
Add tomatoes, basil, oregano and paprika, stir and cook for 1 minute
Add beans; 6 cups water, close the lid and cook at High for 10 minutes
Quick release the pressure; open the instant pot lid, add pasta, yeast, kale, salt and pepper, stir and set the pot on Sauté mode again
Cook for 5 minutes more, divide into bowls and serve.

601. Kidney Beans Dish
Cooking Time:35 minutes
Servings:8
Ingredients:
1 lb. red kidney beans, soaked for 8 hours and drained
8 oz. smoked Cajun Tasso; chopped.
1 celery rib; chopped.
2 tbsp. garlic; minced.
1 green bell pepper; chopped.
2 tsp. thyme; dried
4 green onions; chopped.

2 yellow onions; chopped.
3 tbsp. extra virgin olive oil
2 bay leaves
Cajun seasoning to the taste
Hot sauce to the taste
Directions:
Set your instant pot on Sauté mode; add oil and heat it up
Add Tasso; then stir well. cook for 5 minutes and transfer to a bowl
Add onions and Cajun seasoning to the pot; stir and cook for 10 minutes
Add garlic, stir and cook 5 minutes.
Add bell pepper and celery; stir and cook 5 minutes.
Add beans, water to cover everything, bay leaves, thyme, close the lid and cook at High for 15 minutes.
Quick release the pressure, open the instant pot lid, add Tasso and leave aside for 5 minutes
Divide beans and Tasso mix on plates, garnish with green onions and serve with hot sauce to the taste.

602. Lentils Tacos
Cooking Time:25 minutes
Servings:4
Ingredients:
2 cups brown lentils
4 cups water
1 tsp. salt
1 tsp. garlic powder
4 oz. tomato sauce
1/2 tsp. cumin
1 tsp. chili powder
1 tsp. onion powder
Taco shells for serving
Directions:
In your instant pot, mix lentils with water, tomato sauce, cumin, garlic powder, chili powder and onion powder; then stir well. close the lid and cook at High for 15 minutes
Quick release the pressure, open the instant pot lid; divide lentils mix into taco shells and serve.

603. Couscous with Veggies and Chicken
Cooking Time:25 minutes
Servings:4
Ingredients:
8 chicken thighs; skinless
15 oz. canned stewed tomatoes; chopped.
3/4 cup couscous
1 zucchini; chopped
1 ½ cups mushrooms; cut into halves
1 ½ cups carrots; chopped.
1/2 cup chicken stock
1 green bell pepper; chopped.
1 yellow onion; chopped
2 garlic cloves; minced.
Salt and black pepper to the taste
A handful parsley; chopped.
Directions:
In your instant pot; mix chicken with mushrooms, carrots, bell pepper, onion, garlic, tomatoes and stock; then stir well. close the lid and cook at High for 8 minutes

Quick release the pressure, open the instant pot lid, add couscous, zucchini, salt and pepper; then stir well. close the lid again and cook on Low for 6 minutes
Release the pressure again, open the instant pot lid; add parsley, stir gently, divide into bowls and serve.

604. Mediterranean Lentils
Cooking Time: 40 minutes
Servings: 3
Ingredients:
1 cup brown or green lentils
1 tomato; diced
2 ½ cups Vegetable Stock
1 bay leaf
1 small sweet or yellow onion; diced
1 garlic clove; diced
1 tbsp. olive oil
1 tsp. dried oregano
1/2 tsp. ground cumin
1/2 tsp. dried parsley
1/2 tsp. salt or as your liking
1/4 tsp. freshly ground black pepper; or more as needed
Directions:
Select the "Sauté" Low mode on your instant pot. When the display reads "Hot," add the oil and heat until it shimmers.
Add the onion. Cook for 3 to 4 minutes until soft.
Turn off the Instant Pot and add the garlic; oregano, cumin, parsley, salt and pepper. Cook until fragrant, about 1 minute
Stir in the tomato, lentils, stock and bay leaf. Lock the lid and turn the steam release handle to Sealing. Using the Manual function, set the cooker to High Pressure for 18 minutes
After completing the cooking time, let the pressure release naturally for 10 minutes; quick release any remaining pressure
Remove the lid carefully and remove and discard the bay leaf.
Taste and season with more salt and pepper, as needed. If there's too much liquid remaining, select Sauté Medium or High and cook until it evaporates.

605. Asian Rice
Cooking Time: 22 minutes
Servings: 5
Ingredients:
2 cups basmati rice; rinsed well, drained and dried
2 ½ cups water
1 tbsp. chili oil
1/2 tsp. ground cardamom
2 tsp. cumin seeds
1 tsp. salt as your liking
Directions:
Select the "Sauté" Low mode on your instant pot. When the display reads "Hot," add the oil and heat until it shimmers.
Add the cumin seeds and cardamom. Cook until fragrant, stirring frequently. Add the salt, rice and water and stir well

Lock the lid and turn the steam release handle to Sealing. Using the Manual function, set the cooker to High Pressure for 6 minutes
After completing the cooking time, let the pressure release naturally for 10 minutes; quick release any remaining pressure. Remove the lid carefully and fluff the rice.

606. Black Beans

Cooking Time: 1 hour 5 minutes
Servings: 7
Ingredients:
2 cups dried black beans; rinsed but not soaked
4 garlic cloves; diced
1 small onion; diced
3 cups Vegetable Stock
1/4 cup fresh cilantro leaves, chopped
1 cup diced roasted green chiles
2 tbsp. freshly squeezed lime juice
1 to 2 tbsp. olive oil
1 tbsp. ground cumin
1 tsp. dried oregano
1 tsp. chili powder
1 tsp. salt; or more as your liking
Directions:
Select the "Sauté" Low mode on your instant pot. When the display reads "Hot," add the oil and onion. Sauté for 1 to 2 minutes, turning off the Instant Pot after about 1 minute
Add the garlic. Sauté for 30 seconds. Stir in the cumin; oregano and chili powder and cook for another 30 seconds or so until the spices "bloom"
Add the green chiles, stock and black beans, stirring well. Lock the lid and turn the steam release handle to Sealing.
Using the Manual function, set the cooker to High Pressure for 35 minutes
After completing the cooking time, let the pressure release naturally for 20 minutes; or until the pin drops.
Remove the lid carefully and stir. Add the salt, lime juice and cilantro. Stir again and serve.

607. Cilantro Lime Brown Rice

Cooking Time: 34 minutes
Servings: 5
Ingredients:
2 cups brown rice; rinsed and drained
⅓ cup fresh cilantro, chopped
2 ½ cups water
Juice of 1 lime
Zest of 1 lime
Dash ground cumin
Salt as your liking
Directions:
In the Instant Pot, combine the rice and water. Lock the lid and turn the steam release handle to Sealing. Using the Manual function, set the cooker to High Pressure for 22 minutes
After completing the cooking time, let the pressure release naturally for 10 minutes while the Instant Pot goes into Keep Warm mode; quick release any remaining pressure.
Remove the lid carefully and stir in the cilantro, lime juice and zest and cumin. Season to taste with salt.

608. Black Beans and Chorizo

Cooking Time:55 minutes
Servings:6
Ingredients:
1 lb. black beans, soaked for 8 hours and drained
6 oz. chorizo; chopped
1 yellow onion; cut into half
6 garlic cloves; minced.
1 tbsp. vegetable oil
2 bay leaves
1 orange; cut into half
2 quarts' chicken stock
Salt to the taste
Chopped cilantro; chopped.for serving
Directions:
Set your instant pot on Sauté mode; add oil and heat it up.
Add chorizo, stir and cook for 2 minutes
Add onion, beans, garlic, bay leaves, orange, salt and stock; then stir well. close the lid and cook at High for 40 minutes.
Release the pressure naturally, carefully open the lid; discard bay leaves, onion and orange, add more salt and cilantro; then stir well. divide into bowls and serve

609. Green Chile and Baked Beans

Cooking Time: 1 hour 25 minutes
Servings: 5
Ingredients:
1 pound dried navy beans, soaked in water overnight; rinsed and drained
1/4 cup maple syrup
1 ½ cups diced roasted green chiles
1/4 cup blackstrap molasses
1/4 cup packed light brown sugar
1 small sweet onion; cut into large dice
3 garlic cloves; minced
2 tbsp. ketchup
1 tbsp. vegan Worcestershire sauce
1 tbsp. olive oil
1 tsp. salt or as your liking
1 tsp. apple cider vinegar
Directions:
In a small bowl, whisk the molasses, maple syrup, brown sugar, ketchup and Worcestershire sauce. Set aside.
Select the "Sauté" Low mode on your instant pot. When the display reads "Hot," add the oil and heat until it shimmers.
Add the onion and garlic. Turn off the Instant Pot and sauté the veggies for 1 to 2 minutes, stirring frequently. Add the salt, beans and molasses mix, stirring well
Lock the lid and turn the steam release handle to Sealing. Using the Manual function, set the cooker to High Pressure for 35 minutes
After completing the cooking time, let the pressure release naturally for 20 minutes; or until the pin drops.

Remove the lid carefully and stir. Select Sauté Medium. Stir in the green chiles and simmer the beans for 5 to 10 minutes; or until the sauce thickens. Stir in the vinegar and serve.

610. Green Chile Chickpeas
Cooking Time: 1 hour 15 minutes
Servings: 5
Ingredients:
2 cups dried chickpeas; rinsed
1 small tomato; diced
6 cups water
1 cup diced roasted green chiles or from a can
2 tsp. freshly squeezed lemon juice
1 tsp. ground cumin
1/2 tsp. chili powder; or more as your liking
1/2 tsp. onion powder
1/4 tsp. dried oregano
1/2 tsp. garlic powder
1/2 tsp. red pepper flakes
1/2 tsp. smoked paprika
1/4 tsp. freshly ground black pepper
1 tsp. salt or as your liking
Directions:
In the Instant Pot, combine the chickpeas and water. Lock the lid and turn the steam release handle to Sealing. Using the Manual function, set the cooker to High Pressure for 45 minutes
After completing the cooking time, let the pressure release naturally for 20 minutes; quick release any remaining pressure.
Remove the lid carefully and drain the chickpeas, reserving 1 to 2 tbsp. of the cooking water. Return the chickpeas to the Instant Pot
Stir in the tomato, green chiles, lemon juice, cumin, chili powder, salt, garlic powder, red pepper flakes, paprika, onion powder; oregano and black pepper. If they're too dry, add the reserved cooking water.
Select the "Sauté" Low mode on your instant pot and cook for 3 to 4 minutes. You may need to turn the Instant Pot off if anything starts to burn at the bottom
Put the lid back on and turn on the Keep Warm function. Let the chickpeas sit in all that goodness for 5 minutes, then they're ready.

611. Red Beans and Rice
Cooking Time: 1 hour 15 minutes
Servings: 5
Ingredients:
5 cups cooked white rice
2 celery stalks, sliced
5 garlic cloves; minced
2 cups dried red beans
4 cups Vegetable Stock
2 bay leaves
1 red onion; diced
1 bell pepper, any color; diced
1 tbsp. olive oil
2 tsp. Cajun seasoning
1/2 tsp. dried oregano
1/2 tsp. dried parsley
Salt as your liking
Freshly ground black pepper
Chopped fresh parsley; for garnishing
Hot sauce; for serving
Directions:
Select the "Sauté" Low mode on your instant pot. When the display reads "Hot," add the oil and heat until it shimmers.
Add the red onion, bell pepper and celery. Cook for 3 to 4 minutes, stirring frequently.
Turn off the Instant Pot and add the garlic, bay leaves, Cajun seasoning; oregano and dried parsley.
Continue to cook for 1 minute more, stirring
Stir in the beans and stock. Lock the lid and turn the steam release handle to Sealing. Using the Manual function, set the cooker to High Pressure for 40 minutes
After completing the cooking time, let the pressure release naturally for about 25 minutes; or until the pin drops.
Remove the lid carefully and remove and discard the bay leaves
Taste and season with salt and pepper, as needed.
Serve with rice and top with parsley and hot sauce.

612. Spicy Lentils
Cooking Time: 34 minutes
Servings: 5
Ingredients:
2 Roma tomatoes; diced
2 cups Vegetable Stock
1 cup green; rinsed and drained
1 cup well chopped kale
1 small onion; diced
1 or 2 garlic cloves, finely diced
1 bell pepper, any color; diced
1 tbsp. olive oil
1 tsp. smoked paprika
1 tsp. chili powder
1 tsp. ground cumin
1 tsp. salt; or more as your liking
Freshly ground black pepper
Directions:
Select the "Sauté" Low mode on your instant pot. When the display reads "Hot," add the oil and heat until it shimmers.
Add the onion. Sauté for 1 to 2 minutes and then turn off the Instant Pot. Add the garlic. Cook for about 30 seconds, stirring (don't let it burn
Add the bell pepper, tomatoes, stock, lentils, salt, cumin, chili powder and paprika.
Lock the lid and turn the steam release handle to Sealing. Using the Manual function, set the cooker to High Pressure for 15 minutes
After completing the cooking time, let the Instant Pot go into Keep Warm mode and let the pressure release naturally for 10 minutes; quick release any remaining pressure
Remove the lid carefully and stir in the kale, which will wilt after 1 to 2 minutes. Taste and season with salt and pepper, as needed.

613. Butternut Lentils
Cooking Time: 30 minutes
Servings: 5
Ingredients:

3 cups butternut squash, peeled and cubed
1 ¾ cups water; or Vegetable Stock,
1/2 onion; diced
1 cup red lentils; rinsed
1 tbsp. olive oil
1 garlic clove; minced
1 tsp. smoked paprika
1/2 tsp. salt or as your liking
1/2 tsp. ground cumin
Pinch chili powder
Directions:
Select the "Sauté" Low mode on your instant pot. When the display reads "Hot," add the oil and heat until it shimmers.
Add the onion. Cook for 2 to 3 minutes, stirring frequently. Turn off the Instant Pot and add the garlic. Cook for 30 seconds, stirring
Stir in the squash, water, lentils, paprika, salt, cumin and chili powder.
Lock the lid and turn the steam release handle to Sealing. Using the Manual function, set the cooker to High Pressure for 10 minutes
After completing the cooking time, let the pressure release naturally for 10 minutes; quick release any remaining pressure
Remove the lid carefully and stir. The lentils and butternut will break down quickly, no need to mash. Just stir and, when they're smooth, taste and adjust the seasonings, as needed.

614. Shrimp and White Beans
Cooking Time:45 minutes
Servings:8
Ingredients:
1 lb. white beans; soaked for 8 hours and drained
1 garlic clove; minced
1 green bell pepper; chopped.
1 celery rib; chopped
4 parsley springs; chopped.
2 yellow onions; chopped.
2 cups seafood stock
1 lb. shrimp; peeled and deveined
2 bay leaves
3 tbsp. canola oil
Creole seasoning to the taste
Cooked rice for serving
Hot sauce for serving
Directions:
Set your instant pot on Sauté mode; add oil and heat it up
Add onions and Creole seasoning to the taste; stir and cook for 5 minutes
Add garlic; stir and cook 5 minutes more
Add bell pepper and celery; stir and cook for 5 minutes
Add beans, stock and some water to cover everything in the pot.
Add bay leaves and parsley; then stir well. close the lid and cook at High for 15 minutes.
Quick release the pressure, open the instant pot lid, add shrimp, close the lid and leave it aside for 10 minutes
Divide beans and shrimp among plates on top of cooked rice and serve with hot sauce

615. Mushroom and Leek Risotto
Cooking Time: 20 minutes
Servings: 5
Ingredients:
12 ounces baby bella mushrooms, sliced
1 leek, white and lightest green parts only, halved and sliced
2 garlic cloves; minced
1 cup Arborio rice; rinsed and drained
2 ¾ cups Vegetable Stock
4 tbsp. vegan butter; divided
1 tsp. dried thyme
1/2 tsp. salt; or as your liking
Juice of 1/2 lemon
Freshly ground black pepper
Chopped fresh parsley; for garnishing
Directions:
Select the "Sauté" Low mode on your instant pot. When the display reads "Hot," add 2 tbsp. of butter to melt.
Add the leek and mushrooms. Sauté for about 2 minutes, stirring frequently
Add the garlic. Cook for about 30 seconds, stirring, turn off the Instant Pot if it starts to burn. Add the rice and toast it for 1 minute. Turn off the Instant Pot
Stir in the stock, thyme and salt. Lock the lid and turn the steam release handle to Sealing. Using the Manual function, set the cooker to High Pressure for 8 minutes.
After completing the cooking time, quick release the pressure
Remove the lid carefully and stir in the lemon juice and remaining 2 tbsp. of vegan butter. Taste and season with more salt and pepper, as needed.
Garnish with fresh parsley.

616. Italian Lentils Dinner
Cooking Time:25 minutes
Servings:4
Ingredients:
3/4 cup green lentils; soaked overnight and drained
1/2 cup brown rice; soaked overnight and drained
1 cup mozzarella cheese; shredded.
1 cup green and red bell pepper; chopped.
2 cups chicken; already cooked and shredded.
3 carrots; chopped.
2 ½ cups chicken stock
1 cup tomato sauce
3/4 cup onion; chopped.
3 tsp. Italian seasoning
2 garlic cloves; crushed.
A handful greens
Salt and black pepper to the taste
Directions:
In your instant pot; mix lentils with rice, salt, pepper, stock, tomato sauce, onion, red and green pepper, chicken, carrots, greens, Italian seasoning and garlic; then stir well. close the lid and cook on High for 15 minutes
Quick release the pressure, carefully open the lid; add cheese; then stir well. divide among bowls and serve.

617. Veggies Rice Pilaf

Cooking Time: 28 minutes
Servings: 5
Ingredients:
1/2 cup frozen peas
1/2 cup sliced almonds
1/2 sweet onion, chopped
1 carrot, halved lengthwise and sliced
1 celery stalk, sliced
1 cup basmati rice; rinsed and drained
1 cup Vegetable Stock
1 cup broccoli florets
1/2 cup sliced white mushrooms
2 garlic cloves; minced
1 tbsp. olive oil; or avocado oil
Salt as your liking
Freshly ground black pepper
Directions:
Select the "Sauté" Low mode on your instant pot. When the display reads "Hot," add the oil and heat until it shimmers.
Add the onion, carrot, celery, broccoli and mushrooms. Sauté for 2 to 3 minutes, stirring frequently. Add the garlic and turn off the Instant Pot. Sauté the garlic for 30 seconds, stirring frequently
Stir in the rice and stock and season to taste with salt and pepper
Lock the lid and turn the steam release handle to Sealing. Using the Manual function, set the cooker to High Pressure for 3 minutes.
After completing the cooking time, let the pressure release naturally for 15 minutes; quick release any remaining pressure
Remove the lid carefully and stir in the frozen peas. Replace the cover (no need to seal itand let sit for a few minutes. When ready to serve, stir in the almonds.

618. Black Bean Soup
Cooking Time: 1 hour 25 minutes
Servings: 4
Ingredients:
1/2 cup chopped scallions, for garnish
4 slices bacon, diced
1 green bell pepper; chopped
1 jalapeño; chopped
4 garlic cloves; minced
1/2 bunch fresh cilantro, finely chopped
1 yellow onion, diced
1 cup dried black beans
3 cups chicken broth
2 bay leaves
1 tsp. dried thyme
2 tsp. dried oregano
2 tsp. ground cumin
2 tsp. salt or as your liking
Directions:
In your Instant Pot, combine the beans, broth, bacon, onion, bell pepper, jalapeño, garlic, cilantro, salt, oregano, thyme, cumin and bay leaves. Stir well to combine
Now secure the lid on the pot and close the valve. Now Press "Manual" and set the pot at "High" pressure for 45 minutes.
After completing the cooking time, allow the pot to sit undisturbed for 10 minutes, then release any remaining pressure
Using an immersion blender, puree some of the soup to thicken it while leaving some beans intact. Garnish with the scallions and serve.

619. Chickpea Basil Salad
Cooking Time: 1 hour 10 minutes
Servings: 3
Ingredients:
1 cup dried chickpeas; rinsed
1 cup fresh basil leaves; chopped or sliced
1 ½ cups grape tomatoes, halved
water, enough to cover the chickpeas by 3 to 4 inches
3 tbsp. balsamic vinegar
1/2 tsp. garlic powder
1/2 tsp. salt; or more as your liking
Directions:
In the Instant Pot, combine the chickpeas and water. Lock the lid and turn the steam release handle to Sealing. Using the Manual function, set the cooker to High Pressure for 45 minutes.
After completing the cooking time, let the pressure release naturally for 20 minutes; quick release any remaining pressure
Remove the lid carefully and drain the chickpeas. Refrigerate to cool (unless you want to serve this warm, which is good, too
While the chickpeas cool, in a large bowl, stir together the basil, tomatoes, vinegar, garlic powder and salt. Add the beans, stir to combine and serve.

620. Re-fried Pinto Beans
Cooking Time: 1 hour
Servings: 7
Ingredients:
1 pound dried pinto beans; rinsed
2 quarts Vegetable Stock
1 onion, quartered
3 garlic cloves, peeled
1 tbsp. freshly squeezed lime juice
1 tbsp. olive oil
1 tbsp. salt or as your liking
1/2 tsp. chili powder
1 tsp. ground cumin
1 tsp. dried Mexican oregano
1/4 tsp. freshly ground black pepper
Directions:
In the Instant Pot, combine the oil, onion, garlic, beans, stock, cumin; oregano, chili powder and pepper.
Lock the lid and turn the steam release handle to Sealing. Using the Manual function, set the cooker to High Pressure for 38 minutes
After completing the cooking time, let the pressure release naturally for about 20 minutes; or until the pin drops
Remove the lid carefully and use a ladle to remove most of the remaining liquid, saving it.
Using an immersion blender, blend the beans until smooth, adding the cooking water back in as needed. Stir in the lime juice and salt.

621. Coconut Jasmine Rice

Cooking Time: 20 minutes
Servings: 5
Ingredients:
1 (14-ouncecan lite coconut milk
2 cups jasmine rice; rinsed and drained
1/2 cup water
1/2 tsp. sea salt or as your liking
Directions:
In the Instant Pot, combine the rice, coconut milk, water and salt.
Lock the lid and turn the steam release handle to Sealing. Using the Manual function, set the cooker to High Pressure for 4 minutes
After completing the cooking time, let the pressure release naturally for 10 minutes; quick release any remaining pressure
Remove the lid carefully and fluff the rice. Taste and season with more salt, as needed.

622. Pepper Lemon Quinoa
Cooking Time: 20 minutes
Servings: 5
Ingredients:
1 ½ cups quinoa; rinsed
1 ½ cups water
1 tbsp. vegan butter
1/4 tsp. garlic powder
1/4 tsp. dried basil
1 tsp. salt; or more as your liking
1/2 tsp. freshly ground black pepper
Juice of 1 lemon
Zest of 1 lemon
Directions:
In the Instant Pot, combine the quinoa, water, salt, pepper, garlic powder and basil.
Lock the lid and turn the steam release handle to Sealing. Using the Manual function, set the cooker to High Pressure for 8 minutes
After completing the cooking time, let the pressure release naturally for 10 minutes; quick release any remaining pressure.
Remove the lid carefully and stir in the butter, lemon juice and zest. Taste and season with more salt and pepper, as needed

623. Chinese Fried Rice
Cooking Time: 22 minutes
Servings: 5
Ingredients:
1 small onion; diced
1 ¾ cups jasmine rice; rinsed and drained
1/4 cup lite soy sauce
1 ¾ cups water
2 cups frozen mixed vegetable; peas, carrots, corn
1 tbsp. sesame oil
3/4 tsp. garlic powder
3/4 tsp. ground ginger
Directions:
Select the "Sauté" Low mode on your instant pot. When the display reads "Hot," add the oil and heat until it shimmers.
Add the onion. Cook for 1 minute, stirring frequently.
Turn off the Instant Pot and add the rice, ginger, garlic powder, soy sauce and water

Lock the lid and turn the steam release handle to Sealing. Using the Manual function, set the cooker to High Pressure for 5 minutes
After completing the cooking time, turn off the Instant Pot and let the pressure release naturally for 10 minutes; quick release any remaining pressure.
Remove the lid carefully and stir in the frozen vegetables
Rest the lid back on "no need to lock it" and select the Keep Warm function. Let the veggies warm for 3 to 4 minutes before serving.

624. Barley and Mushroom Risotto
Preparation time: 10 minutes
Cooking time: 30 minutes
Servings: 4
Ingredients:
2 cups yellow onions, peeled and chopped
1 tablespoon olive oil
1 cup pearl barley
1 teaspoon fennel seeds
2 tablespoons black barley
3 cups chicken stock
⅓ cup dry sherry
1½ cups water
ounce dried mushrooms
Salt and ground black pepper, to taste
¼ cup Parmesan cheese, grated
Directions:
Set the Instant Pot on Sauté mode, add the oil, and heat it up. Add the fennel and onions, stir, and cook for 4 minutes. Add the barley, sherry, mushrooms, stock, water, salt, and pepper and stir well. Cover the Instant Pot, cook on the Rice setting for 18 minutes, release the pressure, uncover the Instant Pot, and set it on Manual mode. Add more salt and pepper, if needed, stir and cook for 5 minutes. Divide into bowls, add the cheese on top, and serve.
Nutrition Values:
Calories: 200
Fat: 5
Fiber: 6.1
Carbs: 31
Protein: 7.6

625. Barley with Vegetables
Preparation time: 10 minutes
Cooking time: 25 minutes
Servings: 4
Ingredients:
1 tablespoon extra virgin olive oil
1 tablespoon butter
1 white onion, peeled and chopped
1 garlic clove, peeled and minced
1½ cups pearl barley, rinsed
1 celery stalk, chopped
⅓ cup mushrooms, chopped
4 cups vegetable stock
2¼ cups water
Salt and ground black pepper, to taste
3 tablespoons fresh parsley, chopped
1 cup Parmesan cheese, grated
Directions:

Set the Instant Pot on Sauté mode, add the oil and butter and heat them up. Add the onion and garlic, stir, and cook for 4 minutes. Add the celery and barley and toss to coat. Add the mushrooms, water, stock, salt, and pepper, stir, cover the Instant Pot and cook on the Multigrain setting for 18 minutes. Release the pressure, uncover the Instant Pot, add the cheese and parsley and more salt and pepper, if needed, stir for 2 minutes, divide into bowls, and serve.
Nutrition Values:
Calories: 170
Fat: 6
Fiber: 4.5
Carbs: 30
Protein: 8

626. Cracked Wheat and Vegetables
Preparation time: 10 minutes
Cooking time: 15 minutes
Servings: 4
Ingredients:
½ cup cracked whole wheat
1½ cups water
2 tomatoes, cored and chopped
2 small potatoes, cubed
5 cauliflower florets, chopped
Salt and ground black pepper, to taste
¼ teaspoon mustard seeds
¼ teaspoon cumin seeds
1 teaspoon ginger, grated
1 tablespoon yellow split peas, rinsed
2 garlic cloves, peeled and minced
1 yellow onion, peeled and chopped
2 curry leaves
3 teaspoons vegetable oil
¼ teaspoon garam masala
Cilantro leaves, chopped, for serving
Directions:
Set the Instant Pot on Sauté mode, add the oil and heat it up. Add the cumin and mustard seeds, stir, and cook for 1 minute. Add the onion, garlic, split peas, garam masala, ginger, and curry leaves, stir, and cook for 2 minutes. Add the cauliflower, potatoes, and tomatoes, stir, and cook for 4 minutes. Add the wheat, salt, pepper, and water, stir, cover, and cook on Multigrain mode for 5 minutes. Release the pressure, uncover the Instant Pot, transfer the wheat and vegetables to plates, sprinkle cilantro on top, and serve.
Nutrition Values:
Calories: 145
Fat: 2
Fiber: 4
Carbs: 16
Protein: 7

627. Cracked Wheat Surprise
Preparation time: 5 minutes
Cooking time: 17 minutes
Servings: 2
Ingredients:
2 cups cracked wheat
1 teaspoon fennel seeds
2½ cups butter
2 cups light brown sugar
3 cloves
1 cup milk
Salt
3 cups water
Almonds, chopped
Directions:
Set the Instant Pot on Sauté mode, add the butter and heat it up. Add the cracked wheat, stir, and cook for 5 minutes. Add the cloves and fennel seeds, stir, and cook for 2 minutes. Add the sugar, a pinch of salt, milk, and water, stir, cover, and cook on the Multigrain setting for 10 minutes. Release the pressure, uncover the Instant Pot, divide into bowls, and serve with chopped almonds on top.
Nutrition Values:
Calories: 120
Fat: 1
Fiber: 1
Carbs: 4
Protein: 8

628. Barley Salad
Preparation time: 10 minutes
Cooking time: 20 minutes
Servings: 4
Ingredients:
1 cup hulled barley, rinsed
2½ cups water
¾ cup jarred spinach pesto
1 green apple, chopped
¼ cup celery, chopped
Salt and ground white pepper, to taste
Directions:
Put the barley, water, salt, and pepper into the Instant Pot, stir, cover and cook on the Multigrain setting for 20 minutes. Release the pressure, uncover the Instant Pot, strain the barley, and put in a bowl. Add the celery, apple, spinach pesto, and more salt and pepper, toss to coat, and serve.
Nutrition Values:
Calories: 170
Fat: 7
Fiber: 7
Carbs: 0
Protein: 5

629. Wheat Berry Salad
Preparation time: 10 minutes
Cooking time: 35 minutes
Servings: 6
Ingredients:
1½ cups wheat berries
1 tablespoon extra virgin olive oil
Salt and ground black pepper, to taste
4 cups water
For the salad:
1 tablespoon balsamic vinegar
1 tablespoon extra virgin olive oil
1 cup cherry tomatoes, cut into halves
2 green onions, chopped
2 ounces feta cheese, crumbled
½ cup Kalamata olives, pitted and chopped

½ cup fresh basil leaves, chopped
½ cup fresh parsley, chopped
Directions:
Set the Instant Pot on Sauté mode, add the tablespoon oil and heat it up. Add the wheat berries, stir, and cook for 5 minutes. Add the water, salt, and pepper, cover the Instant Pot, and cook on Multigrain mode for 30 minutes. Release the pressure for 10 minutes, uncover the Instant Pot, drain the wheat berries, and put them in a salad bowl. Add the salt and pepper, 1 tablespoon oil, balsamic vinegar, tomatoes, green onions, olives, cheese, basil, and parsley, toss to coat, and serve.
Nutrition Values:
Calories: 240
Fat: 11
Fiber: 6.3
Carbs: 31
Protein: 5

630. Bulgur Salad
Preparation time: 15 minutes
Cooking time: 12 minutes
Servings: 4
Ingredients:
Zest from 1 orange
Juice from 2 oranges
2 garlic cloves, minced
2 teaspoons canola oil
2 tablespoons ginger, grated
1 cup bulgur, rinsed
1 tablespoon soy sauce
⅔ cup scallions, chopped
⅓ cup almonds, chopped
Salt, to taste
2 teaspoons brown sugar
½ cups water
Directions:
Set the Instant Pot on Sauté mode, add the oil and heat it up. Add the ginger and garlic, stir, and cook for 1 minutes. Add the bulgur, sugar, water, and orange juice, stir, cover, and cook on the Multigrain setting for 5 minutes. Release the pressure naturally, uncover the Instant Pot, and set the bulgur aside. Heat up a pan over medium heat, add the almonds, stir, and toast them for 3 minutes. Add the orange zest, salt, soy sauce and scallions, stir, and cook for 1 minute. Add this to bulgur mix, stir with a fork, transfer to a bowl, and serve.
Nutrition Values:
Calories: 232
Fat: 7
Fiber: 6
Carbs: 38
Protein: 7

631. Bulgur Pilaf
Preparation time: 10 minutes
Cooking time: 21 minutes
Servings: 6
Ingredients:
2 cups red onions, peeled and chopped
2 tablespoons extra virgin olive oil
Salt and ground black pepper, to taste

2 teaspoons ginger, grated
¼ cup dill, chopped
1 garlic clove, peeled and minced
1½ cups bulgur
¼ cup fresh mint, chopped
¼ cup fresh parsley, chopped
3 tablespoons lemon juice
½ teaspoon cumin
½ teaspoons turmeric
2 cups vegetable stock
1½ cups carrot, chopped
½ cup walnuts, toasted and chopped
Directions:
Set the Instant Pot on Sauté mode, add the oil and heat it up. Add the onion, stir, and cook on Multigrain temperature for 12 minutes. Add the garlic, stir, and cook for 1 minute. Add the cumin, turmeric, and bulgur, stir, and cook for 1 minute. Add the ginger, stock, carrots, salt, and pepper, stir, cover and cook on the Manual setting for 5 minutes. Release the pressure, uncover the Instant Pot, add the mint, dill, parsley, lemon juice, and more salt and pepper, if needed, and stir gently. Divide among plates, and serve with almonds on top.
Nutrition Values:
Calories: 270
Fat: 12
Fiber: 8
Carbs: 38
Protein: 7

632. Israeli Couscous
Preparation time: 10 minutes
Cooking time: 8 minutes
Servings: 4
Ingredients:
½ cup red onion, chopped
½ teaspoon sesame oil
¼ cup red bell pepper, seeded and chopped
1 cup couscous, rinsed
1½ cups vegetable stock
½ teaspoon ground cinnamon
¼ teaspoon coriander
Salt and ground black pepper, to taste
2 tablespoons red wine vinegar
Directions:
Set the Instant Pot on Sauté mode, add the oil, and heat it up. Add the bell pepper and onion, stir, and cook for 5 minutes. Add the couscous, coriander, stock, cinnamon, salt, pepper, and vinegar, stir, cover, and cook on the Multigrain setting for 3 minutes. Release the pressure, uncover the Instant Pot, divide the couscous into bowls, and serve.
Nutrition Values:
Calories: 150
Fat: 1
Fiber: 5
Carbs: 33
Protein: 6

633. Millet with Vegetables
Preparation time: 10 minutes
Cooking time: 25 minutes
Servings: 4

Ingredients:
1 cup onion, chopped
2 garlic cloves, peeled and minced
½ cup oyster mushrooms, sliced
½ cup green lentils, rinsed
1 cup millet
2¼ cups vegetable stock
½ cup bok choy, sliced
1 cup snow peas
2 tablespoons parsley, chopped
2 tablespoons chives, chopped
1 cup asparagus, chopped
1 tablespoon lemon juice
Salt and ground black pepper, to taste
Directions:
Set the Instant Pot on Sauté mode, add the onions, garlic, and mushrooms, stir, and cook for 2 minutes. Add the millet and lentils, stir, and cook for 1 minute. Add the stock, stir, cover, and cook on the Multigrain setting for 10 minutes. Release the pressure naturally, uncover the Instant Pot, add the asparagus, bok choy, and peas, stir, cover, and cook on the Manual setting for 3 minutes. Release the pressure again, uncover, add the lemon juice, salt, pepper, parsley, and chives, stir gently, divide into bowls, and serve.
Nutrition Values:
Calories: 100
Fat: 1.2
Fiber: 7
Carbs: 20
Protein: 10

634. Buckwheat Porridge
Preparation time: 10 minutes
Cooking time: 6 minutes
Servings: 4
Ingredients:
3 cups rice milk
1 cup buckwheat groats
1 banana, sliced
¼ cup raisins
1 teaspoon ground cinnamon
½ teaspoon vanilla extract
Chopped nuts, for serving
Directions:
Put the buckwheat into the Instant Pot, add the milk, raisins, banana, vanilla, and cinnamon, stir, cover, and cook on Porridge mode for 6 minutes. Release the pressure for 15 minutes, uncover the Instant Pot, stir porridge, divide into bowls, and serve with chopped nuts on top.
Nutrition Values:
Calories: 400
Fat: 3
Fiber: 13
Carbs: 30
Protein: 13

635. Couscous with Chicken and Vegetables
Preparation time: 10 minutes
Cooking time: 15 minutes
Servings: 4
Ingredients:
8 chicken thighs, skinless
1½ cups mushrooms, cut into halves
1½ cups carrots, chopped
1 green bell pepper, seeded and chopped
1 yellow onion, peeled and chopped
2 garlic cloves, peeled and minced
15 ounces canned stewed tomatoes, chopped
Salt and ground black pepper, to taste
¾ cup couscous
1 zucchini, chopped
½ cup chicken stock
½ cup fresh parsley, chopped
Directions:
In the Instant Pot, mix chicken with mushrooms, carrots, bell pepper, onion, garlic, tomatoes and stock, stir, cover and cook on the Manual setting for 8 minutes. Release the pressure fast, uncover the Instant Pot, add couscous, zucchini, salt and pepper, stir, cover again and cook on Low for 6 minutes. Release the pressure again, uncover the Instant Pot, add parsley, stir gently, divide into bowls, and serve.
Nutrition Values:
Calories: 300
Fat: 10
Fiber: 3
Carbs: 35
Protein: 20

636. Creamy Millet
Preparation time: 10 minutes
Cooking time: 20 minutes
Servings: 4
Ingredients:
1 cup split mung beans
1 bay leaf
1 cup carrot, chopped
1 cup millet, chopped
1 cup celery, chopped
4 cardamom pods
6 cups water
1½ cups fresh peas
1 tablespoon lime juice
¼ cup fresh cilantro, chopped
1 tablespoon butter
1 teaspoon coriander seeds, ground
1 teaspoon fennel seeds, ground
½ teaspoon cumin seeds, ground
½ teaspoon turmeric
Salt and ground black pepper, to taste
½ teaspoon ginger, grated
Directions:
Set the Instant Pot on Sauté mode, add the mung beans, stir, and cook until they are golden. Add the millet, carrot, bay leaf, celery, cardamom, water, salt, and pepper, stir, cover, and cook on the Multigrain setting for 10 minutes. Release the pressure, uncover the Instant Pot, and set it on simmer mode. Heat up a pan with the butter over medium heat, add the coriander, fennel, cumin, turmeric, and ginger, stir, and cook for 2 minutes. Add this to the Instant Pot, stir, add more salt and pepper, peas, and lime juice, simmer for 5 minutes, divide among plates, sprinkle with cilantro, and serve.
Nutrition Values:

Calories: 231
Fat: 2
Fiber: 8
Carbs: 41
Protein: 11

637. Oats and Vegetables
Preparation time: 10 minutes
Cooking time: 15 minutes
Servings: 4
Ingredients:
1 cup steel-cut oats
1½ cups water
1 carrot, peeled and chopped
½ green bell pepper, seeded and chopped
1-inch ginger piece, peeled and grated
1 Thai green chili, chopped
2 curry leaves
¼ teaspoon mustard seeds
½ teaspoon black lentils
Onion powder
1½ tablespoons canola oil
Turmeric
Salt, to taste
Directions:
Put oats into the Instant Pot, add the water, cover, and cook on the Multigrain setting for 7 minutes. Heat up a pan with the oil over medium heat, add the mustard seeds, lentils, chili pepper, curry leaf, ginger, carrot, bell pepper, and a pinch of onion powder and turmeric, stir, and cook for 5 minutes. Release the pressure from the Instant Pot, uncover, add the oats to the pan with some salt, stir, divide into bowls, and serve.
Nutrition Values:
Calories: 211
Fat: 6.3
Fiber: 5.6
Carbs: 32
Protein: 7.5

638. Cranberry Beans and Pasta
Preparation time: 10 minutes
Cooking time: 20 minutes
Servings: 8
Ingredients:
2 cups dried cranberry beans, soaked for 8 hours and drained
7 garlic cloves, peeled and minced
6 cups water
2 celery ribs, chopped
1 yellow onion, peeled and chopped
1 teaspoon rosemary, chopped
¼ teaspoon red pepper flakes
26 ounces canned diced tomatoes
3 teaspoons dried basil
½ teaspoon smoked paprika
2 teaspoons dried oregano
Salt and ground black pepper, to taste
2 cups small pasta
3 tablespoons nutritional yeast
10 ounces kale leaves
Directions:
Set the Instant Pot on Sauté mode, add the onion, celery, garlic, red pepper flakes, rosemary, and a pinch of salt, stir, and brown for 2 minutes. Add the tomatoes, basil, oregano and paprika, stir and cook for 1 minute. Add the beans, and water, cover the Instant Pot and cook on the Bean/Chili setting for 10 minutes. Release the pressure, uncover the Instant Pot, add the pasta, yeast, kale, salt, and pepper, stir ,and set the Instant Pot on Sauté mode. Cook for 5 minutes, divide into bowls, and serve.
Nutrition Values:
Calories: 330
Fat: 14
Fiber: 10
Carbs: 32
Protein: 18

639. Cranberry Beans Mixture
Preparation time: 10 minutes
Cooking time: 15 minutes
Servings: 6
Ingredients:
1½ cups cranberry beans, soaked for 8 hours and drained
4-inch dried seaweed, sliced
4 bacon slices, chopped
Salt and ground black pepper, to taste
8 cups kale, chopped
4 ounces shiitake mushrooms, chopped
½ teaspoon garlic powder
1 teaspoon extra virgin olive oil
Directions:
Put the beans into the Instant Pot, add 2 inches water, salt, pepper, seaweed, cover and cook on the Bean/Chili setting for 8 minutes. Release the pressure, uncover the Instant Pot, transfer the beans and cooking liquid to a bowl and set the dish aside. Set the Instant Pot on Sauté mode, add the oil and heat it up. Add the garlic powder, bacon, mushrooms, salt, pepper, ¾ cup of the cooking liquid from the Instant Pot, stir well, and cook for 1 minute. Cover the Instant Pot, cook on the Manual setting for 3 minutes, and release pressure. Add the beans and kale, stir, and divide into bowls.
Nutrition Values:
Calories: 228
Fat: 2
Fiber: 14
Carbs: 41
Protein: 9

640. Quinoa and Vegetables
Preparation time: 10 minutes
Cooking time: 2 minutes
Servings: 4
Ingredients:
1½ cups quinoa
1 red bell pepper, seeded and chopped
3 celery stalks, chopped
Salt, to taste
4 cups spinach
2 tomatoes, cored and chopped
1½ cups chicken stock
½ cup black olives, pitted and chopped

½ cup feta cheese, crumbled
⅓ cup jarred pesto sauce
¼ cup almonds, sliced
Directions:
In the Instant Pot, mix the quinoa with the bell pepper, celery, spinach, stock, and salt, stir gently, cover, and cook on the Multigrain setting for 2 minutes. Release the pressure for 10 minutes, uncover the Instant Pot, add the tomatoes, pesto, and olives, stir, and transfer to plates. Add the cheese and almonds on top, toss to coat, and serve.
Nutrition Values:
Calories: 249
Fat: 7
Fiber: 5.4
Carbs: 20
Protein: 7.4

641. Mexican Cranberry Beans
Preparation time: 10 minutes
Cooking time: 20 minutes
Servings: 6
Ingredients:
1 pound cranberry beans, soaked for 8 hours and drained
3¼ cups water
4 garlic cloves, peeled and minced
1 yellow onion, peeled and chopped
1½ teaspoons cumin
⅓ cup fresh cilantro, chopped
1 tablespoon chili powder
1 teaspoon dried oregano
Salt and ground black pepper, to taste
Cooked rice, for serving
Directions:
Put the beans into the Instant Pot, add the water, garlic, and onion, cover, and cook on the Bean/Chili setting for 20 minutes. Release the pressure, uncover the Instant Pot, add the cumin, cilantro, oregano, chili powder, salt, and pepper, stir well, mash a bit using a fork, divide among plates on top of rice, and serve.
Nutrition Values:
Calories: 100
Fat: 1
Fiber: 4
Carbs: 10
Protein: 6

642. Cranberry Bean Chili
Preparation time: 10 minutes
Cooking time: 40 minutes
Servings: 8
Ingredients:
1 pound cranberry beans, soaked in water for 7 hours and drained
5 cups water
14 ounces canned tomatoes with green chilies, chopped
¼ cup millet
½ cup bulgur
1½ teaspoons cumin
2 tablespoons tomato paste
1 teaspoon chili powder
1 teaspoon garlic, minced
½ teaspoon liquid smoke
1 teaspoon dried oregano
½ teaspoon ancho chili powder
Salt and ground black pepper, to taste
Hot sauce, for serving
Pickled jalapeños, for serving
Directions:
Put the beans and 3 cups water into the Instant Pot, cover, and cook on the Bean/Chili setting for 25 minutes. Release the pressure, add the rest of the water, tomatoes with chilies, millet, bulgur, cumin, tomato paste, chili powders, garlic, liquid smoke, oregano, salt, and pepper, stir, cover, and cook on Manual for 10 minutes. Release the pressure, uncover, divide into bowls, and serve with hot sauce on top and pickled jalapeños on the side.
Nutrition Values:
Calories: 200
Fat: 13
Fiber: 4
Carbs: 14
Protein: 15

643. Lentil Tacos
Preparation time: 10 minutes
Cooking time: 15 minutes
Servings: 4
Ingredients:
4 ounces tomato sauce
½ teaspoon cumin
1 teaspoon salt
1 teaspoon garlic powder
1 teaspoon chili powder
1 teaspoon onion powder
4 cups water
2 cups brown lentils
Taco shells, for serving
Directions:
In the Instant Pot, mix the lentils with the water, tomato sauce, cumin, garlic powder, chili powder, and onion powder, stir, cover, and cook on the Bean/Chili setting for 15 minutes. Release the pressure, uncover the Instant Pot, divide the lentils into taco shells, and serve.
Nutrition Values:
Calories: 157
Fat: 4
Fiber: 8
Carbs: 24
Protein: 6.4

644. Indian Lentils
Preparation time: 10 minutes
Cooking time: 20 minutes
Servings: 4
Ingredients:
3 teaspoons butter
1 teaspoon extra virgin olive oil
1 cup red lentils
1 yellow onion, peeled and chopped
2 teaspoons cumin
¼ teaspoon coriander
¼ teaspoon garlic powder
¼ teaspoon turmeric

¼ teaspoon paprika
¼ teaspoon red pepper flakes
Salt and ground black pepper, to taste
3 cups chicken stock
Directions:
Set the Instant Pot on Sauté mode, add the butter and oil and heat up. Add the onions, stir, and cook for 4 minutes. Add the cumin, coriander, garlic powder, turmeric, paprika, and pepper flakes, stir, and cook for 2 minutes. Add the lentils and stock, stir, cover, and cook on the Bean/Chili setting for 15 minutes. Release the pressure, uncover the Instant Pot, divide into bowls, and serve.
Nutrition Values:
Calories: 198
Fat: 6
Fiber: 8.7
Carbs: 26
Protein: 10.4

645. Lentils Salad
Preparation time: 10 minutes
Cooking time: 8 minutes
Servings: 4
Ingredients:
2 cups chicken stock
1 cup lentils
1 bay leaf
½ teaspoon dried thyme
¼ cup red onion, chopped
½ cup celery, chopped
¼ cup red bell pepper, chopped
2 tablespoons extra virgin olive oil
1 tablespoon garlic, minced
½ teaspoon dried oregano
Juice of 1 lemon
2 tablespoons fresh parsley
Salt and ground black pepper, to taste
Directions:
Put the lentils into the Instant Pot. Add the bay leaf, stock and thyme, stir, cover, and cook on the Bean/Chili setting for 8 minutes. Release the pressure, uncover the Instant Pot, drain the lentils and put them in a bowl. Add the celery, onion, bell pepper, garlic, parsley, oregano, lemon juice, olive oil, salt and pepper, toss to coat, and serve.
Nutrition Values:
Calories: 165
Fat: 5
Fiber: 10
Carbs: 20
Protein: 9

646. Italian Lentils
Preparation time: 10 minutes
Cooking time: 15 minutes
Servings: 4
Ingredients:
½ cup brown rice, soaked overnight and drained
¾ cup green lentils, soaked overnight and drained
2½ cups chicken stock
1 cup tomato sauce
¾ cup onion, chopped
1 cup green and red bell pepper, chopped
2 cups chicken, already cooked and shredded
3 carrots, peeled and chopped
½ cup greens
Salt and ground black pepper, to taste
3 teaspoons Italian seasoning
2 garlic cloves, peeled and crushed
1 cup mozzarella cheese, shredded
Directions:
In the Instant Pot, mix the lentils with the rice, salt, pepper, stock, tomato sauce, onion, red and green pepper, chicken, carrots, greens, Italian seasoning and garlic, stir, cover and cook on Rice mode for 15 minutes. Release the pressure, uncover the Instant Pot, add the cheese, stir, divide among bowls, and serve.
Nutrition Values:
Calories: 186
Fat: 2
Fiber: 3.3
Carbs: 28
Protein: 14.4

647. Lentils and Tomato Sauce
Preparation time: 10 minutes
Cooking time: 20 minutes
Servings: 4
Ingredients:
1 tablespoon olive oil
1 green bell pepper, seeded and chopped
1 yellow onion, peeled and chopped
1 celery stalk, chopped
1½ cups tomatoes, chopped
Salt and ground black pepper, to taste
1 teaspoon curry powder
2 cups water
1½ cups lentils
Directions:
Set the Instant Pot on Sauté mode, add the oil and heat it up. Add the celery, bell pepper, onion, and tomatoes, stir, and cook for 4 minutes. Add the curry, salt, pepper, lentils, and water, stir, cover and cook on the Bean/Chili setting for 15 minutes. Release the pressure, uncover the Instant Pot, divide the lentils among bowls, and serve.
Nutrition Values:
Calories: 105
Fat: 3
Fiber: 4.6
Carbs: 1.7
Protein: 6

648. Chickpeas Curry

Preparation time: 10 minutes
Cooking time: 21 minutes
Servings: 6
Ingredients:
4 teaspoons cumin seeds
8 teaspoons olive oil
4 teaspoons garlic, minced
1 yellow onion, diced
2 teaspoons garam masala
2 teaspoons coriander
2 teaspoons turmeric
3 cups chickpeas, already cooked, drained and rinsed
28 ounces canned diced tomatoes
3 potatoes, cubed
½ cup water
Salt and ground black pepper, to taste
Basmati rice, already cooked, for serving
Cilantro, chopped, for serving
Directions:
Set the Instant Pot on Sauté mode, add the oil and heat it up. Add the cumin seeds, stir, and cook for 30 seconds. Add the onion, stir, and cook for 5 minutes. Add the garlic, garam masala, coriander, turmeric, tomatoes, potatoes, chickpeas, water, salt, and pepper, stir, cover and cook on the Bean/Stew setting for 15 minutes. Release the pressure, uncover the Instant Pot, divide the chickpeas onto plates, and serve with rice on the side and cilantro on top.
Nutrition Values:
Calories: 384
Fat: 8.3
Fiber: 12
Carbs: 69
Protein: 11.5

SOUPS AND STEWS

649. Creamy Kale Soup
Servings: 4
Preparation time: 10mins
Ingredients
4 stalks celery, trimmed and chopped
8 cloves garlic, peeled and minced
1 tablespoon butter
1 package (16 ouncesfrozen chopped kale
1 package (16 ouncesfrozen cauliflower florets
4 cups beef or chicken stock
1 tablespoon balsamic vinegar
Salt and freshly ground pepper, to taste
½ cup heavy cream
4 tablespoons finely grated Parmesan cheese
1 onion, diced
Directions
In Instant Pot on sauté setting, cook onion, celery and garlic in butter until slightly softened, about 2 minutes.
Add kale, cauliflower, stock and balsamic vinegar to pot and season to taste with salt and pepper.
Secure pot lid, close pressure valve and cook on high for 3 minutes. Let pressure release naturally.
Slowly pour cream into soup, stirring constantly.
Mash some of the cauliflower if desired for a thicker consistency.
Ladle soup into bowls and garnish with Parmesan cheese to serve.
Enjoy!
Nutrition Values: Calorie 175, Fats 15g, Carbs 24g, Protein 10g

650. Broccoli Cheese Soup
Servings: 8
Preparation time: 25mins
Ingredients
2 tablespoons butter
1 medium onion, diced
4 cloves garlic, peeled and minced
4 cups chicken stock
4 cups broccoli florets
1 cup heavy cream
8 ounces Colby cheese, shredded
Directions
In Instant Pot on sauté setting, melt butter and cook onion and garlic until translucent, about 5 minutes.
Add broccoli and chicken stock to pot and season to taste with salt and pepper. Secure pot lid, close pressure valve and cook on high setting for 5 minutes. When cooking time ends, carefully turn venting knob from sealing to venting position for a quick pressure release.
Add heavy cream and Colby cheese to soup and stir until cheese is melted.
Season soup to taste with salt and pepper, serve and enjoy!
Nutrition Values: Calorie 268, Fats 22g, Carbs 5g, Protein 8g

651. Broccoli Cauliflower Soup
Servings: 6
Preparation time: 40mins
Ingredients
1 small onion, diced
3 cloves garlic, peeled and minced
1 package (10 ouncesfrozen broccoli
1 package (10 ouncesfrozen cauliflower
4 cups chicken stock
1 package (3 ouncescream cheese, softened
¼ teaspoon ground nutmeg
6 ounces sharp cheddar cheese, shredded
Salt and freshly ground black pepper, to taste
1 tablespoon butter stalks celery, trimmed and diced
Directions
In Instant Pot on sauté setting, melt butter and cook celery, onion and garlic until translucent, about 5 minutes.
Add broccoli, cauliflower, chicken stock, cream cheese and nutmeg to pot and season to taste with salt and pepper.
Secure pot lid, close pressure valve and cook on high setting for 30 minutes. When cooking time ends, let pressure release naturally.
For chunky soup, serve immediately; otherwise puree soup with an immersion blender to desired texture.
Garnish servings of soup with grated cheese and enjoy!
Nutrition Values: Calorie 228, Fats 16g, Carbs 7g, Protein 9g

652. Clam and Cauliflower Chowder
Servings: 6
Preparation Time: 20 minutes
Ingredients:
3 (6.5-ouncecans chopped clams
3 tablespoons butter
1 small yellow onion
4 cups chopped cauliflower
1 ½ cups heavy cream
½ teaspoon dried thyme
Salt and pepper
Directions:
Drain the clams into a bowl and add water to the juice to make 2 cups of liquid.
Turn the Instant Pot on to the Sauté setting then add the butter and onion.
Cook for 2 minutes then add the cauliflower and clam juice.
Close and lock the lid then push the Manual button and set the timer for 5 minutes.
When the timer goes off, let the pressure vent for 3 minutes then press Cancel and do a Quick Release by switching the steam valve to "venting". When the pot has depressurized, stir in the clams and heavy cream.
Cook on the Sauté setting until heated through then season with thyme, salt, and pepper. Serve hot.
Nutrition Values: calories 250, fat 17g, protein 17g, carbs 9g

653. Turkey Soup
Servings: 4
Preparation time: 30mins
Ingredients
1 medium red bell pepper, diced

4 stalks celery, trimmed and diced
2 cloves garlic, peeled and minced
2 tablespoons butter
1-pound boneless skinless turkey thighs
Salt and freshly ground black pepper, to taste
4 cups chicken stock ½ teaspoon dried oregano
½ teaspoon dried basil
½ teaspoon dried thyme
1 large bay leaf
2 small zucchinis, diced
1 cup frozen peas
1 tablespoon fresh cilantro, minced
1 onion, diced
Directions
In Instant Pot on sauté setting, cook onion, bell pepper, celery and garlic in butter until onion is translucent, about 5 minutes. Move onion mixture to sides of pot.
Season turkey thighs to taste with salt and pepper, add to pot and cook on both sides until lightly browned, 2-3 minutes per side.
Add chicken stock, oregano, basil, thyme and bay leaf to pot and season soup to taste with salt and pepper. Secure pot lid, close pressure valve and cook on high setting for 15 minutes. When cooking time ends, carefully turn venting knob from sealing to venting position for a quick pressure release.
Remove turkey thighs from pot and dice or shred as desired. Return turkey to pot and add zucchini and peas.
Cover pot and let soup stand until zucchini and peas are warmed, about 5 minutes. Remove bay leaf from soup.
Ladle soup into bowls and garnish with cilantro. Serve and enjoy!
Nutrition Values: Calorie 259, Fats 11g, Carbs 5g, Protein 33g

654. Buffalo Chicken Soup
Servings: 6
Preparation Time: 15 minutes
Ingredients:
1 tablespoon olive oil
½ cup diced yellow onion
1-pound boneless chicken thighs, chopped (cooked
4 cups chicken broth
3 tablespoons hot sauce
6 ounces cream cheese, chopped
½ cup heavy cream
Directions:
Turn the Instant Pot on to the Sauté setting and let it heat up.
Add the oil then stir in the onion and cook for 3 to 4 minutes. Stir in the chicken, chicken broth, and hot sauce.
Close and lock the lid then press the Soup button and adjust the timer to 5 minutes. When the timer goes off, let the pressure vent for 5 minutes then do a Quick Release by pressing the Cancel button and switching the steam valve to "venting". When the pot has depressurized, open the lid.
Spoon a cup of the soup into a blender and add the cream cheese. Blend smooth then stir the mixture back into the pot with the heavy cream.
Stir until smooth then serve hot.
Nutrition Values: calories 345, fat 28g, carbs 2.5g, protein 19g

655. Ham & Asparagus Soup
Servings: 6
Preparation time: 80mins
Ingredients
1 onion, diced
4 stalks celery, trimmed and diced
2 cloves garlic, peeled and minced
1 meaty ham bone
4 cups chicken stock
2 pounds asparagus stalks
1 bay leaf
½ teaspoon dried thyme
Salt and ground black pepper, to taste
1 tablespoon butter
Directions
Melt butter in instant pot on sauté setting and cook onion, celery and garlic until softened, about 5 minutes.
Add ham bone and stock to pot and simmer for 3 minutes.
Peel and trim asparagus stalks as necessary, cut in half and add to pot with thyme. Season soup to taste with salt and pepper.
Secure pot lid, close pressure valve and cook on soup setting for about 45 minutes. When cooking time ends, let pressure release naturally.
Remove ham bone and shred ham with a fork. If desired, blend soup with an immersion blender to desired consistency.
Stir ham into soup, serve and enjoy!
Nutrition Values: Calorie 296, Fats 17g, Carbs 10g, Protein 22g

656. Hearty Beef and Bacon Chili
Servings: 4
Preparation time: 40mins
Ingredients
6 slices bacon, chopped
2 small red peppers, chopped
1-pound ground beef (80% lean
1 cup diced tomatoes
1 cup low-carb tomato sauce
2 tablespoons chili powder
1 teaspoon garlic powder
Salt and pepper
Directions:
Turn on the Instant Pot to the Sauté setting and add the chopped bacon. Let the bacon cook until it is crisp then remove it with a slotted spoon.
Add the red peppers to the pot. Cook for 5 minutes, stirring, then add the rest of the ingredients.
Close and lock the lid then press the Bean/Chili button to cook for 30 minutes. When the timer goes off, let the pressure vent for 10 minutes then press Cancel to do a Quick Release by switching the steam valve to "venting".
Open the lid when the pot has depressurized and stir in the bacon.
Season with salt and pepper to taste then serve hot.

Nutrition Values: calories 470 fat 30g, protein 38g, carbs 12g

657. Chicken Tomato Sausage Stew
Servings: 6
Preparation time: 30mins
Ingredients
1 tablespoon coconut oil
1-pound Andouille pork sausage
1 medium white onion, thinly sliced
6 cups tomatoes, chopped
4-pound chicken thighs, boneless, skinless
3 bell peppers, diced
2 celery stalks, chopped
2 cups water or bone broth
2 large carrots, chopped
6 garlic cloves, minced
/4 cup parsley, minced
1 teaspoon thyme
1 teaspoon salt
1/2 teaspoon red chili flakes, crushed
1/2 teaspoon smoked paprika
1/4 teaspoon cayenne
1/4 teaspoon black pepper hot sauce (if desired
1 bay leaf
Directions
Put coconut oil into Instant Pot. Press "Sauté" button, put sausage and chicken into Instant Pot and sauté till the meat is evenly cooked. Take out cooked meat and set aside.
Put celery, onions, bell peppers, and carrots into Instant Pot.
Press "Sauté" button and stir from time to time.
Put minced garlic into Instant Pot and continue sautéing.
Put chopped tomatoes and broth into Instant Pot. Continue sautéing until simmering.
Once cooled, slice sausage and chicken into small chunks.
Put sausage, chicken, spices and the minced parsley into Instant Pot, stir until evenly mixed.
Close the lid, and turn the vent to "Sealed".
Press "Soup" button, set the timer for 5-10 minutes and set "Pressure" to high.
Once the timer is up press "Cancel" button and turn the steam release handle to "Venting" position for quick release, until the float valve drops down.
Open the lid.
Serve warm, topped with hot sauce (if desired.
Nutrition Values: Calories 280, Fat 15g, Carb 5g, Protein 18g

658. Green Beans Soup
Preparation time: 25 minutes
Servings: 4
Ingredients:
2 tablespoons olive oil
1 shallot, chopped
1 teaspoon garlic, minced
1 red bell pepper, chopped
8 cups chicken stock
1 and ½ pounds green beans, trimmed and halved
1 cup tomatoes, chopped
1 tablespoon chili powder

1 cup coconut cream
Directions:
Set your instant pot on sauté mode, add the oil, heat it up, add the shallot and the garlic and sauté for 2 minutes.
Add the rest of the ingredients, put the lid on and cook on High for 13 minutes.
Release the pressure naturally for 10 minutes, divide the soup into bowls and serve.
Nutrition Values: calories 242, fat 22.9g, fiber 2.8g, carbs 8.9g, protein 3.7g

659. Bay Leaves Carrots Kale Chicken Soup
Servings: 4
Preparation time: 9mins
Ingredients
2 tablespoons olive oil or butter
3 carrots, peeled & cut into small bite-sized pieces
1 medium onion, chopped
2 bay leaves
4 celery stalks, cut into small bite-sized pieces
1/2 teaspoon black pepper
1 teaspoon salt
1/4 teaspoon oregano, dried
1/2 teaspoon thyme, dried
1-pound chicken breast, cooked, shredded
4 cups chicken broth + 1 cup water
1/2 teaspoon Worcestershire sauce or fish sauce
1 cup kale, chopped
Directions
Put butter or oil into Instant Pot. Press "Sauté" and add onions. Sauté for 5 minutes with the lid open, until soft.
Add oregano, thyme, pepper, salt, bay leaves, celery and carrots into Instant Pot. Keep sautéing for 1 more minute, until fragrant.
Add water and broth into Instant Pot. Close the lid and turn the vent to "Sealed".
Press "Soup", set the timer for 4 minutes and set "Pressure" to high. Once the timer is up press "Cancel" button and turn the steam release handle to "Venting" position for quick release, until the float valve drops down.
Open the lid.
Add kale and chicken into Instant Pot and let sit for 1 minute until kale turns bright green.
Add pepper, salt and fish sauce and stir to incorporate.
Nutrition Values: Calories 240, Fat 29g, Carb 4g, Protein 14g

660. Broccoli and Zucchini Soup
Preparation time: 25 minutes
Servings: 4
Ingredients:
1 shallot, chopped
2 teaspoons avocado oil
1-pound broccoli florets
1-pound zucchinis, sliced
4 cups chicken stock
1 teaspoon basil, dried
1 tablespoon cilantro, chopped
Directions:

Set your instant pot on sauté mode, add the oil, heat it up, add the shallot and sauté for 2 minutes.
Add the broccoli and the rest of the ingredients, put the lid on and cook on High for 12 minutes.
Release the pressure naturally for 10 minutes, ladle the soup into bowls and serve.
Nutrition Values: calories 70, fat 11.3g, carbs 6.7g, protein 5.3g

661. Healthy Creamy Mushroom Stew
Servings: 6
Preparation time: 40mins
Ingredients
1 celery stalk, chopped
2 Tablespoons green onions, chopped
2 garlic cloves, minced
2 cups beef stock
½ cup heavy cream
5 ounces cream cheese, softened
1 Tablespoon unsalted butter, melted
1 Tablespoon lemon juice
1 teaspoon fresh or dried thyme
2 Tablespoons fresh sage, chopped
1 bay leaf
1 teaspoon salt
1-pound cremini mushrooms, sliced
1 teaspoon fresh ground black pepper
Directions
Rinse the mushrooms, pat dry.
Press Sauté button on Instant Pot and melt the butter.
Add green onions, garlic. Cook for 1 minute.
Add mushrooms, celery, and garlic. Sauté until vegetables are softened.
Press Keep Warm/Cancel setting to stop Sauté mode.
Add remaining ingredients. Stir well.
Close and seal lid. Select Meat/Stew button. Set cooking time to 20 minutes. Once done, Instant Pot will switch to Keep Warm mode.
Remain on Keep Warm for 10 minutes.
When done, use Quick Release setting; turn valve from sealing to venting to release pressure quickly.
Open lid carefully.
Stir ingredients and serve.
Garnish with green onion, grated parmesan cheese.
Nutrition Values: Calories 150, Fat 13g, Carb 6g, Protein 17g

662. Beef Soup
Preparation time: 35 minutes
Servings: 4
Ingredients:
A pinch of salt and black pepper
1 and ½ pound beef meat, cubed
1 cup scallions, chopped
2 tablespoons olive oil
1 tablespoon sweet paprika
6 cups veggie stock
1 tablespoon parsley, chopped
Directions:
Set your instant pot on sauté mode, add the oil, heat it up, add the meat and the scallions and brown for 5 minutes.
Add the rest of the ingredients, put the lid on and cook on High for 20 minutes.
Release the pressure naturally for 10 minutes, ladle the soup into bowls and serve
Nutrition Values: calories 73, fat 7.3g, carbs 2.9g, protein 0.8g

663. Creamy Artichoke Spinach Soup
Servings: 4
Preparation time: 25mins
Ingredients
4 cups spinach
1-ounce jar artichoke hearts, drained and chopped
4 cups low-sodium chicken broth
¼ cup cheddar cheese, shredded
¼ cup mozzarella cheese, shredded
1 Tablespoon butter, melted
1 Tablespoon Italian seasoning
2 teaspoons fresh parsley, chopped
1 teaspoon salt
1 bunch of kale, stemmed and chopped
1 teaspoon fresh ground black pepper
Directions
Place all ingredients in Instant Pot. Stir well.
Close and seal lid. Press Manual setting. Cook for 15 minutes.
When done, use Quick-Release setting. Open lid carefully. Stir ingredients.
Serve.
Nutrition Values: Calories 80, Fat 9g, Carb 3g, Protein 9g

664. Spinach Soup
Preparation time: 30 minutes
Servings: 4
Ingredients:
2 teaspoons olive oil
scallion, chopped
1 celery stalk, chopped
4 cups baby spinach
4 garlic cloves, minced
teaspoons cumin, ground
6 cups veggie stock
1 teaspoon basil, dried
Directions:
Set your instant pot on sauté mode, add the oil, heat it up, add the scallion and garlic and sauté for 5 minutes.
Add the celery, cumin and the basil and sauté for 4 minutes more.
Add the spinach and the stock, put the lid on and cook on High for 10 minutes.
4.Release the pressure naturally for 10 minutes, ladle the soup into bowls and serve.
Nutrition Values: calories 37, fat 3.1g, carbs 3g, protein 1.4g

665. Cilantro Avocado Chicken Soup
Servings: 4
Preparation time: 40mins
Ingredients
4 chicken breasts, boneless, skinless
1 tablespoon coconut oil
4 avocados, peeled and chopped
4 cups chicken broth

Zest and juice from 1 lime
1 Tablespoon fresh cilantro, chopped
1 teaspoon salt
1 teaspoon fresh ground black pepper
2 tomatoes, chopped
2 garlic cloves, minced
Directions
Rinse the chicken, pat dry. Cut into strips.
Press Sauté button on Instant Pot. Melt the coconut oil.
Add chicken strips. Sauté until chicken no longer pink.
Add garlic and tomatoes. Stir well.
Press Keep Warm/Cancel setting to stop Sauté mode.
Add chopped avocados, chicken broth, lime juice, lime zest, cilantro, salt, and black pepper. Stir well.
Close and seal lid. Press Meat/Stew button on Instant Pot. Cook for 20 minutes.
Once done, Instant Pot will switch to Keep Warm mode.
Remain in Keep Warm mode for 10 minutes.
When done, use Quick-Release. Open lid carefully.
Stir ingredients. Serve.
Nutrition Values: Calories 300, Fat 20g, Carb 9g, Protein 20g

666. Broccoli Coconut Beef Curry Stew
Servings: 6
Preparation time: 50mins
Ingredients
2 1/2-pound beef stew chunks, chopped into small cubes
3 zucchinis, chopped
1-pound broccoli florets
2 tablespoons curry powder
½ cup water or chicken broth
1 tablespoon garlic power
14 oz. can coconut milk
salt to taste
Directions
Put every ingredient into Instant Pot, and stir until evenly mixed.
Close the lid, and turn the vent to "Sealed"
Press "Manual" button, set the timer for 45 minutes and set "Pressure" to high.
Once the timer is up press "Cancel" button and turn the steam release handle to "Venting" position for quick release, until the float valve drops down. Open the lid.
Add coconut milk and stir with a wooden spoon until evenly mixed. Salt to taste.
Nutrition Values: Calories 380, Fat 25g, Carb 6g, Protein 30g

667. Cabbage Soup
Preparation time: 20 minutes
Servings: 4
Ingredients:
1-pound green cabbage, shredded
1 shallot, chopped
12 cups chicken stock
1 celery stalk, chopped
1 tablespoon olive oil

A pinch of salt and black pepper
2 tablespoons dill, chopped
Directions:
Set your instant pot on sauté mode, add oil, heat it up, add the shallot and sauté for 2 minutes.
Add the rest of the ingredients, put the lid on and cook on High for 13 minutes. Release the pressure fast for 6 minutes, ladle the soup into bowls and serve.
Nutrition Values: calories 92, fat 5.4g, carbs 5.7g, protein 3.9g

668. Mouth Watering Smoked Sausage Stew & Chicken
Servings: 6
Preparation time: 30mins
Ingredients
1 tablespoon coconut oil
1 pound Andouille pork sausage
medium white onion, thinly sliced
6 cups tomatoes, chopped
3 bell peppers, diced
2 celery stalks, chopped
2 cups water or bone broth
2 large carrots, chopped
1 pound chicken thighs, boneless, skinless
6 garlic cloves, minced
1/4 cup parsley, minced
1 teaspoon thyme 1 teaspoon salt
1/2 teaspoon red chili flakes, crushed
1/2 teaspoon smoked paprika
1/4 teaspoon cayenne
1/4 teaspoon black pepper hot sauce (if desired
1 bay leaf
Directions
Put coconut oil into Instant Pot. Press "Sauté" button, put sausage and chicken into Instant Pot. Sauté till the meat is evenly cooked. Take out cooked meat and set aside.
Put celery, onions, bell peppers, and carrots into Instant Pot. Press "Sauté" button and stir from time to time. Put minced garlic into Instant Pot and continue sautéing.
Put chopped tomatoes and broth into Instant Pot. Continue sautéing until simmering. Once cooled, slice sausage and chicken into small chunks. Put sausage, chicken, spices and the minced parsley into Instant Pot, stir until evenly mixed. Close the lid, and turn the vent to "Sealed".
Press "Soup" button, set the timer for 5-10 minutes and set "Pressure" to high. Once the timer is up press "Cancel" button and turn the steam release handle to "Venting" position for quick release, until the float valve drops down. Open the
Serve warm, topped with hot sauce (if desired.
Nutrition Values: Calories 280, Fat 15g, Carb 5g, Protein 8g

669. Pomodoro Soup with Basil
Servings: 4
Preparation time: 30mins
Ingredients
2 tbsps. olive oil
½ onion, diced

tbsps. tomato paste
3 cups vegetable broth
8 ounces diced tomatoes
A handful of basil, chopped
1 tsp. balsamic vinegar
½ cup shredded Cheddar cheese
Directions
Set your Instant Pot on SAUTÉ and heat the oil in it.
Add the onions and sauté for 3–4 minutes.
Stir in the tomato paste and cook for 30–60 seconds.
Pour the broth over and stir in the tomatoes.
Close the lid and cook on SOUP for 10 minutes.
Release the pressure naturally.
Stir in half of the basil and the balsamic vinegar.
Blend the mixture with a hand blender, until smooth.
Top with the remaining basil and serve. Enjoy!
Nutrition Values: Calories 196, Fat 13.2g, Carb 8.8g, Protein 9.4g

670. Fish Stew
Servings: 6
Preparation time: 20mins
Ingredients
3 cups fish stock
1 onion, diced
1 cup chopped broccoli
2 celery stalks, chopped
1½ cups cauliflower, diced
1 carrot, sliced optional
1 pound white fish fillets, chopped
1 cup heavy cream
1 bay leaf 2 tbsps. butter
¼ tsp. pepper
½ tsp. salt
¼ tsp. garlic powder
Directions
Set your Instant Pot to SAUTÉ and melt the butter in it. Add onion and carrots (if using, and cook for 3 minutes.
Stir in the remaining ingredients.
Close the lid and hit MANUAL. Cook for 4 minutes on HIGH.
Do a natural pressure release. Discard the bay leaf. Serve and enjoy!
Nutrition Values: Calories 294, Fat 18g, Carb 6.1g, Protein 24.2g

671. Bolognese Soup
Servings: 4
Preparation time: 40mins
Ingredients
1 cup onion, chopped
½ tsp. oregano
½ tsp. thyme
1 pound ground beef
¼ cup tomato puree
14 ounces canned diced tomatoes
2 tsps. minced garlic
2 cups cauliflower, diced
3 cups chicken broth
½ tsp. pepper
½ tsp. salt
4 tbsps. olive oil
1 tbsp. chopped basil

Directions
Set the Instant Pot to SAUTÉ and heat the olive oil in it.
Add the onions and cook for about 3 minutes.
Stir in the garlic and cook for 1 more minute.
Add the beef and cook until browned.
Stir in the tomatoes and tomato puree. Cook for about 2 minutes.
Add the broth, salt, and pepper, and stir to combine, and close the lid.
Cook at high pressure for 5 minutes.
Do a quick pressure release and stir in the cauliflower.
Cook at high pressure for another 5 minutes.
Let the pressure drop naturally.
Serve topped with chopped basil. Enjoy!
Nutrition Values: Calories 411, Fat 22.5g, Carb 8.5g, Protein 40.7g

672. Keto Chili
Servings: 4
Preparation time: 45mins
Ingredients
2 tbsp. olive oil
½ tsp. cumin
2 tbsp. tomato paste
2 pounds ground beef
2 cup tomatoes, diced
1 tsp. chili powder
1 onion, diced
1 cup beef broth
1 tsp. minced garlic
Salt and pepper, to taste
Directions
Set the Instant Pot to SAUTÉ and heat the olive oil in it.
Cook the onions for about 2 minutes. Add the garlic and cook for 1 more minute.
Add the beef and cook until it is browned, breaking it with a spatula.
Stir in the tomato paste and spices and cook for 1 more minute.
Stir in the broth and tomatoes.
Close the lid and cook for 30 minutes on MEAT/STEW.
Do a quick pressure release.
Serve and enjoy!
Nutrition Values: Calories 505, Fat 33.5g, Carb 5.1g, Protein 42.7g

673. Mexican Chicken Soup
Servings: 8
Preparation time: 15mins
Ingredients
2 cups cooked and shredded chicken
4 tbsps. olive oil
½ cup chopped cilantro
8 cups chicken broth
1/3 cup salsa
1 tsp. onion powder
½ cup chopped scallions
4 ounces canned and chopped green chilies
½ tsp. minced habanero
1 cup chopped celery root

1 tsp. cumin
1 tsp. garlic powder
Salt and pepper, to taste
Directions
Place everything in the Instant Pot. Give it a good stir to combine.
Close the lid and set the Instant Pot to SOUP. Cook for 10 minutes.
When cooking is complete, use a natural pressure release.
4.Serve and enjoy!
Nutrition Values: Calories 204, Fat 14g, Carb 4.2g, Protein 14.4g

674. Pressure-Cooked Beef Stew
Servings: 4
Preparation time: 40mins
Ingredients
3 tbsps. olive oil
1 pound beef, cubed
3cups beef broth
½ onion, diced
28 ounces canned diced tomatoes
2 tsp. minced garlic
1 carrot, sliced optional
1 red bell pepper, chopped
2 tbsps. chopped parsley
1 tsp. thyme
1 bay leaf
Directions
Set your Instant Pot to SAUTÉ and heat the olive oil in it.
Add onions and cook for 3 minutes, or until softened.
Add the garlic and thyme and cook until they become fragrant, about one minute.
Add the beef and cook it until browned on all sides.
Dump the rest of the ingredients into the Instant Pot and stir to combine.
Close the lid and set the Instant Pot to MANUAL.
Cook on HIGH for 20 minutes.
When cooking is complete, wait for five minutes before releasing the pressure quickly.
Serve and enjoy!
Nutrition Values: Calories 382, Fat 25g, Carb 10.6g, Protein 26.6g

675. Lentil Spinach Stew
Servings: 4
Preparation time: 40mins
Ingredients
4 cups chicken stock
½ cup red lentils, soaked
2 cups fresh spinach, torn
2 large carrots, sliced
1 tbsp. fresh ginger, grated
2 garlic cloves, crushed
1 tbsp. oil
1 celery stalk, chopped
2 small onions, chopped
¼ cup chickpeas, drained
Salt and pepper to taste
½ tsp. garlic powder
½ tsp. onion powder
1 tsp. smoked paprika

Directions
Heat up the oil in the Sauté mode and add onions, garlic, and celery stalk.
Cook for 3-4 minutes, stirring constantly. Add carrots and season with salt, pepper, garlic powder, onion powder, and smoked paprika. Stir all well and continue to cook for another 5 minutes.
Finally, add the remaining ingredients and seal the lid. Set the steam release handle to the Sealing position and press the Manual mode.
Cook for 20 minutes on High pressure.
When done, release the pressure naturally and open the lid.
Spoon into bowls and serve immediately.
Nutrition Values: Calories 210, Fat 20g, Carb 5.2g, Protein 11.6g

676. Veal Bean Soup
Servings: 6
Preparation time: 44mins
Ingredients
2 tsps. olive oil
1 lb. black beans, soaked overnight
8 oz. lean veal tenderloin, cut into bite-sized pieces
1 cup tomatoes, diced
1 small onion, chopped
2 garlic cloves, minced
1 tsp. cumin, ground
1 tsp. tomato paste
½ tsp. cayenne pepper, ground
½ tsp. Italian seasoning
Salt Black pepper
Directions
Place the beans in a large colander and rinse thoroughly. Drain and set aside.
Cut the meat into bite-sized pieces and place in a large bowl.
Sprinkle with cumin, Italian seasoning, salt, and pepper. Mix with your hands and set aside.
Plug in the Instant Pot and grease the stainless steel insert with olive oil. Add onions and garlic.
Stir-fry for 3-4 minutes, or until translucent. Add meat and cook for 5 minutes, or until golden brown. Now, add beans and tomatoes.
Pour enough water to cover and stir in the cayenne pepper and tomato paste. Cover with a lid and adjust the steam release handle.
Press the Manual button and set the timer for 30 minutes.
Cook on High pressure. When done, perform a quick pressure release and open the pot. Optionally, garnish with some finely chopped parsley or chives before serving.
Nutrition Values: Calories 210, Fat 5.2g, Carb 2.2g, Protein 30.6g

677. Purple Cabbage Stew
Servings: 6
Preparation time: 44mins
Ingredients
1 tsp. olive oil
10 oz. purple cabbage, shredded
10 oz. beef stew meat
1 small zucchini, chopped

2 small onion, chopped
1 garlic clove, crushed
2 baby carrots, sliced
½ dried marjoram, ground
½ tsp. dried oregano, ground
1 cup beef broth
½ tsp. salt
½ tsp. red pepper flakes
Directions
Plug in the Instant Pot and grease the stainless steel insert with olive oil.
Add zucchini, onions, and garlic. Cook for 5 minutes, stirring occasionally. Now, add meat, cabbage and carrots.
Sprinkle with marjoram, oregano, salt, and red pepper flakes. Stir well and pour in the beef broth. Bring it to a boil and cook for 5 more minutes.
Add water enough to cover all and securely lock the lid. Adjust the steam release handle and press the Manual button.
Set the timer for 25 minutes and cook on High pressure. When done, perform a quick pressure release and open the pot.
Optionally, stir in 2 tbsps. Tomato paste and cook using Sauté heat setting for 5 more minutes to get a thicker stew.
Sprinkle with some grated Parmesan cheese before serving for some extra taste.
Nutrition Values: Calories 114, Fat 10g, Carb 4g, Protein 15.5g

678. Garbanzo Turkey Soup
Servings: 6
Preparation time: 50mins
Ingredients
3 cups chicken broth, reduced sodium
1 tsp. olive oil
1 lb. turkey breasts, skinless and boneless
1 cup chickpeas, soaked overnight
½ cup corn, drained and rinsed
1 cups tomatoes, diced
1 small green chili pepper, chopped
1 small carrot, sliced
1 tbsp. Taco seasoning
¼ tsp. dried thyme, ground
Salt Black pepper
Directions
Rinse the turkey breasts under running water and pat dry with a kitchen paper.
Transfer to a cutting board and trim off any excess fat. Cut into bite-sized pieces and place in a large bowl.
Sprinkle with Taco seasoning and mix well with your hands to coat. Plug in the Instant Pot and grease the stainless steel insert with olive oil.
Add turkey and cook for 5 minutes, or until golden brown.
Add chickpeas, corn, green chili pepper, and carrot. Sprinkle all with some thyme, salt, and pepper to taste and stir well.
Securely lock the lid and adjust the steam release handle and press the Manual button. Set the timer for 30 minutes and cook on High pressure.

When done, perform a quick pressure release and open the pot. Transfer to serving bowls and optionally, serve with a slice of buckwheat bread or Wasa crackers. Enjoy!
Nutrition Values: Calories 251, Fat 22g, Carb 5g, Protein 22g

679. Green Bean Soup with Beef
Servings: 6
Preparation time: 50mins
Ingredients
2 cups beef broth
1 tsp. olive oil
1 lb. green beans, chopped
6 oz. lean beef tenderloin, cut into bite-sized pieces
1 small carrot, sliced
1 medium-sized red onion, chopped
2 cups cauliflower, chopped
1 tbsp. fresh parsley, finely chopped
1 tbsp. tomato paste
¼ tsp. dried thyme, ground
½ tsp. dried basil, ground
1 tsp. salt
½ tsp. black pepper, ground
Directions
Plug in the Instant Pot and add oil to the stainless steel insert. Press the Sauté button and heat.
Add meat and cook for 5 minutes, or until browned. Now, add green beans, carrot, onion, cauliflower, and parsley.
Pour in the broth and add 2 cups of water. Stir in the thyme, basil, salt, and pepper. Securely lock the lid and set the steam release handle by moving the valve to the Sealing position.
Set the timer for 40 minutes and cook on High pressure. When done, perform a quick pressure release and open the pot.
Stir in the tomato paste and continue to cook for 5 more minutes over Sauté mode. For a creamy version, add ¼ cup of sour cream and bring it to a boil. Cook for additional 5 minutes. Enjoy!
Nutrition Values: Calories 117, Fat 6.1g, Carb 3.2g, Protein 12.7g

680. Trout Stew
Servings: 5
Preparation time: 35mins
Ingredients
2 cups fish stock
1 lb. trout fillets, cut into bite-sized pieces
1 small zucchini, cut into cubes
3 cups tomatoes, diced
¼ cup dry red wine
1 tbsp. fresh parsley, finely chopped
1 small onion, chopped
1 tbsp. all-purpose flour
½ tsp. dried oregano, ground
1 tsp. fresh basil, finely chopped
tsp. cayenne pepper
½ tsp. dried rosemary, ground
Sea salt
Black pepper
Directions

Rinse the fish and cut into bite-sized pieces. Sprinkle with salt and rosemary.
Stir well to coat all. Set aside. Plug in your Instant Pot and place the fish on the bottom of your Instant Pot. Add zucchini, parsley, and onion. Stir well and pour in the wine. Bring it to a boil and simmer for 5 minutes.
Now, add tomatoes and pour in the fish stock. Season with oregano, cayenne pepper, and black pepper. Stir well and close the lid.
Set the steam release handle and press the Manual button. Set the timer for 15 minutes and cook on High pressure.
When you hear the cooker's end signal, perform a quick pressure release and open the pot. Press the Sauté button and stir in the flour.
Cook for the next 4-5 minutes, or until the stew thickens as desired.
Transfer to a serving bowl and sprinkle with basil.
Nutrition Values: Calories 233, Fat 8.7g, Carb 6g, Protein 27.9g

681. Brisket Broccoli Stew
Servings: 6
Preparation time: 60mins
Ingredients
4 cups beef broth
1 tsp. olive oil
1 lb. lean beef brisket, boneless and chopped
2 cups broccoli, chopped
1 small onion, chopped
1 yellow bell pepper, chopped
1 medium-sized carrot, sliced
1 medium-sized potato, chopped
2 tbsps. heavy cream
1 tsp. balsamic vinegar
1 tsp. dried thyme, ground
1 tsp. smoked paprika, ground
½ tsp. Italian seasoning
½ tsp. red pepper chili flakes
Salt to taste
Directions
Plug in the Instant Pot and grease the stainless steel insert with olive oil. Press the Sauté button and add onions.
Stir-fry for 3-4 minutes, or until the onions translucent. Add meat and sprinkle with smoked paprika and salt.
Stir well and cook for 5 more minutes, stirring occasionally. Now, add broccoli, bell pepper, potato, and carrot.
Stir well and pour in the broth. Securely lock the lid and adjust the steam release handle. Press the Manual button and set the timer for 30 minutes.
Cook on High pressure. When done, perform a quick pressure release and open the pot.
Press the Sauté button and stir in the heavy cream, balsamic vinegar, thyme, paprika, Italian seasoning, red pepper chili flakes, and salt. Bring it to a boil and simmer for 5 more minutes.
Optionally, sprinkle with some finely chopped parsley before serving. Enjoy!
Nutrition Values: Calories 248, Fat 10.8g, Carb 8.6g, Protein 28.6g

682. Instant Pot Spiced Coconut Fish Stew
Servings: 4
Preparation Time: 5 Mins
Cooking Time: 30 Mins
Ingredients:
1 1/2 lb. fish fillets
1 cup coconut milk
2 tbsp. coconut oil
1 cup onion chopped
1 tbsp. garlic
1 tbsp. ginger
1/2 serrano or jalapeno
1 cup tomato chopped
1 tsp ground coriander
1/4 tsp ground cumin
1/2 tsp turmeric
1 tsp lime juice
1/2 tsp black pepper and salt
Directions
Set your instant pot on sauté mode; heat in oil and cook onion, garlic and ginger until fragrant. Add in fish and cook for 5 Mins per side or until browned and then stir in the remaining ingredients. Lock lid. Cook on meat/stew setting for 20 Mins and then let pressure come down on its own.
Nutrition Information Nutrition Values:
Calories: 190; Total Fat: 11.5 g; Carbs: 6 g; Dietary Fiber: 2 g; Sugars: 3 g; Protein: 16g; Cholesterol: 33 mg; Sodium: 458 mg

683. Instant Pot Chicken and Vegetable Stew
Servings: 4-6
Preparation Time: 15 Mins
Cooking Time: 30 Mins
Ingredients:
4 tablespoons olive oil
2 red onions, chopped
1 pound diced chicken
1 pound curly kale, torn
12 ounces baby spinach
3 cups plus 2 tablespoons water
4 cups homemade vegetable broth
1 tablespoon fresh lemon juice
1 large pinch of cayenne pepper
Salt, to taste
Directions:
In an instant pot, heat oil on sauté setting and then sauté onion and salt until fragrant. Add in diced chicken and cook for 5 Mins or until browned. Stir in the remaining ingredients; lock lid and cook on high pressure for 20 Mins. Release pressure naturally.
Nutrition Values:
Calories: 202; Total Fat: 17.4 g; Carbs: 8.3g; Dietary Fiber: 3.1g; Sugars: 2.8 g; Protein: 3.1 g; Cholesterol: 0 mg; Sodium: 109 mg

684. Ground Beef and Vegetable Stew
Servings: 6
Preparation Time: 10 Mins
Cooking Time: 30 Mins

Ingredients:
2 tablespoons olive oil
1 ½ pounds ground beef
1 onion, thinly sliced
3 cloves garlic, minced
1 bell pepper, thinly sliced
1 can roasted crushed tomatoes
1/2 cup water
2 cups bone broth
1/2 tsp smoked paprika
1 tsp oregano
1 tbsp. chili powder
1 tbsp. cumin
1/2 tsp sea salt
1/2 tsp pepper
Directions:
In an instant pot, heat oil on sauté setting and then sauté onion and garlic until fragrant. Add in beef and cook for 5 Mins or until browned. Stir in the remaining ingredients; lock lid and cook on high pressure for 20 Mins. Release pressure naturally.
Nutrition Values:
Calories: 313; Total Fat: 15.5 g; Carbs: 8.9 g; Dietary Fiber: 3.9 g; Sugars: 2.6 g; Protein: 34.4 g; Cholesterol: 101 mg; Sodium: 290 mg

685. Instant Pot Spiced and Creamy Vegetable Stew with Cashews
Servings: 4
Preparation Time: 10 Mins
Cooking Time: 19 Mins
Ingredients:
2 tablespoons olive oil
1 cup diced red onion
⅔ cups diced carrot
2 cups diced cauliflower
⅛ teaspoons dried thyme
1 ⅓ tablespoons curry powder
2 ⅔ cups vegetable broth
½ cup coconut cream
⅛ teaspoons salt
⅛ teaspoons pepper
Toasted cashews for serving
Directions
Heat oil in your instant pot and sauté red onion, cauliflower and carrots for 4 Mins; stir in spices and stock and lock lid. Cook on manual for 10 Mins and then let pressure come down naturally. Stir in coconut cream and cook on manual high for 5 Mins. Serve the stew topped with toasted cashews.
Nutrition Values:
Calories: 318; Total Fat: 27 g; Carbs: 15 g; Dietary Fiber: 4 g; Sugars: 5 g; Protein: 5 g; Cholesterol: 0 mg; Sodium: 182 mg

686. Coconut Fish Stew with Spinach
Servings: 2
Preparation Time: 5 Mins
Cooking Time: 20 Mins
Ingredients:
300g firm white fish, cubed
450g spinach, roughly chopped
100g coconut cream
2 ½ tbsp. Thai curry paste
2 tbsp. coconut oil
100ml water
Kosher salt and pepper, to taste
Directions:
Add the oil to an instant pot set on manual high. Stir in the curry paste and cook for 3 Mins to bring the spices to life.
Pour in the coconut cream and water and bring the sauce to a boil.
Add in the fish cubes and lock lid. Cook on high for 15 Mins and then let pressure come down on its own. Gently stir in the spinach and cook for 3 Mins until it wilts.
Serve hot!
Nutrition Values:
Calories: 550; Total Fat: 49.5 g; Carbs: 15.9g; Protein: 20.3g

687. Filling Herbed Turkey Stew
Servings: 2
Preparation Time: 10 Mins
Cooking Time: 25 Mins
Ingredients:
6 ounces ground turkey, cooked
2 (15-ouncecan crushed or skewed tomatoes
3 cloves garlic, crushed
2 teaspoons red wine vinegar
Pinch of parsley
Pinch of cumin
Pinch of basil
Pinch of rosemary
Pinch of red pepper flakes
1 Avocado for serving
Directions:
Set your instant pot on manual high, add in vinegar, tomatoes, and seasonings; cook for about 5 Mins. Stir in ground turkey and cook on high for 20 Mins and the let pressure come down on its own. Serve warm.
Nutrition Values:
Calories: 251; Total Fat: 30.9 g; Carbs: 10.1g; Protein: 18.

688. Low Carb Bouillabaisse Fish Stew
Servings: 6
Preparation Time: 10 Mins
Cooking Time: 40 Mins
Ingredients
1 cup dry white wine
Juice and zest of 1 orange
2 tbsp. olive oil
1 large onion, diced
2 cloves garlic, minced
1 tsp dried basil
1/2 tsp dried thyme
1/2 tsp salt
1/4 tsp ground black pepper
4 cups fish stock, chicken stock can also be used
1 can diced tomatoes, drained
1 bay leaf
400g boneless, skinless white fish fillet (ex. cod
400g prawns peeled and deveined
400g mussels in their shells
Juice of 1/2 lemon

1/4 cup fresh Italian (flat leafparsley
Directions:
Set your instant pot on manual high and heat oil; add the onion and fry all the vegetables until almost tender; add the garlic, basil, thyme, salt, and pepper. Pour in the wine and bring to a boil. Add the fish stock, orange zest, tomatoes, and bay leaf and stir to combine.
Lock lid and cook on high for 1 hour. Quick release the pressure and set on manual high; toss the fish and prawns with the lemon juice and stir into the broth in the pot. Cook for about 20 Mins and then add in the mussels right at the end and allow to steam for 20 Mins with the lid on.
Nutrition Values:
Calories: 310: Fat: 30.7g; Carbs: 4.8g; Protein: 3.7g

689. Instant Pot Thai Nut Chicken
Servings: 4
Preparation Time: 10 Mins
Cooking Time: 2 Hours
Ingredients
8 boneless skinless chicken thighs (about 2 pounds
½ cup coconut flour
3/4 cup creamy nut butter
1/2 cup orange juice
1/4 cup diabetic apricot jam
2 tablespoons sesame oil
2 tablespoons soy sauce
2 tablespoons teriyaki sauce
2 tablespoons hoisin sauce
1 can coconut milk
3/4 cup water
1 cup chopped roasted almonds or any of the other nuts on green list
Directions
Place coconut flour in a large resealable plastic bag. Add chicken, a few pieces at a time, and shake to coat. Transfer to a greased instant pot. In a small bowl, combine the nut butter, orange juice, jam, oil, soy sauce, teriyaki sauce, hoisin sauce and 3/4 cup coconut milk; pour over chicken. Lock lid and cook on high for 2 hours. Let pressure come down on its own Sprinkle with nuts before serving.
Nutrition Values:
Calories: 363: Fat: 18.2g; Carbs: 11.6g; Protein: 38.7g

690. Tasty Instant Pot Greek Fish Stew
Servings: 5
Preparation Time: 10 Mins
Cooking Time: 20 Mins
Ingredients:
5 large white fish fillets
1 large red onion, chopped
4 cloves of garlic
1 leek, sliced
1 carrot, chopped
3 sticks celery, chopped
1 can tomatoes
1/2 tsp. saffron threads
8 cups fish stock
2 tbsp. fresh lemon juice
1 tbsp. lemon zest
handful parsley leaves chopped
handful mint leaves chopped
Directions:
Combine all ingredients in your instant pot and lock lid; cook on high for 20 Mins and then release pressure naturally. Serve with gluten-free bread.
Nutrition Values:
Calories: 443; Total Fat: 18.4 g; Carbs: 9.7 g; Dietary Fiber: 1.8 g; Sugars: 3.5 g; Protein: 58.8 g; Cholesterol: 153 mg; Sodium: 871 mg

691. Pressure Cooker Vegetable and Fish Stew
Servings: 4
Preparation Time: 15 Mins
Cooking Time: 19 Mins
Ingredients
2 tbsp. extra-virgin olive oil
1 red onion, sliced
2 jalapeño peppers, seeds removed and diced
4 cups sliced green cabbage
1 carrot, peeled and chopped
4 cups crushed tomatoes
2 cup diced white fish filet
4 cup vegetable broth
3 tbsp. apple cider vinegar
2 tsp. Stevia
½ tsp. salt
¼ tsp. black pepper
Directions
Heat extra virgin olive oil in an instant pot set on sauté mode and stir in red onion, jalapenos, cabbage, and carrot; sauté for about 7 Mins or until almost tender.
Stir in tomatoes, fish, broth, apple cider vinegar, and Stevia, salt and pepper until well combined. Lock lid and cook on high pressure for 12 Mins. Let pressure come down naturally. Serve hot.
Nutrition Values:
Calories: 222; Total Fat: 19.7 g; Carbs: 13.7 g; Dietary Fiber: 5.9 g; Sugars: 6.3 g; Protein: 18.9 g; Cholesterol: 0 mg; Sodium: 112 mg

692. Easy Cheesy Turkey Stew
Servings: 5
Preparation Time: 5 Mins
Cooking Time: 25 Mins
Ingredients:
2 tbsp. coconut oil
1/2 red onion
1 lb. ground turkey
2 cups coconut milk
2 garlic cloves
1 tbsp. mustard
2 cups riced cauliflower
1 tsp salt
1 tsp. black pepper
1 tsp. thyme
1 tsp. celery salt
1 tsp. garlic powder
Directions
Melt coconut oil in an instant pot, add garlic and onion and cook until fragrant. Stir in ground turkey until crumbled.

Stir in cauliflower and spices until well mixed. Cook until meat is browned. Stir in coconut milk and lock lid. Cook on high for 20 Mins and then let pressure come down on its own. Stir in shredded cheese and serve.
Nutrition Values:
Calories: 475; Total Fat: 39 g; Carbs: 10.5g; Protein: 22.7g

693. Instant Pot Beef and Sweet Potato Stew
Servings: 6
Preparation Time: 10 Mins
Cooking Time: 25 Mins
Ingredients:
4 tablespoons olive oil
2 pounds ground beef
3 cups beef stock
2 sweet potatoes, peeled and diced
1 clove garlic, minced
1 onion, diced
1 (14-ozcan petite minced tomatoes
1 (14-ozcan tomato sauce
3-4 tbsp. chili powder
¼ tsp. oregano
2 tsp. salt
½ tsp. black pepper
Cilantro, optional, for garnish
Directions
Brown the beef in a pan over medium heat; drain excess fat and then transfer it to an instant pot. Stir in the remaining ingredients and lock lid; cook on high for 25 Mins and then release pressure naturally. Garnish with cilantro and serve warm.
Nutrition Values:
Calories: 240; Total Fat: 21.6 g; Carbs: 12 g; Dietary Fiber: 3.5 g; Sugars: 4.2 g; Protein: 30.3 g; Cholesterol: 81 mg; Sodium: 1201 mg

694. Instant Pot Coconut Fish Stew
Servings: 1 Serving
Preparation Time: 10 Mins
Cooking Time: 42 Mins
Ingredients:
1 tablespoon olive oil
1 red onion
1 tablespoon onion powder
150g tilapia filet
¼ cup coarsely chopped celery
2 cloves garlic
1 ½ cups vegetable broth
½ teaspoon parsley
½ teaspoon basil
White pepper
Sea salt
Directions:
Heat oil in your instant pot set over manual high heat; sauté onion until fragrant and then add in the fish. Cook for about 6 Mins per side or until browned. Add in the remaining ingredients and lock lid; cook on high for 30 Mins and then let pressure come down on its own.
Nutrition Values:
Calories: 237; Fat: 18.4g; Carbs: 5.4g; Protein: 23.6g

695. Instant Pot Loaded Protein Stew
Yields: 2
Preparation Time: 5 Mins
Cooking Time: 1 Hour
Ingredients:
1-pound ground chicken
2 minced cloves garlic
2 large carrots, grated
1 medium red bell pepper, diced
1 teaspoon Stevia
1/4 cup low-sodium soy sauce
1/4 tsp. crushed red pepper flakes
1/4 cup ketchup
Directions:
Combine all ingredients in your instant pot and cook on high setting for 1 hour. Shred the chicken and return to the pot.
Nutrition Values:
Calories: 262; Total Fat: 8.6 g; Carbs: 11.1g; Dietary Fiber: 1.4 g; Sugars: 7.7 g; Protein: 34.8 g; Cholesterol: 101 mg; Sodium: 1170 mg

696. Instant Pot Low Carb Mussel Stew
Servings: 4
Preparation Time: 10 Mins
Cooking Time: 1 Hour 30 Mins
Ingredients:
1kg fresh or frozen, cleaned mussels
3 tbsp. olive oil
4 cloves garlic, minced
1 Large onion, finely diced
1 punnet mushrooms, diced
2 cans diced tomatoes
2 tbsp. oregano
½ tbsp. basil
½ tsp. black pepper
1 tsp. paprika
dash red chili flakes
3/4 cup water
Directions:
Set your instant pot on manual high and fry in onions, garlic, shallots and mushrooms; stir in the remaining ingredients, except mussels. Lock lid and cook on high for 1 hour; let pressure come down and then set on manual high. Add cleaned mussels to the pot and cook for 30 more Mins
Ladle your mussels into bowls with plenty of broth. If any mussels didn't open up during cooking, toss those as well. Enjoy!
Nutrition Values:
Calories: 228; Total Fat: 9.9g; Carbs- 32.1g; Protein: 4.69g

697. Scrumptious Beef Stew
Servings: 6
Preparation Time: 5 Mins
Cooking Time: 25 Mins
Ingredients:
2 pounds beef stew meat
4 tbsp. extra virgin olive oil
3 cloves garlic, minced
1/4 cup tomato paste
4 large carrots, diced

2 medium potatoes, diced
2/3 cup chopped red onion
1 tsp. oregano
1 cup beef broth
1 ½ cups cooked peas
Directions
Heat oil u sauté mode in your instant pot; stir in meat and garlic and cook until browned. Add tomato paste, carrots, potato, onion, oregano and broth and lock lid. Cook on manual for 20 Mins and then release pressure naturally. Stir in cooked peas to serve.
Nutrition Values:
Calories: 422; Total Fat: 22.3 g; Carbs: 25.2 g; Dietary Fiber: 5.6 g; Sugars: 7.3 g; Protein: 51 g; Cholesterol: 135 mg; Sodium: 277 mg

698. Turkish Split Pea Stew
Servings: 4
Preparation Time: 10 Mins
Cooking Time: 15 Mins
Ingredients:
1 red onion, chopped
1½ tablespoons olive oil
4-5 cloves garlic, chopped
½ cup chopped tomatoes
2 cups split peas, rinsed
1 celery stick, chopped
1 medium carrot, chopped
1½ teaspoons cumin powder
1 teaspoon paprika powder
¼ teaspoon chili powder
¼ teaspoon cinnamon
6 cups vegetable stock
2 tablespoons lemon juice
1 bay leaf
½ teaspoon sea salt
Chopped scallions and chives for garnish
Directions
Turn your instant pot on sauté mode and heat oil; add onion, celery and carrots and sauté for 4 Mins. Stir in the remaining ingredients and press the cancel or warm button. Lock lid and press manual high for 10 Mins. When done, let pressure release naturally and then serve topped with chopped scallions or chives and lemon wedge.
Nutrition Values:
Calories: 205; Total Fat: 19.7 g; Carbs: 15.9 g; Dietary Fiber: 6.8 g; Sugars: 7.3 g; Protein: 5.9 g; Cholesterol: 0 mg; Sodium: 465 mg

699. Delicious Seafood Stew
Servings: 6
Preparation Time: 15 Mins
Cooking Time: 20 Mins
Ingredients:
3 tablespoons olive oil
2 pounds seafood (1 pound large shrimp & 1 pound scallops
1/2 cup chopped white onion
3 garlic cloves, minced
1 tbsp. tomato paste
1 can (28 oz.crushed tomatoes
4 cups vegetable broth
1 pound yellow potatoes, diced
1 tsp. dried basil
1 tsp. dried thyme
1 tsp. dried oregano
1/8 tsp. cayenne pepper
1/4 tsp. crush red pepper flakes
1/2 tsp. celery salt
salt and pepper
handful of chopped parsley
Directions:
Mix all ingredients, except seafood, in your instant pot and lock lid; cook on high for about 15 Mins. Quick release the pressure and then stir in seafood and continue; lock lid and cook on high for five Mins and then let pressure come down on its own. Serve hot with crusty gluten-free bread and garnished with parsley.
Nutrition Values:
Calories: 323; Total Fat: 15.3 g; Carbs: 7.7 g; Dietary Fiber: 0.8 g; Sugars: 1.9 g; Protein: 57.1 g; Cholesterol: 478 mg; Sodium: 1323 mg

700. Curried Chicken Stew
Servings: 2
Preparation Time: 20 Mins
Cooking Time: 1 Hour 40 Mins
Ingredients:
2 bone-in chicken thighs
2 tbsp. olive oil
3 carrots, diced
1 sweet onion, chopped
1 cup coconut milk
1/4 cup hot curry paste
Toasted almonds
Coriander
Sour cream to serve
Directions:
Set your instant pot to manual high setting; heat oil and cook chicken for 8 Mins or until browned. Stir in carrots and onion and cook for about 3 Mins.
In a bowl, combine curry paste and coconut milk; whisk until well blended and pour over chicken mixture.
Lock lid and cook on high for 1 ½ hours and then let pressure come down naturally.
Serve the stew topped with toasted almonds, coriander, fresh chili and a dollop of sour cream.
Nutrition Values:
Calories: 409; Total Fat: 15.5 g; Carbs: 10.7 g; Dietary Fiber: 1.9 g; Sugars: 3.4 g; Protein: 55.3 g; Cholesterol: 231 mg; Sodium: 609 mg

701. Beef Chuck & Green Cabbage Stew
Servings: 2
Preparation Time: 20 Mins
Cooking Time: 3 Hours
Ingredients:
1 packet frozen baby carrots
2 onions, roughly chopped
1 cup chopped cabbage
4 garlic cloves, smashed
2 bay leaves
4 pieces of beef chuck with marrow
Salt & pepper

1 thin diced tomato, drained
1 cup chicken stock
Directions
Place the baby carrots and chopped onions into the bottom of your instant pot. Layer the cabbage wedges on top and add the crushed garlic cloves and bay leaves.
Season the beef shanks generously with salt and pepper then add them on top of the veggies.
Pour in the diced tomatoes and broth before putting on the lid. Set the pot on high for 3 hours. Let pressure come down naturally.
Once ready, allow to cool then pack in freezer friendly bags or jars and freeze until when you are ready to eat.
Nutrition Values:
Calories: 394; Total Fat: 11.4 g; Carbs: 13.1 g; Dietary Fiber: 4.1 g; Sugars: 6.8 g; Protein: 54.6 g; Cholesterol: 152 mg; Sodium: 509 mg

702. Madras Lamb Stew
Servings: 2
Preparation Time: 25 Mins
Cooking Time: 2 Hours
Ingredients:
3 fatty lamb chops
3 tbsp. coconut milk
2 cups water
3 tbsp. Red Curry Paste
2 tbsp. Thai fish sauce
1 tbsp. dried onion flakes
2 tbsp. fresh red chilies, minced
1 tbsp. sugar
1 tbsp. ground cumin
1 tbsp. ground coriander
1/8 tsp. ground cloves
1/8 tsp. ground nutmeg
1 tbsp. ground ginger
Toppings when ready to serve:
2 tbsp. coconut milk powder
1 tbsp. red curry paste
2 tbsp. sugar
1/4 cup cashews, roughly chopped
1/4 cup fresh cilantro, chopped
Directions:
Place the raw lamb chops in an instant pot; add the coconut milk, water, red curry paste, fish sauce, onion flakes, chilies, cumin, coriander, cloves, nutmeg, and ginger.
Cover and cook on high for 2 hours.
Let the lamb curry cool completely then pack in freezer friendly bags or jars.
After thawing and heating, just before serving, whisk the coconut milk powder, curry paste and sweetener into the sauce
Break the meat into pieces and stir into the sauce together with the chopped cashews.
Garnish with fresh coriander.
Nutrition Values:
Calories: 484; Total Fat: 19.4 g; Carbs: 10.7 g; Dietary Fiber: 1.8 g; Sugars: 4.5 g; Protein: 48.8 g; Cholesterol: 223 mg; Sodium: 987 mg

703. Curried Goat Stew
Servings: 4
Preparation Time: 5 Mins
Cooking Time: 1 Hour
Ingredients:
4 goat chops
2 tbsp. olive oil
3 carrots, cut in 2-inch pieces
1 sweet onion, cut in thin wedges
1/2 cup unsweetened coconut milk
1/4 cup mild curry paste
Toasted almond
Fresh green or red chili
Directions:
Combine all ingredients in an instant pot and lock lid. Cook on high for 1 hour and let pressure come down on its own.
Serve topped with toasted almonds and a dollop yogurt.
Nutrition Values:
Calories: 423; Total Fat: 17.2 g; Carbs: 8.8 g; Dietary Fiber: 4.9 g; Sugars: 2.3 g; Protein: 31.2 g; Cholesterol: 128 mg; Sodium: 1012 mg

704. Instant Pot Lemon Chicken Stew
Servings: 2
Preparation Time: 10 Mins
Cooking Time: 1 Hour 30 Mins
Ingredients:
2 carrots, chopped
2 ribs celery, chopped
1 onion, chopped
10 large green olives
4 cloves garlic, crushed
2 bay leaves
½ tsp. dried oregano
¼ tsp. salt
¼ tsp. pepper
6 boneless skinless chicken thighs
¾ cup chicken stock
¼ cup almond flour
2 tbsp. lemon juice
½ cup chopped fresh parsley
grated zest of 1 lemon
Directions:
In your instant pot, combine carrots, celery, onion, olives, garlic, bay leaves, oregano, salt and pepper. Arrange chicken pieces on top of vegetables. Add broth and ¾ cup water. Lock lid and cook on high setting for 1 ½ hours. Let pressure come down naturally. Discard bay leaves.
In a small bowl, whisk together a cup of cooking liquid and flour until very smooth; whisk in lemon juice and pour the mixture into your pot. Cook on manual high for about 15 Mins or until thickened.
In a small bowl, mix together lemon zest and chopped parsley; sprinkled over the chicken mixture and serve. Enjoy!
Nutrition Values:
Calories: 392; Total Fat: 19.4 g; Carbs: 11.2 g; Dietary Fiber: 6.7 g; Sugars: 2.4 g; Protein: 31.2 g; Cholesterol: 103 mg; Sodium: 1213 mg

705. Hearty Lamb & Cabbage Stew
Servings: 4

Preparation Time: 15 Mins
Cooking Time: 2 hours 30 Mins
Ingredients:
2 tbsp. coconut oil
200g lamb chops, bone in
1 lamb or beef stock cube
2 cups water
1 cup shredded cabbage
1 onion, sliced
2 carrots, chopped
2 sticks celery, chopped
1 tsp. dried thyme
1 tbsp. balsamic vinegar
1 tbsp. almond flour
Directions:
Set your instant pot to manual high and heat in oil; brown in the lamb chops and then add in the remaining ingredients. Cook on high for 2 hours and then let pressure come down naturally. Remove bones from the meat.
To thicken your sauce, ladle ¼ cup of sauce into a bowl and whisk in almond flour. Return to the pot and stir well; lock lid and cook for 30 Mins on manual high.
Nutrition Values:
Calories: 384; Total Fat: 19.4 g; Carbs: 6.8 g; Dietary Fiber: 4.8 g; Sugars: 1.5 g; Protein: 38.4 g; Cholesterol: 223 mg; Sodium: 822 mg

706. Rosemary-Garlic Beef Stew
Servings: 2
Preparation Time: 15 Mins
Cooking Time: 2 Hours
Ingredients:
3 medium carrots
3 sticks celery
1 medium onion
2 tbsp. olive oil
4 cloves garlic, minced
200g beef chuck
Salt and pepper
¼ cup almond flour
2 cups beef stock
2 tbsp. Dijon mustard
1 tbsp. Worcestershire sauce
1 tbsp. soy sauce
1 tbsp. xylitol
½ tbsp. dried rosemary
½ tsp. thyme
Directions
Combine all ingredients in an instant pot and cook on high setting for 2 hours. Let pressure come down naturally.
Nutrition Values:
Calories: 419; Total Fat: 21.6 g; Carbs: 13.9 g; Dietary Fiber: 4.6 g; Sugars: 8.4 g; Protein: 39.6 g; Cholesterol: 89 mg; Sodium: 1626 mg

707. Instant Pot Oxtail Stew
Servings: 2
Preparation Time: 10 Mins
Cooking Time: 2 Hours
Ingredients:
½ pound oxtail
1 cup grated cabbage
1/2 cup grated carrots
2 large red onions, chopped
1 large bunch celery, chopped
1/2 cup diced tomatoes
2 jelly stock cubes
4 cups water
1 tbsp. crushed garlic
1 branch rosemary
2 bay leaves
Grated cheese to serve
Directions
Place all ingredients except cheese into an instant pot and cook on high setting for 2 hours. Let pressure come down naturally. Serve sprinkled with grated cheese.
Nutrition Values:
Calories: 414; Total Fat: 14.3 g; Carbs: 9.1 g; Dietary Fiber: 7.6g; Sugars: 1.4 g; Protein: 20.2 g; Cholesterol: 96 mg; Sodium: 812 mg

708. Pressure Cooked Lamb-Bacon Stew
Servings: 2
Preparation Time: 20 Mins
Cooking Time: 2 Hours
Ingredients:
2 cloves garlic, minced
1 leek, sliced
2 celery ribs, diced
1 cup sliced button mushrooms
2 Vidalia onions, thinly sliced
2 tbsp. butter
2 cups chicken stock
200g lamb, cut in cubes
4 oz. cream cheese
1 cup heavy cream
1 packet bacon – cooked crisp, and crumbled
1 tsp. salt
1 tsp. pepper
1 tsp. garlic powder
1 tsp. thyme
Directions
Set your instant pot on manual high setting and melt in butter; sear lamb meat until browned. Add in garlic, leeks, celery, mushrooms, onions, and cook for about 5 Mins; stir in the remaining ingredients and lock lid. Cook on high for 2 hours and then let pressure come down on its own.
Nutrition Values:
Calories: 365; Total Fat: 19.2 g; Carbs: 12.9 g; Dietary Fiber: 6.6 g; Sugars: 4.3 g; Protein: 21.1 g; Cholesterol: 91 mg; Sodium: 843 mg

709. Instant Pot Low Carb Vegetable Stew
Servings: 1 Serving
Preparation Time: 5 Mins
Cooking Time: 10 Mins
Ingredients
1 medium cauliflower
8 cups water
1 tsp. lemon juice
3 tsp. ground flax seeds

3 cups spinach
1 tsp. cayenne pepper
1 tsp. black pepper
1 tsp. soy sauce
Directions:
Core cauliflower and cut the florets into large pieces; reserve stems for juicing.
Add cauliflower to an instant pot and add water; lock lid and cook on high pressure for 10 Mins. Release pressure naturally and then transfer the cauliflower. Stir in the remaining ingredients and serve hot or warm.
Nutrition Values:
Calories: 198; Total Fat: 11.2 g; Carbs: 11.1 g; Dietary Fiber: 6.3 g; Sugars: 2.9 g; Protein: 1.8 g; Cholesterol: 0 mg; Sodium: 213 mg

710. Best Beef Stew for a King!
Servings: 2
Preparation Time: 15 Mins
Cooking Time: 2 Hours 10 Mins
Ingredients:
200g beef meat, cubed
1 tsp. Salt
1 tsp. pepper
1 medium onion, finely chopped
2 celery ribs, sliced
2 cloves of garlic, minced
1 can tomato paste
3 cups beef stock
2 tbsp. Worcestershire sauce
1 cup frozen mixed veggies
1 tablespoon almond flour
1 tablespoon water
Directions
Combine all ingredients except flour, frozen veggies, and water in your instant pot.
Cook on high setting for 2 hours. Let pressure come down on its own.
Stir together water and flour; stir into the pot and then add in veggies; lock lid and cook for 10 Mins.
Nutrition Values:
Calories: 368; Total Fat: 14.3 g; Carbs: 13.6 g; Dietary Fiber: 5.8 g; Sugars: 6.9 g; Protein: 44.6 g; Cholesterol: 89 mg; Sodium: 2691 mg

DESSERTS

711. Keto Mocha Brownies
Preparation Time: 45 Minutes
Servings: 6
Ingredients:
For the base:
6 eggs; separated
3 tbsp butter; unsalted
2 tsp baking powder
1 ½ cup swerve
1 ½ cups of almond flour
1/4 tsp salt
For the topping:
1 ½ cup swerve or stevia crystal
2 butter sticks; unsalted
1/4 cup black coffee; unsweetened
5 egg yolks
Directions:
Place egg whites in a large mixing bowl and beat on medium speed until light and fluffy. Add swerve, almond glour, melted butter, baking powder, and salt. Beat well on medium-high speed until completely incporporated
Line a small cake pan with some parchment paper and add the batter. Tightly wrap with aluminum foil and set aside
Plug in the instant pot and position a trivet at the bottom of the inner pot. Pour in some water and add the cake pan
Securely seal the lid and set the steam release handle to the *Sealing* position. Press the *Manual* button and set the timer for 15 minutes on high pressure
When done; perform a quick pressure release and open the lid. Remove the pan from the pot and set aside to cool
Now place a steam basket in the stainless steel insert and pour in some more water, Set aside
In a large mixing bowl, combine together the filling ingredients. With a whisking attachment on, beat well on medium-high speed for 2 - 3 minutes
Pour the mixture into an oven-safe bowl and wrap with aluminum foil. Place the bowl in the steam basket and seal the lid.
Set the steam release handle and cook for 4 minutes on the *Manual* mode
When you hear the cooker's end signal, perform a quick pressure release and open the lid. Remove the bowl from the pot and chill for a while
Pour the mixture over the crust and cool to a room temperature. Refrigerate for at least an hour before serving.
Nutrition Values: Calories: 236; Total Fats: 21.1g; Net Carbs: 2.3g; Protein: 9.4g; Fiber: 0.8g

712. Keto Raspberry Cheesecake
Preparation Time: 2 hours 20 Minutes
Servings: 6
Ingredients:
1 cup almond flour
1/4 cup almond butter
5 eggs
3 tsp stevia powder
1/4 cup sunflower seeds
1/4 tsp salt
For the filling:
4 tbsp stevia powder
3 cups cream cheese
1 tsp raspberry extract
1/2 cup heavy cream
1 tsp agar powder
Directions:
Line a fitting springform pan with some parchment paper and grease the walls with some cooking spray, Set aside
In a large mixing bowl, combine almond flour, sunflower seeds, stevia, and salt. Using a spatula, mix until well incorporated, Set aside
In a separate bowl, combine eggs and butter. With a whisking attachment on, beat with a hand mixer for 3 - 4 minutes.
Now; pour egg mixture into dry ingredients. With a paddle attachment on, beat until combined.
Transfer the dough mixture to the springform pan and spread evenly, Set aside
In a large mixing bowl, combine all filing ingredients and beat for 3 minutes with a hand mixer. Pour the filling over the crust
Plug in the instant pot and pour 1 cup of water in the stainless steel insert. Set the trivet on the bottom. Place the springform pan on the top and seal the lid. Adjust the steam release handle and press the *Slow Cook* button. Set the timer for 2 hours and cook on *Low* pressure
When you hear the cooker's end signal, perform a quick pressure release and open the pot. Transfer the pan to a wire rack and let it chill for at least an hour. Refrigerate for 30 minutes before serving.
Optionally, top with some fresh raspberries.
Nutrition Values: Calories: 535; Total Fats: 51.4g; Net Carbs: 4.5g; Protein: 15.1g; Fiber: 0.7g

713. Choco Cinnamon Cake
Preparation Time: 45 Minutes
Servings: 8
Ingredients:
1 cup coconut flour
1/2 cup granulated stevia
1/2 cup almonds; minced
4 tbsp almond butter
1/2 cup cream cheese
1 tbsp unsweetened cocoa powder
2 large eggs
1/4 tsp apple pie spice
1/4 tsp cinnamon; ground
1/4 tsp salt
Directions:
Combine coconut flour, almonds, granulated stevia, salt, cinnamon, and apple pie spice in a large mixing bowl. Using a spatula, mix until combined
Gradually, add eggs, butter, and cream cheese. Beat with a hand mixer until well incorporated.
Plug in your instant pot and pour 1 cup of water in the stainless steel insert. Set the trivet on the bottom. Line a fitting springform pan with some parchment paper and grease the walls with some cooking spray.

Pour in the mixture and cover the top with some aluminum foil
Set the pan on top of the trivet and close the lid. Adjust the steam release handle and press the *Manual* button. Set the timer for 35 minutes on *High* pressure
When you hear the cooker's end signal, perform a quick pressure release and open the pot. Using oven mitts, remove the pan to a wire rack and let it cool completely
Sprinkle with cocoa and enjoy!
Nutrition Values: Calories: 285; Total Fats: 20.5g; Net Carbs: 7.9g; Protein: 10.4g; Fiber: 10.4g

714. Delicious Raspberry Muffins with Chocolate Topping
Preparation Time: 45 Minutes
Servings: 6
Ingredients:
1 cup fresh raspberries
1/4 cup coconut butter; melted
1 cup almond flour
1/4 cup granulated stevia
2 large eggs
1 tsp vanilla extract
1/4 cup whole milk
1 tsp baking powder
1/4 tsp salt
For the topping:
1/4 tsp cinnamon; ground
1/4 cup dark chocolate chips; melted
1/4 cup butter
Directions:
In a large mixing bowl, combine almond flour, stevia, baking powder, and salt. Mix until combined and set aside
In a separate bowl, combine eggs, milk, and vanilla extract. Beat with a hand mixer until fluffy
Now; add the wet ingredients to the bowl with dry ingredients. Mix until you get a thick batter. Add raspberries and stir with a spatula
Pour the mixture in silicone muffin molds and set aside
Plug in the instant pot and pour 1 cup of water in the stainless steel insert. Set the trivet on the bottom and place molds on top.
Close the lid and adjust the steam release handle. Press the *Manual* button and set the timer for 30 minutes. Cook on *High* pressure
Meanwhile; combine all topping ingredients in a mixing bowl. Beat with a mixer until all well combined and creamy, Set aside
When you hear the cooker's end signal, perform a quick pressure release and open the pot.
Carefully transfer the muffins to a wire rack and let it cool completely
Using a pipping bag, swirl the mixture over each muffin. Refrigerate for 15 minutes before serving.
Nutrition Values: Calories: 193; Total Fats: 14.7g; Net Carbs: 4.2g; Protein: 7.1g; Fiber: 4.4g

715. Amazing Keto Almond Coffee Cups
Preparation Time: 45 Minutes
Servings: 4
Ingredients:
For the crust:
1 cup almonds; minced
2 large eggs
1/2 cup shredded coconut
1 tbsp butter; softened
1/2 tsp vanilla extract
For the filling:
2 tsp stevia powder
1 tsp xanthan gum
1 cup heavy whipping cream
1 tsp instant black coffee; unsweetened
Directions:
First, prepare the topping. Plug in the instant pot and combine all filling ingredients in the stainless steel insert. Press the *Saute* button and gently stir. Cook for 2 - 3 minutes without boiling. Turn off the pot and transfer all to a large bowl. Refrigerate for 30 minutes. Clean the pot and set aside
Now; combine almonds and coconut in a large bowl. Mix with a spatula and add eggs. Using a hand mixer, beat until well combined. Add butter and vanilla extract. Beat again ntil well combined
Divide the mixture evenly between silicone muffin molds. Press with your fingers to form cups.
Pour 1 cup of water in the stainless steel insert and set the trivet on the bottom. Place the silicone molds on top and close the lid. Adjust the steam release handle and press the *Manual* button. Set the timer for 30 minutes and cook on *High* pressure
When done; perform a quick release of the pressure and open the pot. Transfer to a wire rack to cool completely. Spoon the filling onto each crust and refrigerate for 1 hour before serving.
Optionally, top with some fresh raspberries.
Nutrition Values: Calories: 339; Total Fats: 31.7g; Net Carbs: 3.8g; Protein: 9.2g; Fiber: 3.9g

716. Keto Cherry Mousse
Preparation Time: 15 Minutes
Servings: 6
Ingredients:
1 ½ cup whipping cream
1/4 cup erythritol
5 large egg yolks; beaten
1/2 cup whole milk
1/2 cup coconut cream
1 tbsp pecans; minced
2 tsp cherry extract
1/2 tsp salt
Directions:
Combine whipping cream, egg yolks, erytthritol, milk, salt, and coconut cream in a medium-sized saucepan over a medium-high heat. Stir well and heat up without boiling. Remove from the heat and pour the mixture into oven-safe ramekins. Sprinkle with minced pecans and wrap each ramekin with aluminum foil, Set aside
Plug in your instant pot and pour 1 cup of water in the stainless steel insert. Set the trivet on the bottom and place the ramekins on top

Securely lock the lid and adjust the steam release handle by moving the valve to the *Sealing* position. Set the timer for 7 minutes on *Manual* mode
When you hear the cooker's end signal, perform a quick pressure release and open the pot. Transfer the ramekins to a wire rack and let it cool completely
Refrigerate for at least an hour before serving.
Nutrition Values: Calories: 223; Total Fats: 21.8g; Net Carbs: 13.2g; Protein: 4.5g; Fiber: 0.9g

717. Chocolate Chip Pudding
Preparation Time: 10 Minutes
Servings: 4
Ingredients:
1 cup unsweetened almond milk
2 tbsp chocolate chips; sugar-free
1 tbsp agar powder
1 ¼ cup whipping cream
1/2 cup coconut cream
1/4 cup swerve
1/4 cup almonds; finely chopped.
2 tbsp cocoa powder; unsweetened
1 tsp vanilla extract
Directions:
Plug in the instant pot and pour in the milk. Press the *Saute* button and heat up. Add swerve, cocoa powder, coconut cream, and vanilla extract.
Bring it to a boil, stirring constantly, and then add agar powder. Continue to cook for 1 - 2 minutes.
Press the *Cancel'* button and stir in finely chopped almonds
Transfer the mixture to a large mixing bowl and pour in the whipping cream. Beat well on high speed for 2 - 3 minutes.
Finally, divide the mixture between serving bowls and cool completely before serving.
Nutrition Values: Calories: 257; Total Fats: 24.5g; Net Carbs: 6.5g; Protein: 3.9g; Fiber: 2.9g

718. Tasty Crumbled Lemon Muffin Parfait
Preparation Time: 40 Minutes
Servings: 6
Ingredients:
1/4 cup almond flour
4 tbsp unsweetened raw cocoa
1/2 tsp baking powder
3 tbsp granulated stevia
1 tsp vanilla extract
2 large eggs
1/4 cup almond butter
For the creamy filling:
1 tsp lemon extract
1 tsp stevia powder
1 cup cream cheese
1/4 cup whipping cream
Directions:
In a large mixing bowl, combine almond flour, stevia, cocoa, and baking powder. Stir well and set aside
In a separate bowl, combine eggs, butter, and vanilla extract. Beat with a hand mixer until well combined.
Now; add this mixture to the dry ingredients and mix well. Divide the mixture evenly between muffin molds and set aside

Plug in the instant pot and pour 1 cup of water in the stainless steel insert. Set the trivet on the bottom and place the molds on top. Close the lid and adjust the steam release handle. Press the *Manual* button and set the timer for 20 minutes on *High* pressure
Meanwhile; combine all filling ingredients in a large bowl. Beat with a hand mixer until smooth and creamy, Set aside
When you hear the cooker's end signal, perform a quick pressure release and open the pot. Transfer the molds to a wire rack and let it cool completely
Crumble the muffins into small pieces. Make a 1-inch thick layer with a muffin crumbles and top with 1-inch thick creamy filling. Repeat the process with the remaining mixture. Optionally, sprinkle the top with lemon zest.
Refrigerate for 1 hour before serving.
Nutrition Values: Calories: 216; Total Fats: 19.8g; Net Carbs: 3g; Protein: 6.9g; Fiber: 1.7g

719. Sweet Potato & Cinnamon Patties
Preparation Time: 30 Minutes
Servings: 4
Ingredients:
1 small sweet potato; cubed
1 tbsp psyllium husk powder
1/2 cup Mascarpone
1/2 cup almond flour
3 tbsp granulated stevia
1/4 cup flaxseed meal
3 tbsp coconut oil; softened
1/2 tsp cinnamon powder
1 tsp vanilla extract
Directions:
Plug in the instant pot and add potatoes. Pour in enough water to cover and seal the lid. Set the steam release handle and cook for 3 minutes on the *Manual* mode
When done; perform a quick pressure release and open the lid
Remove potatoes from the pot and drain. Cool for a while and transfer to a food processor along with the remaining ingredients. Process until smooth.
Now press the *Saute* button and grease the inner pot with some oil. Add about 1/4 cup of the potato mixture and cook for 3 - 4 minutes on one side
Gently turn over and continue to cook for another 2 minutes.
Repeat the process with the remaining mixture
Optionally, sprinkle with some granulated stevia before serving.
Nutrition Values: Calories: 213; Total Fats: 18.1g; Net Carbs: 4g; Protein: 5.8g; Fiber: 2.8g

720. Keto Coconut Bars
Preparation Time: 25 Minutes
Servings: 6
Ingredients:
2 cups shredded coconut
1 tbsp chia seeds
1/4 cup flaxseed meal
1/2 cup coconut oil
1 tbsp sesame seeds

1/4 cup almonds; finely chopped.
2 tbsp almond butter
3 large eggs
2 tbsp granulated stevia
1 tsp vanilla extract
1/4 tsp salt

Directions:
Combine the ingredients in a large bowl and mix until a lightly sticky mixture forms. Optionally, add some more stevia and set aside
Line a small baking pan with some parchment paper and lightly grease with some coconut oil. Add the mixture and press well with the palms of your hands to flatten the surface as evenly as possible
Loosely cover with aluminum foil and set aside
Plug in the instant pot and set the trivet at the bottom of the inner pot. Pour in two cups of water and place the baking pan
Seal the lid and set the steam release handle to the *Sealing* position. Cook for 15 minutes on the *Manual* mode
When done; perform a quick pressure release and open the lid. Remove the pan and cool to a room temperature before slicing into bars.
Refrigerate for one hour before serving.
Nutrition Values: Calories: 376; Total Fats: 36.8g; Net Carbs: 2.9g; Protein: 7.2g; Fiber: 4.9g

721. Chocolate Bounties
Preparation Time: 20 Minutes
Servings: 5
Ingredients:
1 cup shredded coconut
1/2 cup heavy whipping cream
2 tbsp unsweetened cocoa powder
4 tbsp butter
1 tbsp hazelnuts; minced
1 tsp vanilla extract
1 tsp stevia powder
1/4 tsp salt
For the coating:
1 tsp lemon zest; freshly grated
1 tbsp shredded coconut
1 cup dark chocolate; 80% cocoa
2 tbsp heavy cream

Directions:
Plug in your instant pot and add butter to the stainless steel insert. Press the *Saute* button and stir with a wooden spatula until melts.
Add heavy whipping cream, cocoa, vanilla extract, and stevia powder. Heat up without boiling. Stir constantly
Turn off the pot and transfer all to a large mixing bowl. Add shredded coconut, salt, and hazelnuts. Mix until well combined and set aside
Clean the stainless steel insert and pour in 1 cup of water. Set the trivet on the bottom.
Combine chocolate, heavy cream, and lemon zest in an oven-safe ramekin. Place the ramekin on the top of the trivet and close the lid. Adjust the steam release handle and press the *Manual* button. Cook for 2 minutes on *High* pressure
When done; perform a quick pressure release and open the pot

Coat the walls of your ice tray with some chocolate. Fill with coconut mixture and then top with the remaining chocolate. Sprinkle with cconut and set aside to cool completely
Refrigerate for 2 hours before serving.
Nutrition Values: Calories: 236; Total Fats: 22.7g; Net Carbs: 6.4g; Protein: 2.1g; Fiber: 2.9g

722. Lemon Cake
Preparation Time: 45 Minutes
Servings: 8
Ingredients:
For the cake:
3 cups almond flour
3 tsp baking powder
2 tsp lemon extract
1/4 cup butter; softened
5 large eggs
3 tbsp stevia powder
1/4 cup coconut milk; full-fat
1 tbsp coconut cream
1/4 tsp salt
For the syrup:
1 tbsp lemon juice; freshly squeeze
1/4 cup granulated stevia
1/4 cup raspberries
1/4 cup blueberries

Directions:
In a large mixing bowl, combine together almond flour, stevia powder, baking powder, and salt.
Mix well and add eggs, one at the time, beating constantly
Now add coconut milk, coconut cream, butter, and lemon extract. Using a paddle attachment beat for 3 minutes on medium speed
Grease a small cake pan with some oil and line with parchment paper. Pour the mixture in it and tightly wrap with aluminum foil.
Plug in the instant pot and set the trivet at the bottom of the inner pot. Place the cake pan on top and pour in one cup of water.
Seal the lid and set the steam release handle to the *Sealing* position. Press the *Manual* button and cook for 25 minutes
When done; perform a quick pressure release and open the lid. Carefully remove the pan and set aside
Now press the *Saute* button. Add berries and pour in one cup of water and granulated stevia. Gently simmer for 5 - 6 minutes, stirring constantly
Finally, add agar powder and give it a good stir. Cook until the mixture thickens.
Pour the syrup over chilled cake and refrigerate for 2 hours before serving.
Nutrition Values: Calories: 186; Total Fats: 16g; Net Carbs: 3.8g; Protein: 6.4g; Fiber: 1.3g

723. Choco Orange Muffins
Preparation Time: 45 Minutes
Servings: 5
Ingredients:
1/2 cup almond flour
5 large eggs
1/4 cup almonds; roughly chopped.
1 tbsp chia seeds

1 tbsp flaxseed meal
1/2 cup whole milk
1 tbsp butter
1 tbsp dark chocolate chips
1/2 tsp baking powder
1/4 tsp bicarbonate of soda
1/4 tsp cinnamon; ground
1 tsp orange extract
2 tsp stevia powder
Directions:
In a large mixing bowl, combine almond flour, almonds, chia seeds, flaxseed meal, baking powder, and bicarbonate of soda. Mix until well combined. Add eggs, butter, milk, orange extract, stevia, and cinnamon. With a paddle attachment on, beat with a hand mixer for 2 - 3 minutes, or until well incorporated
Divide the mixture evenly between greased silicone muffin molds. Tuck in the chocolate chips and set aside
Plug in the instant pot and set the trivet on the bottom. Place the molds on top and close the lid. Adjust the steam release handle and press the *Manual* button. Set the timer for 30 minutes and cook on *High* pressure
When done; perform a quick pressure release and open the pot. Transfer the molds to a wire rack and let it cool to a room temperature
Nutrition Values: Calories: 246; Total Fats: 18.3g; Net Carbs: 4.9g; Protein: 11.8g; Fiber: 4.2g

724. Rum Cheesecake
Preparation Time: 30 Minutes
Servings: 10
Ingredients:
2 cups almond flour
3 cups Mascarpone
4 large eggs; separated
1/4 cup coconut cream
1 cup plain Greek yogurt
2 - 3 drops stevia
2 tbsp almond butter
1/4 cup cocoa powder; unsweetened
1/4 cup swerve
3 tsp baking powder
1/2 tsp cinnamon powder
2 tsp rum extract
Directions:
Plug in the instant pot and position a trivet. Pour in one cup of water in the stainless steel insert and set aside
Beat egg whites and swerve with a hand mixer until light foam appears. Add egg yolks, coconut cream, almond butter, baking powder, and cocoa powder, beating constantly
Finally, add almond flour and continue to beat until completely combined
Pour the mixture into lightly greased cake pan and cook for 15 minutes on the *Manual* mode
When done; perform a quick pressure release and open the lid. Remove the cake from the pan and cool for a while

Now combine Mascarpone and Greek yogurt. Add rum extract, cinnamon powder, and stevia. Using a hand mixer, mix well until completely combined
Pour the mixture over the crust and refrigerate for a couple of hours before slicing.
Nutrition Values: Calories: 247; Total Fats: 18.1g; Net Carbs: 5.6g; Protein: 15.6g; Fiber: 1.7g

725. Yummy Vanilla Mint Cake
Preparation Time: 45 Minutes
Servings: 6
Ingredients:
1/2 cup almond flour
3 tbsp granulated stevia
1/2 tsp vanilla extract
5 large eggs yolks
1/4 cup butter
1 tbsp unsweetened cocoa powder
1/2 tsp baking powder
1/4 tsp salt
For the icing:
1 tsp mint extract
1 tbsp shredded dark chocolate; 80% cocoa
2 tbsp butter; softened
5 large egg whites
1/4 cup raspberries; for topping
Directions:
First, line a fitting springform pan for your instant pot with some parchment paper. Grease the inside walls with some cooking spray and set aside
Combine almond flour, granulated stevia, cocoa powder, baking powder, and salt in a large bowl. Using a kitchen spatula, stir to combine, Set aside
In a separate mixing bowl, combine butter, egg yolks, and vanilla extract. Beat using a stand mixer for 3 minutes
Now; stir in the wet ingredients into dry ingredients. Continue to beat until all well incorporated. Pour the mixture into previously prepared pan.
Plug in the instant pot and pour 1 cup of water in the stainless steel insert. Set the trivet on the bottom and place the pan on top
Securely lock the lid and adjust the steam release handle. Press the *Manual* button and set the timer for 30 minutes. Cook on *High* pressure
Meanwhile; combine icing ingredients in a large bowl. Whisk for 3.4 minutes, or until smooth and creamy. Fill the pipping bag with this mixture and set aside
When you hear the cooker's end signal, perform a quick pressure release and open the pot. Transfer the cake to wire rack and let it cool completely
Decorate the cake with icing and top with raspberries.
Nutrition Values: Calories: 274; Total Fats: 24.1g; Net Carbs: 3.2g; Protein: 10.1g; Fiber: 1.7g

726. Strawberry Pancakes
Preparation Time: 45 Minutes
Servings: 3
Ingredients:
1 cup cream cheese
5 large eggs
1/2 tbsp psyllium husk powder
1 tsp vanilla extract

1/4 cup coconut flour
2 tbsp butter
1/4 tsp salt
For the topping:
1/2 tsp stevia powder
1/2 strawberry extract
1 cup whipped cream
Directions:
In a large mixing bowl, combine coconut flour, psyllium husk powder, and salt. Mix well and then gradually add eggs. Beat with an electric mixer for 3 minutes
Now; add butter, cream cheese, and vanilla extract. Continue to beat until all well combined, Set aside
Plug in the instant pot and grease the stainless steel insert with some cooking spray. Pour about 1/3 of the mixture in the pot and close the lid. Adjust the steam release handle and press the *Manual* button. Set the timer for 3 minutes. Cook on *High* pressure
When done; perform a quick pressure release and carefully transfer to a large plate. Repeat the process with the remaining mixture
Now; prepare the topping. Combine all ingredients in a large bowl and mix until well combined. Divide the mixture evenly and top each pancake
Nutrition Values: Calories: 618; Total Fats: 156.3g; Net Carbs: 6.7g; Protein: 18.6g; Fiber: 4g

727. Keto Vanilla Cherry Panna Cotta
Preparation Time: 15 Minutes
Servings: 2
Ingredients:
For the vanilla layer:
1 cup heavy whipping cream
1/2 tsp vanilla extract
1 tbsp walnuts; roughly chopped.
2 tbsp whole milk
1 tsp agar powder
For the cherry layer:
1 tbsp almonds; roughly chopped.
2 tsp cherry extract
1 cup heavy whipping cream
1 tsp agar powder
Directions:
Plug in the instant pot and combine all vanilla layer ingredients in the stainless steel insert. Press the *Saute* button and stir constantly. Bring it to a light simmer and then press *Cancel'* button. Transfer to a large bowl and set aside
Clean the pot and pat-dry with a kitchen paper. Now; add all cherry layer ingredients and stir well. Again, bring it to a light simmer, stirring constantly
Pour about 1/2-inch thick vanilla layer in a medium-sized glass. Now; add the second layer of the cherry mixture. Repeat the process until you have used both mixtures
Optionally, garnish with some fresh mint and refrigerate for at least 1 hour before serving.
Nutrition Values: Calories: 467; Total Fats: 48.7g; Net Carbs: 4.6g; Protein: 4.5g; Fiber: 0.8g

728. Delicious Vanilla Cream with Raspberries
Preparation Time: 10 Minutes
Servings: 4
Ingredients:
1 ½ cup coconut milk; full-fat
1 tbsp almond flour
2 tbsp butter
1/4 cup raspberries
3 egg yolks
3 tbsp swerve
1 tbsp agar powder
1 vanilla bean
2 tsp vanilla extract
Directions:
Using a sharp paring knife, slice the vanilla bean lengthwise and remove the seeds, Set aside
Plug in the instant pot and press the *Saute* button. Grease the inner pot with butter and add coconut milk. Warm up, stirring constantly, and then add egg yolks, swerve, and vanilla extract
Cook for 3 - 4 minutes, stirring constantly
Finally, add agar powder, and vanilla seeds. Give it a good stir and continue to cook for another couple of minutes, or until the mixture thickens.
Press the *Cancel'* button and remove the cream from the pot. Divide between serving bowls and optionally top with some whipped cream or fresh strawberries.
Plug in the instant pot and pour in the milk. Press the *Saute* button and heat up. Add swerve, cocoa powder, coconut cream, and vanilla extract.
Bring it to a boil, stirring constantly, and then add agar powder. Continue to cook for 1 - 2 minutes. Press the *Cancel'* button and stir in finely chopped almonds.
Transfer the mixture to a large mixing bowl and pour in the whipping cream. Beat well on high speed for 2 - 3 minutes.
Finally, divide the mixture between serving bowls and top each with raspberries. Serve cold.
Nutrition Values: Calories: 302; Total Fats: 30.7g; Net Carbs: 3.9g; Protein: 4.2g; Fiber: 2.7g

729. Keto Mocha de Creme
Preparation Time: 25 Minutes
Servings: 4
Ingredients:
2 large eggs; separated
1 cup coconut milk; full-fat
3 tbsp brewed espresso
3 tbsp stevia powder
¾ cup heavy cream
2 tbsp cocoa powder; unsweetened
1 tsp vanilla extract
1/4 tsp salt
Directions:
In a small bowl, whisk together eggs, cocoa powder, espresso, stevia powder, vanilla, and salt, Set aside
Plug in the instant pot and press the *Saute* button. Pour in the coconut milk and heavy cream. Give it a good stir and warm up
Press the *Cancel* button and slowly pour the warm milk mixture over the egg mixture, whisking constantly
Divide the mixture between 4 ramekins and loosely cover with aluminum foil.

Position a trivet at the bottom of your pot and pour in 2 cups of water. Gently place the ramekins on top and seal the lid
Set the steam release handle to the *Sealing* position and press the *Manual* button.
Cook for 15 minutes.
When done; perform a quick pressure release and open the lid. Remove the ramekins and transfer to a wire rack. Cool to a room temperature and then refrigerate for about an hour.
Nutrition Values: Calories: 257; Total Fats: 25.5g; Net Carbs: 3.5g; Protein: 5.5g; Fiber: 2.1g

730. Keto Mint Brownies
Preparation Time: 35 Minutes
Servings: 6
Ingredients:
¾ cup almond flour
2 tbsp butter
1/2 cup Mascarpone
1/2 cup flaxseed meal
4 large eggs
1/4 cup swerve
3 tbsp hazelnuts; finely chopped.
1 tsp mint extract
1/4 tsp salt
Directions:
Combine the ingredients in a large mixing bowl and beat well on medium speed until fully incorporated and smooth.
Line a small cake pan with parchment paper and brush with some oil. Pour in the batter and loosely cover with aluminum foil
Plug in the instant pot and set the trivet in the inner pot. Pour in about one cup of water and place the cake pan on top
Seal the lid and set the steam release handle to the *Sealing* position. Press the *Manual* button and set the timer for 25 minutes.
When done; perform a quick pressure release and open the lid. Carefully remove the pan from the pot and chill for a while
Slice into 8 brownies and serve
Nutrition Values: Calories: 203; Total Fats: 15.8g; Net Carbs: 1.6g; Protein: 9.4g; Fiber: 3.1g

731. Creamy Keto Coconut Cake
Preparation Time: 35 Minutes
Servings: 10
Ingredients:
2 cups coconut flour
1/4 cup granulated stevia
2 cups whipping cream; sugar-free
3 tsp baking powder
1 cup coconut cream
5 large eggs
3 tbsp hazelnuts; finely chopped.
1/4 cup almond flour
3 tbsp shredded coconut
2 tsp vanilla extract
Directions:
Plug in the instant pot and pour in one cup of water. Position a trivet at the bottom of the inner pot and set aside,
In a large mixing bowl, combine all dry ingredients and mix well. Add eggs, one at the time, and beat well on medium-high speed
Now add coconut cream and vanilla extract. Continue to beat for 2 more minutes on medium speed
Grease a small springform pan with some coconut oil and pour in the mixture. Place in the pot and seal the lid. Set the steam release handle and press the *Manual* button. Set the timer for 20 minutes on high pressure
Meanwhile; beat well the whipping cream until light and fluffy. Add chopped hazelnuts and optionally some finely chopped almonds
Refrigerate until use
When you hear the cooker's end signal, perform a quick pressure release and open the lid. Remove the pan from the pot and cool for a while
Top with whipped cream and refrigerate for 2 - 3 hours before serving.
Nutrition Values: Calories: 217; Total Fats: 18.2g; Net Carbs: 5.1g; Protein: 5.8g; Fiber: 4.5g

732. Almond Vanilla Brownies
Preparation Time: 35 Minutes
Servings: 6
Ingredients:
¾ cup almond flour
1/4 cup cocoa powder; unsweetened
1/3 cup coconut cream
1/4 cup raw almonds; finely chopped.
4 tbsp granulated stevia
2 tsp baking powder
1/4 cup flaxseed meal
3 large eggs
2 tbsp butter; melted
2 tsp vanilla extract
Directions:
In a medium-sized bowl, combine together almond flour, flaxseed meal, cocoa powder, stevia, and baking powder. Mix well and then add eggs, butter, vanilla extract, chopped almonds, and coconut cream. Using a hand mixer beat well until fully incorporated
Line a fitting cake pan with some parchment paper. Pour in the batter and shake the pan a couple of times to flatten the surface. Tightly wrap with aluminum foil and set aside
Now plug in the instant pot and position a trivet at the bottom of the inner pot. Pour in two cups of water and carefully place the pan on the trivet.
Seal the lid and set the steam release handle. Press the *Manual* button and cook for 25 minutes on high pressure
When done; perform a quick pressure release and open the lid. Remove the pan and cool completely before slicing.
Nutrition Values: Calories: 158; Total Fats: 13.5g; Net Carbs: 2.7g; Protein: 5.9g; Fiber: 13.5g

733. Special Strawberry Cream Cake
Preparation Time: 2 hours 10 Minutes
Servings: 5
Ingredients:
For the crust:
1 cup almond flour

3 tbsp swerve
1/4 cup almond butter; softened
1 cup shredded coconut
2 tsp baking powder
1 tsp baking soda
4 large eggs
1/4 tsp salt
For the cream layer:
1/4 cup swerve
1 tsp vanilla extract
6 large eggs
1/4 cup heavy cream
¾ cup cream cheese
Directions:
Plug in the instant pot and position a trivet at the bottom of the inner pot. Pour in 2 cups of water and set aside
Now prepare the crust. In a large mixing bowl, combine together all dry ingredients and mix well. Now add eggs and softened almond butter. With a dough hook on, beat until completely smooth.
Line a 6-inch springform pan with some parchment paper and pour the mixture in. flatten the surface with a kitchen spatula and set aside
In a medium-sized bowl, combine all the ingredients for the cream layer. Mix well with kitchen whisker and pour over the crust
Tightly wrap the pan with some aluminum foil and place in the pot. Seal the lid and set the steam release handle to the *Sealing* position.
Press the *Slow Cook* button and set the timer for 2 hours on low pressure
When done; perform a quick pressure release by moving the pressure valve to the *Venting* position. Carefully open the lid and remove the cake. Cool to a room temperature and transfer to the refrigerator overnight.
Nutrition Values: Calories: 154; Total Fats: 12.4g; Net Carbs: 2.8g; Protein: 6.9g; Fiber: 2.2g

734. Yummy Chocolate Cupcakes
Preparation Time: 20 Minutes
Servings: 6
Ingredients:
1 ½ cups of almond flour
1/4 cup swerve
2 tbsp cocoa powder; unsweetened
1 cup shredded coconut
2 large eggs
1/4 cup cream cheese
3 tbsp butter
2 tsp baking powder
1/4 cup blueberries
3 tbsp plain Greek yogurt
1 tsp vanilla extract
Directions:
In a large mixing bowl, combine together eggs and butter. Beat well on high speed until light and fluffy mixture. Then add swerve, cream cheese, and Greek yogurt. Continue to mix until smooth.
Finally, add almond flour, shredded coconut, and baking powder. Mix well again and fold in blueberries.

Divide the mixture between 6 silicone cups and set aside
Plug in the instant pot and position a trivet at the bottom of the inner pot. Pour in 1 cup of water and carefully place cups on the trivet
Seal the lid and set the steam release handle to the *Sealing* position. Set the timer for 10 minutes on the *Manual* mode
Perform a quick pressure release and open the lid. Remove the cups from the pot and cool to a room temperature
Nutrition Values: Calories: 212; Total Fats: 18.9g; Net Carbs: 4.2g; Protein: 6g; Fiber: 2.7g

735. Coconut Flan
Preparation Time: 29 minutes
Servings: 6
Ingredients:
2 tablespoons water
1 cup unsweetened coconut milk
3 large eggs
Pinch salt
1 cup heavy cream
¾ cup powdered erythritol, divided
2 teaspoons vanilla extract
Directions:
Whisk together ½ cup of the powdered erythritol and water in a saucepan over medium heat until it starts to darken. Divide the mixture among six small ramekins and set aside to cool.
Combine the coconut milk and cream in a saucepan and cook over medium heat until it starts to steam then whisk in the rest of the erythritol and the vanilla extract. Beat the eggs in a mixing bowl then pour a few tablespoons of the warmed milk into it while whisking.
Pour the egg mixture into the milk mixture and whisk smooth then pour into the ramekins.
Cover the ramekins with foil and place them in the steamer insert in your Instant Pot. Pour in ½ cup water then close and lock the lid.
Press the Manual button and adjust the timer for 9 minutes.
When the timer goes off, let the pressure vent naturally then press Cancel.
When the pot has depressurized, open the lid. Remove the ramekins and let the flan cool to room temperature then chill until ready to serve.
Nutrition Values:
calories 205 fat 19.5g ,protein 4.5g ,carbs 3g ,fiber 1g ,net carbs 2g

736. Blueberry Mug Cake
Preparation Time: 15 minutes
Servings: 4
Ingredients:
4 large eggs
½ cup fresh blueberries
¼ teaspoon salt
1 1/3 cup almond flour
2 teaspoons vanilla extract
¼ cup sugar-free maple syrup
Directions:

Place the trivet in the Instant Pot and add 1 cup of water.
Whisk together the almond flour, egg, sugar-free maple syrup, vanilla, and salt in a mixing bowl.
Fold in the blueberries then divide the mixture among four 8-ounce jars.
Cover the jars with foil then place on the trivet, close and lock the lid.
Press the Manual button and adjust the timer to 10 minutes.
When the timer goes off, do a Quick Release by pressing Cancel and switching the steam valve to "venting".
When the pot has depressurized, open the lid.
Remove the jars and let them cool a little before serving.
Nutrition Values:
calories 285 fat 23g ,protein 14g ,carbs 9.5g ,fiber 4g ,net carbs 5.5g

737. Ricotta Lemon Cheesecake
Preparation Time:40 minutes
Servings: 6
Ingredients:
1/3 cup whole-milk ricotta cheese
2 large eggs
1 (8-ouncepackage cream cheese, softened
¼ cup powdered erythritol
Juice and zest of 1 lemon
½ teaspoon lemon extract
Directions:
Combine all of the ingredients except the eggs in a mixing bowl.
Beat until the mixture is smooth then adjust sweetener to taste.
Lower the mixer speed and blend in the eggs until they are fully incorporated, being careful not to overmix.
Grease a 6-inch springform pan and pour in the cheesecake mixture.
Cover the pan with foil and place it in the Instant Pot on top of the trivet.
Pour in 2 cups of water then close and lock the lid.
Press the Manual button and adjust the timer for 30 minutes on High Pressure.
When the timer goes off, let the pressure vent naturally.
When the pot has depressurized, open the lid.
Let the cheesecake cool a little then chill for at least 8 hours before serving.
Nutrition Values:
calories 180 fat 16g ,protein 6.5g ,carbs 2g ,fiber 0g ,net carbs 2g

738. Creamy Lemon Curd
Preparation Time:20 minutes
Servings: 6
Ingredients:
2 large eggs
2 large egg yolks
3 ounces butter
2/3 cup lemon juice
1 cup powdered erythritol
Directions:
Combine the butter and erythritol in a mixing bowl and beat for 2 minutes.
Whisk together the eggs and yolks then drizzle them into the bowl while mixing.
Add the lemon juice and mix until well combined.
Divide the mixture among three half-pint jars and loosely cover with the lids.
Place the jars in the Instant Pot on the trivet then pour in 1 ½ cups water.
Close and lock the lid.
Press the Manual button and adjust the timer to 10 minutes on High Pressure.
When the timer goes off, let the pressure vent for 10 minutes then do a Quick Release by pressing Cancel and switching the steam valve to "venting".
When the pot has depressurized, open the lid.
Let the curd thicken for 20 minutes at room temperature then chill.
Nutrition Values:
calories 150 fat 15g ,protein 3g ,carbs 1g ,fiber 0g ,net carbs 1g

739. Chocolate Pudding Cake
Preparation Time:14 minutes
Servings: 8
Ingredients:
2/3 cup stevia-sweetened dark chocolate
½ cup unsweetened applesauce
2 large eggs
½ cup almond flour
1 teaspoon vanilla extract
¼ cup unsweetened cocoa powder
Directions:
Melt the chocolate in a double boiler over low heat until melted.
In a mixing bowl, whisk together the applesauce, eggs, and vanilla extract.
Whisk in the almond flour and cocoa powder then stir in the melted chocolate.
Pour the mixture into a greased 6-inch cake pan.
Place the pan in the Instant Pot on top of the trivet and pour in 2 cups of water.
Close and lock the lid.
Press the Manual button and adjust the timer on High Pressure for 4 minutes.
When the timer goes off, do a Quick Release by pressing Cancel and switching the steam valve to "venting".
When the pot has depressurized, open the lid.
Remove the pan and let the cake cool 10 minutes before removing.
Nutrition Values:
calories 150 fat 11g ,protein 5g ,carbs 16.5g ,fiber 5g ,net carbs 11.5g

740. Mini Vanilla Custards
Preparation Time:29 minutes
Servings: 4
Ingredients:
2 tablespoons water
1 cup unsweetened almond milk
3 large eggs
Pinch salt
1 cup heavy cream

¾ cup powdered erythritol, divided
1 tablespoon vanilla extract
Directions:
Whisk together ½ cup of the powdered erythritol and water in a saucepan over medium heat until the erythritol melts.
Divide the mixture among four small ramekins and set aside to cool.
Combine the almond milk and cream in a saucepan and cook over medium heat until it starts to steam then whisk in the rest of the erythritol and the vanilla extract.
Beat the eggs in a mixing bowl.
Whisk a few tablespoons of the milk mixture into the eggs then whisk in the rest in a steady stream.
Cover the ramekins with foil and place them in the steamer insert in your Instant Pot.
Pour in ½ cup water then close and lock the lid.
Press the Manual button and adjust the timer for 9 minutes.
When the timer goes off, let the pressure vent naturally then press Cancel.
When the pot has depressurized, open the lid.
Remove the ramekins and let the custards cool for 10 minutes then serve warm.
Nutrition Values:
calories 175 fat 16g ,protein 5.5g ,carbs 2g ,fiber 0.5g ,net carbs 1.5g

741. Coconut Almond Cake
Preparation Time:45 minutes
Servings: 8
Ingredients:
½ cup unsweetened shredded coconut
2 large eggs
½ cup heavy cream
¼ cup butter, melted
1 cup almond flour
6 tablespoons powdered erythritol
1 teaspoon baking powder
Directions:
Whisk together the almond flour, coconut, erythritol, and baking powder in a mixing bowl.
Add the eggs, heavy cream, and butter then whisk smooth.
Pour into a greased 6-inch cake pan and cover with foil.
Place the steamer rack in the Instant Pot and add 2 cups of water.
Put the cake pan on the steamer rack then close and lock the lid.
Press the Manual button and adjust the timer to 40 minutes at High Pressure.
When the timer goes off, let the pressure vent for 10 minutes then do a Quick Release by pressing Cancel and switching the steam valve to "venting".
When the pot has depressurized, open the lid.
Remove the cake and let it cool in the pan for 15 minutes before turning out.
Nutrition Values:
calories 290 fat 27.5g ,protein 5.5g ,carbs 7g ,fiber 3.5g ,net carbs 3.5g

742. Maple Almond Cake in a Jar
Preparation Time:15 minutes
Servings: 3
Ingredients:
3 large eggs
¼ teaspoon salt
1 cup almond flour
1 ½ teaspoons vanilla extract
3 tablespoons sugar-free maple syrup
Directions:
Place the trivet in the Instant Pot and add 1 cup of water.
Whisk together the almond flour, egg, sugar-free maple syrup, vanilla, and salt in a mixing bowl.
Divide the mixture among three 8-ounce jars.
Cover the jars with foil then place on the trivet, close and lock the lid.
Press the Manual button and adjust the timer to 10 minutes.
When the timer goes off, do a Quick Release by pressing Cancel and switching the steam valve to "venting".
When the pot has depressurized, open the lid.
Remove the jars and let them cool a little before serving.
Nutrition Values:
calories 275 fat 22.5g ,protein 13.5g ,carbs 7g ,fiber 3.5g ,net carbs 3.5g

743. Easy Chocolate Cheesecake
Preparation Time:40 minutes
Servings: 6
Ingredients:
1/3 cup whole-milk ricotta cheese
2 large eggs
1 (8-ouncepackage cream cheese, softened
¼ cup powdered erythritol
1 teaspoon vanilla extract
¼ cup unsweetened cocoa powder
Directions:
Combine all of the ingredients except the eggs in a mixing bowl.
Beat until the mixture is smooth then adjust sweetener to taste.
Lower the mixer speed and blend in the eggs until they are fully incorporated, being careful not to overmix.
Grease a 6-inch springform pan and pour in the cheesecake mixture.
Cover the pan with foil and place it in the Instant Pot on top of the trivet.
Pour in 2 cups of water then close and lock the lid.
Press the Manual button and adjust the timer for 30 minutes on High Pressure.
When the timer goes off, let the pressure vent naturally.
When the pot has depressurized, open the lid.
Let the cheesecake cool a little then chill for at least 6 hours before serving.
Nutrition Values:
calories 180 fat 16g ,protein 6.5g ,carbs 3.5g ,fiber 1g ,net carbs 2.5g

744. Classic Crème Brulee
Preparation Time:14 minutes

Servings: 6
Ingredients:
6 large egg yolks
2 tablespoons granular erythritol
2 cups heavy cream
3 tablespoons powdered erythritol
1 tablespoon vanilla extract
Directions:
Whisk together the heavy cream, egg yolks, powdered erythritol, and the vanilla in a bowl.
Divide the mixture among 6 small ramekins and cover with foil.
Place the steamer rack in the Instant Pot and add 1 cup water.
Place the ramekins in the steamer rack, offsetting the stacks so they are stable.
Close and lock the lid then press the Manual button and adjust the timer to 9 minutes.
When the timer goes off, let the pressure vent for 15 minutes then do a Quick Release by pressing Cancel and switching the steam valve to "venting".
When the pot has depressurized, open the lid.
Remove the ramekins and chill until they are cold.
Sprinkle the granular erythritol over the crème brulees and place under the broiler until browned.
Let the topping harden before serving.
Nutrition Values:
calories 200 fat 19g ,protein 3.5g ,carbs 2g ,fiber 0g ,net carbs 2g

745. Chili Cauliflower Spread
Preparation Time: 25 minutes,
Servings: 4
Ingredients:
1 (choppedShallot
1 pound Cauliflower florets
¼ cup Chicken stock
2 (choppedRed hot chilies
2 tbsp (mincedGinger
1 tbsp Avocado oil
1 and ¼ tbsp Balsamic vinegar
Directions:
Let your Instant Pot preheat on Sauté mode.
Add oil, ginger, and scallions, then sauté for 2 minutes.
Stir in remaining ingredients and mix well
Seal the pot's lid and cook for 13 minutes on manual mode at High.
Allow the pressure to release in 10 minutes naturally then remove the lid.
Blend the mixture with a hand held blender until smooth.
Serve fresh and enjoy.
Nutrition Values:
Calories 45, Total Fat: 2.5g, Carbs: 2g, Protein: 2.6g, Fiber: 1.3g.

746. Artichokes Spread
Preparation Time: 25 minutes,
Servings: 6
Ingredients:
14 oz. (drainedCanned artichoke hearts
8 oz. (shreddedMozzarella cheese
1 pound (tornSpinach
½ cup Chicken stock
½ cup Coconut cream
1 tsp Garlic powder
a pinch Salt and black pepper
Directions:
Add all the ingredients for the spread to the Instant Pot.
Seal the pot's lid and cook for 15 minutes on manual mode at High.
Allow the pressure to release in 10 minutes naturally then remove the lid.
Blend the mixture with a hand held blender until smooth.
Serve fresh and enjoy.
Nutrition Values:
Calories 204, Total Fat: 11.5g, Carbs: 4.2g, Protein: 5.9g, Fiber: 3.1g.

747. Shrimp and Leeks Appetizer
Preparation Time: 10 minutes,
Servings: 6
Ingredients:
2 lbs. (peeled and deveinedShrimp
2 (slicedLeeks
1 tbsp (choppedChives
2 (mincedGarlic cloves
½ cup Veggie stock
1 tbsp Olive oil
1 tbsp Sweet paprika
Directions:
Let your Instant Pot preheat on Sauté mode.
Add oil, leeks, and garlic, then sauté for 1 minute.
Stir in remaining ingredients except for chives and mix well
Seal the pot's lid and cook for 4 minutes on manual mode at High.
Allow the pressure to release in 5 minutes naturally then remove the lid.
Garnish with chives.
Serve fresh and enjoy.
Nutrition Values:
Calories 224, Total Fat: 5.1g, Carbs: 3.9g, Protein: 35.1g, Fiber: 1g.

748. Easy Italian Asparagus
Preparation Time: 8 minutes,
Servings: 4
Ingredients:
1 cup Water
1 pound (trimmedAsparagus
1 tbsp (choppedCilantro
1 tbsp Lemon juice
1 tsp Olive oil
½ tbsp Italian seasoning
a pinch Salt and black pepper
Directions:
Pour water into the Instant Pot and place steamer basket over it.
Place asparagus in the steamer basket.
Seal the pot's lid and cook for 4 minutes on manual mode at High.
Allow the pressure to release in 4 minutes naturally then remove the lid.

Toss the asparagus with all other ingredients in a platter.
Serve fresh and enjoy.
Nutrition Values:
Calories 39, Total Fat: 2.1g, Carbs: 1.3g, Protein: 2.5g, Fiber: 1.1g.

749. Nutmeg Spiced Endives
Preparation Time: 20 minutes,
Servings: 4
Ingredients:
4 (trimmed and halvedEndives
1 cup Water
1 tsp (groundNutmeg
1 tbsp (choppedChives
2 tbsp Olive oil
Salt and black pepper to the taste
Directions:
Pour water into the Instant Pot and place the steamer basket over it.
Place endives in this steamer basket.
Seal the pot's lid and cook for 10 minutes on manual mode at High.
Allow the pressure to release in 10 minutes naturally then remove the lid.
Toss them with salt, nutmeg, oil, salt, and chives.
Serve fresh and enjoy.
Nutrition Values:
Calories 63, Total Fat: 7.2g, Carbs: 0.3g, Protein: 0.1g, Fiber: 0.1g.

www.ingramcontent.com/pod-product-compliance
Lightning Source LLC
Chambersburg PA
CBHW081109080526
44587CB00021B/3510